The Neuroscience of Everyday Life

By weaving vignettes and case studies throughout, this fascinating and original textbook provides an accessible primer not only on the key principles of neuroscience but, crucially, how they may manifest in the everyday lives of people with neurological conditions.

Each chapter begins with the story of a person or family, including a description of what they want to do in their everyday life, before presenting the neuroscientific principles that underlie this person's situation. Rather than a technical book about neuroanatomy, physiology, or pathology, the spotlight is on understanding the way that neurological differences impact a person's life. Through focusing on a particular condition, each chapter highlights a different aspect of the nervous system, and what happens when things change. A wide range of topics are covered, from conditions such as Parkinson's, dementia, MS, and autism, to conditions resulting from traumatic events such as spinal cord injuries, stroke, and chronic pain. The goal of the book is to trace a thread from neuroscience to how the nervous system affects active participation in daily activities. This approach gives students and professionals a thorough and informed grounding to support problem-solving in practice, improving evidence-based assessment, interventions, and outcomes.

Following current evidence-based teaching practices, this text emphasizes engaged teaching/learning methods throughout each chapter to encourage students' own active discovery. This ground-breaking text will be essential reading for any health science students as well as professionals in practice.

Winnie Dunn, Distinguished Professor, Occupational Therapy, University of Missouri, USA.

Timothy J. Wolf, Associate Dean for Research, Chair Occupational Therapy University of Missouri, USA.

Lorie Gage Richards, Associate Professor, Chair, Occupational Therapy, University of Utah, USA.

Dawn M. Nilsen, Professor and Director, Programs in Occupational Therapy, Columbia University, USA.

The Neuroscience of Everyday Life

An Applied Guide for Health Sciences Students

Edited by Winnie Dunn, Timothy J. Wolf, Lorie Gage Richards, and Dawn M. Nilsen

Routledge
Taylor & Francis Group

NEW YORK AND LONDON

Designed cover image: Getty

First published 2025
by Routledge
605 Third Avenue, New York, NY 10158

and by Routledge
4 Park Square, Milton Park, Abingdon, Oxon, OX14 4RN

Routledge is an imprint of the Taylor & Francis Group, an informa business

ISBN: 978-1-032-90377-4 (hbk)
ISBN: 978-1-63822-126-5 (pbk)
ISBN: 978-1-003-52438-0 (ebk)

DOI: 10.4324/9781003524380

Typeset in Optima
by codeMantra

Access the Instructor and Student Resources: www.routledge.com/9781638221265

We dedicate this book to all the people, families, and communities who taught us that being fully present in their lives at a vulnerable time matters the most.

Contents

Illustrations

Contributors

Antoine Bailliard, Associate Professor, Occupational Therapy, Duke University, USA

Alison Bell, Associate Professor, Occupational Therapy, Thomas Jefferson University, USA

Thomas Bergquist, Associate Professor, Mayo Clinic, USA

Anna Boone, Assistant Professor, Occupational Therapy, University of Missouri, USA

Gaye W. Cronin, Master Clinician, Director of Rehabilitation, Vestibular Atlanta, USA

Jacqueline Daniel, Occupational Therapist, Monmouth University Doctoral Graduate, USA

Katherine Dimitropoulou, Assistant Professor, Occupational Therapy, Columbia University, USA

Timothy Dionne, Assistant Professor, Occupational Therapy, University of New Mexico, USA

Sarah Doerrer, Assistant Professor, Occupational Therapy, George Washington University, USA

Megan Doherty, Associate Professor, Occupational Therapy, University of Missouri, USA

Winnie Dunn, Distinguished Professor, Occupational Therapy, University of Missouri, USA

Batya Engel-Yeger, Professor, Occupational Therapy, University of Haifa, Israel

Valerie Fox, Instructor, Occupational Therapy, Duke University, USA

Andrea L. Garcia, Specialist Professor, Occupational Therapy, Monmouth University, USA

Whitney Henderson, Associate Clinical Professor, Occupational Therapy, University of Missouri, USA

Anne V. Kirby, Associate Professor, Occupational Therapy, University of Utah, USA

Bridget Kraus, Assistant Professor, Occupational Therapy, University of Missouri, USA

Caroline Larson, Assistant Professor, Speech, Language and Hearing Sciences, University of Missouri, USA

Ben Lee, Postdoctoral Diversity and Innovation Scholar, Occupational Therapy, University of New Hampshire, USA

Lauren Little, Associate Professor, Occupational Therapy, Associate Dean of Research Rush University, USA

Rose McAndrew, Assistant Professor, Occupational Therapy, St. Louis Community College, USA

M.J. Mulcahey, Professor, Occupational Therapy, Thomas Jefferson University, USA

Katelyn Mwangi, Assistant Teaching Professor, Occupational Therapy, University of Missouri, USA

Dawn M. Nilsen, Professor and Director, Programs in Occupational Therapy, Columbia University, USA

Calli M. Palmquist, Doctoral Student in Occupational Therapy, University of Minnesota, Rochester, USA

Jessica L. Petersen, Occupational Therapist, Mayo Clinic, USA

Lorie Gage Richards, Associate Professor, Chair, Occupational Therapy, University of Utah, USA

Stephanie N. Ritter, Occupational Therapist, Mayo Clinic, USA

Sarah Schuman, Occupational Therapist, Washington University in St. Louis, USA

Olivia Surgent, Assistant Professor, University of Wisconsin, USA

Sondra Stegenga, Assistant Professor, Special Education, University of Utah, USA

Alexandra L. Terrill, Associate Professor, Occupational Therapy, University of Utah, USA

Melanie Morriss Tkach, Assistant Professor, Occupational Therapy, University of Missouri, USA

Mozhgan Valipour, PhD candidate in Rehabilitation Science, University of Utah, USA

Anna Wallisch, Assistant Professor, Pediatrics University of Kansas Medical Center, USA

Sally Wasmuth, Assistant Professor, Occupational Therapy, Indiana University, USA

Lauren Winterbottom, Research Occupational Therapist, Columbia University, USA

Timothy J. Wolf, Associate Dean for Research, Professor and Chair, Occupational Therapy, University of Missouri, USA

Acknowledgements

Thanks to Pam Duncan, who showed me the best ways to serve people with motor system conditions, and to Steve Nadeau and Jeff Kleim, who furthered my neuroscience knowledge and instilled the idea that the complexity of brain plasticity supports therapeutic interventions.

Lorie

Thanks to Glen Gillen for his mentorship and support.

Dawn

Thanks to Bridget Comparato-Kraus for provided editing support.

Tim

Thanks to Maddie Cook for preparing the illustrations about brain activity for each chapter, to Shelly Crawford for editing the book for consistency, and to Charles Hallenbeck, who fostered my curiosity by his example, and willingly took the path not travelled with me.

Winnie

Introduction

Teachers and learners: Thank you for joining us on a journey of discovery. As Ivan Illich said long ago:

> Most learning is not the result of instruction. It is rather the result of unhampered participation in a meaningful setting. Most people learn best by being "with it."
>
> (Illich, 1971, p. 24)

Collectively all the authors in this book agreed to create a thrilling new way to make sure that *neuroscience is part of your ways of knowing about the people you will serve* (i.e., "being with them"). We fearlessly wove together evidence-based teaching practices, contemporary knowledge about the brain and nervous system, and the way people live their lives into an integrated experience of learning and knowing. We are asking all of you to engage in what Seth Goldenberg calls "radical curiosity":

> Radical Curiosity is fueled by awe--rather than fear—of the unknown … Radical Curiosity is the greatest expression of what it means to be a teacher and a learner, for whom living is synonymous with discovering new knowledge.
>
> (Goldenberg, 2022, p. 10)

We won't be telling you things; we will be inviting you to find out about the nervous system through the experiences of people whose nervous systems are different because of a traumatic event or particular condition. Use your *radical curiosity* to imagine their lives and how you can support them with your burgeoning knowledge about how the nervous system works.

Background for this innovative approach

In this text, we are taking a big leap to create an innovative way to teach practical neuroscience. We surveyed people who taught neuroscience in occupational therapy entry-level programs. In virtually all the cases, faculty told us that they wanted a way to link people's authentic lives to neuroscience. This is an easy thing to say and it is a hard thing to do in a textbook.

Those of us who teach neuroscience really love it. We want to talk about it, think about it, find out more about it every day. Our passion is both our strength in teaching neuroscience and a potentially fatal flaw. Our students see our passion in the animated

DOI: 10.4324/9781003524380-1

way we talk about the brain and its amazing abilities. However, that passion can lead us to telling students so many details that the novice learner cannot sort out the salient points. In essence, students lose sight of the forest by our over focus on teaching them about the trees. We asked ourselves many times during preparation of this book structure.

"What does a novice learner really need to know?"

We decided that they need to know just enough to see the neuroscience within everyday participation.

We recognize that every condition involving the brain has a complex set of implications for participation. However, we also recognize that novice learners need to understand specific examples first before they can integrate the neuroscience information with a complex condition. We have organized each chapter with a person living life, an activity of daily living that they need support to accomplish, and the person's neurological condition along with the neuroscience concepts to be emphasized because of that condition. We have carefully chosen what neuroscience concepts will be emphasized in each chapter, knowing that there are other factors that are also relevant to each condition. By breaking down the important aspects of neuroscience and placing them in the stories of everyday life, we create a context for remembering how neuroscience supports or interferes with participation.

We also include some examples in the last section of the book that provide an integrated look at the complexity of neuroscience factors within a person's life. These integrated examples illustrate how professionals navigate among many factors to support the person's interests and life routines.

Core guiding principles

Below are the *core principles* that guide our thinking to create this innovative approach.

• **The people and their lives are the main event in each chapter.**

Virtually all neuroscience textbooks focus on anatomy and physiology of the nervous system. There are many online resources for diagrams, images, and explanations about the nervous system. All of these resources are necessary and insufficient for applying neuroscience within people's lives.

Novice learners understand living; by using life examples to teach neuroscience, we are attaching new learning to familiar ideas. Looking through the lens of human experiences, we provide learners with a way to organize and remember how the nervous system works and the nervous system's impact on a person's life.

Related to the person's life, *how we refer to people matters*. You will see various ways to reference people's conditions throughout this book. Sometimes you will see *person-first language*; this format would be "Sam is blind" or "Sam, who has Parkinson's disease." Other times you will see *identity-first language*; this format would be "autistic person." We use people's names rather than generic words like "patient" or "client" to remind ourselves that *this person's life* is our central focus. We must always ask people about their interests, preferences and preferred terminology. Terminology changes across time as we understand the human condition more fully. It is your ethical responsibility to keep up with research that informs us about the changing and most respectful, updated language for contemporary practice.

- **Participation is the focus of all discussion.**

In each chapter, we emphasize people doing something that matters to them. Students know what it feels like to learn how to do something; they also have had experiences with something interfering with their preferred activities. We take advantage of their personal experiences by showing examples of other people's challenges with an important life activity. Only then do we link to nervous system operations; we ask them "when the nervous system is different than expected, what will happen to a person's life?" We want this relationship to drive their interest and learning.

- **The neuroscience is explained in everyday language, like talking to a family member or friend in another field.**

There are many new terms when studying neuroscience, in fact, it's like learning a new language. We want students to recognize scientific terms so when they read about a person's condition, they understand what is going on. However, when communicating with families and other professionals without a neuroscience background, it is also critical to explain things with everyday words. In this book, we provide those everyday explanations right along with the terms-of-art for neuroscience so students have examples of how to translate their considerable knowledge into conversational language.

- **The education evidence informs us that students learn and retain information better when they are actively engaged in learning. We embed activities, questions, and other exploratory ideas within boxes in each chapter.**

Another way this book distinguishes itself is by building on the evidence about teaching and learning. Traditionally, neuroscience courses are predominantly lectures and tests. Student retention is low with this format. To maximize retention, we must create engagement with material. Rather than describing all the neuroscience content, we create a structure for students to discover, interact and reflect on neuroscience. For example, within chapters, we invite students to find images in other resources, have debates with each other about the impact of neuroscience operations on life, and create their own graphics for illustrating relationships.

- **Students have a high capacity for finding resources; we take advantage of this by providing structured guidance about what to look for and why it will be helpful, rather than providing the resources directly.**

Students in this decade are digital natives. They have been using the internet to find answers to their questions throughout their lives. We harness this skill set by inviting students to find the resources they need to complete course activities. We structure their search with keywords or authors, so they find the strongest material available. Having students find their own resources, we also take advantage of the most recent knowledge available, which keeps this book current for a longer time.

Book structure

This book is divided into four units:

- Sensorimotor systems
- Social emotional systems
- Cognitive systems
- Integrating systems

Within each unit, there are several chapters. Each chapter addresses a person who wants to do something that matters in their life. Each person has some neurological condition with specific characteristics that may have an impact on the person's life and preferred activities. Through the chapter learners will think deeply about this person and how their nervous system is supporting or interfering with their life. Our goal is to use that person's story to illustrate how that part of the nervous system works, and what happens when things change. Our stories address key nervous system conditions that will highlight the neuroscience principles we want students to learn. Each chapter is organized as follows:

- **Chapter title** [introducing the person and their life activity]
- **Purpose of this chapter** [emphasize the participation area, linking to the neuroscience as background, underpinning, employing scientific reasoning to understand the main event of PARTICIPATION]
- **Neuroscience information** [condition and relevant neuroscience concepts to discover]
- **Daily life routine for this person** [what does the person want/need to do?]
- **Back to the person's life** [now that you know this neuroscience information, what other insights do you have about this person's life?]
- **Larger implications** [What do we know about ourselves and the population at large from this brain condition and this person's story?]
- **Additional resources** [places to go if this area is of particular interest for you]
- **References** [direct references and useful resources; where to go if you want to know more]

By setting an authentic context for learning, we ensure that learners will have neuroscience at their fingertips when they are ready to serve others.

Foundational knowledge about the nervous system

Neuroscience drives and support all our behaviors, so understanding how the nervous system works, and its amazing capacity for adaptation is essential for applying neuroscience within people's lives. People can live satisfying lives with neurological conditions. The professionals that serve them must know enough about the nervous system to make necessary adjustments to support people's interests and priorities.

There are structures and functions that characterize the nervous system. It is important to have this foundation for learning about the people and their circumstances throughout the book.

Major parts of the nervous system

The nervous system is woven into all parts of the body. *Sensory receptors* are housed in the skin, muscles, joints, eyes, ears, nose, mouth, and internal organs. The *spinal cord* holds all the cells that go to and from the brain and is contained within the vertebrae of the back and runs the length of spine. The *brain* is the major processor of input and output and is within the skull. *Nerve cells* (also called neurons) are the special cells of the nervous system; they carry information from the sensory receptors into the spinal cord, brain, are part of the circuitry within the brain, and carry information out to the muscles, joints, and body organs to execute actions.

We say *central nervous system* (CNS) when talking about the brain and spinal cord. We say *peripheral nervous system* (PNS) when talking about the neurons that are within the body traveling to (sensory, or afferent) and from (motor or efferent) the spinal cord. We say *autonomic nervous system* (ANS) when talking about the parts of the nervous system that complete automatic functions, such as breathing and digestion. Within the ANS, we say *parasympathetic* to refer to the everyday automatic functions; we say *sympathetic* to refer to intense responses that occur when there may be a need for protection, i.e., the "fight or flight" response.

Find out what the nervous system looks like

Search the internet for pictures of the parts of the nervous system. Save the links of images you find useful so you have a library you can use throughout the book. Some websites have short videos illustrating the nervous system as well if this multimedia form is a good match for your learning.

Share images with your colleagues; tell each other why certain images are the most helpful to you.

Keywords: lobes (frontal, parietal, occipital, temporal), spinal cord, gray matter, white matter, cranial nerves, brain stem

---

Major functions of the nervous system

The nervous system is a complex set of interconnecting cells that keep track of what is going on (*sensory* input), organize that incoming information to derive meaning from experiences (*perception* and *processing*), and design and implement responses when needed (*response* generation) (Kandel et al., 2013).

Sensory input

The nervous system is highly dependent on *sensory input* to perform its other functions. Without sensory input the nervous system has no information for planning and implementing responses.

There are many different sensory receptors that provide information to the nervous system. Many of us are familiar with hearing and seeing; the *auditory* and *visual* systems keep track of what is going on in the environment. But there are other sensory inputs that are equally important to our well-being. *Taste* and *smell* sensations are more primitive sensory inputs that relate to survival and thriving. There are also sensory receptors within our bodies to keep us apprised of our internal physiological state (called *interoceptors*). Several sensory inputs are designed to keep track of where our bodies are in space, including *touch* (somatosensory), *movement* (vestibular), and *body position* (proprioceptive) sensations. These sensory inputs can operate without our continuous awareness to keep our bodies organized related to gravity and objects in our environment.

If interested

There is a lot of information about sensory deprivation on the web and in journal articles. Sometimes these studies take place within sensory deprivation tanks. Find some reading about what happens when the brain is deprived of sensory input; find some pictures of sensory deprivation tanks.

In the sensory section of this book, you will learn how changes in sensory inputs affect everyday life activities. For example, if a person is sensitive to touch experiences, their reaction to touch can affect social interactions. When a person has difficulty with taste or smell, this can affect one's interest in eating regularly.

See what the sensory receptors look like

The various receptors are quite complex; neuroscientists have studied the receptors so they can tell us just exactly how much input is needed for a particular receptor to respond.

Perception and processing

Once the nervous system receives sensory input, there must be a mechanism to organize and understand the meaning of the input. The *cognitive* and *emotional* parts of the nervous system use one's past experiences to construct the possible meaning of new input. People are gathering new information all the time and so their nervous systems are *creating meaning units* that build and become more complex as people have more experiences.

When people have various neurological conditions, parts of the nervous system that create perception and meaning can become unreliable or inaccurate in their processing. In the cognitive and emotional/ psychosocial sections of this book you will learn how changes in perception and processing can affect everyday life activities. For example, when cognitive systems are changed, people can have difficulty managing money or getting errands run. With changes in the emotional systems, people can misread the cues of other people, leading to errors on work projects or in friendships.

Response generation

After the nervous system has received sensory input and engages in a process of organizing that input, the nervous system *creates responses* when necessary. In the motor, cognitive, and psychosocial sections of this book you will learn how the nervous system generates specifically tailored responses based on circumstances. Any changes in input or processing can affect responses because without accurate information the nervous system will create inaccurate responses. The motor system has many ways to create movement responses including large body movements as well as small precise movements of the mouth, the hands, and the face. The nervous system can also create other body responses (*autonomic*) such as having a sick stomach in reaction to anxiety provoking input.

Each response also generates more input for the nervous system (*feedback*). When you move, the sensations from your muscles and joints return to the nervous system so you can make adjustments as needed. You will learn about neurological conditions that affect what a person does in situations, we will ask you to think about all the ways that responses might be altered because of those conditions.

Find the input/processing/action/feedback cycle

Find an image or animation illustrating the way the nervous system processes input and output. Keep this in your library for reference during the course.

So now you have a general sense of the journey ahead of you. Neuroscience is a key factor in scientific reasoning and supports us to gain insights about how a person's life might be affected when the nervous system is altered by brain injury or other conditions that impact brain function. All the authors and editors continue to be awestruck by the nervous system's capacity to operate and adapt as an underpinning to the human experience. *Stay curious as you travel this path of discovery with us.*

Advanced organizer for your work

Some of you find diagrams and concept maps helpful to your learning. We are providing you with a *concept map* (see Figure 0.1) that illustrates the organization of all the concepts about the nervous system you will encounter in this book. It is *not* anatomically correct, but rather it is an illustration showing the relationships among the parts. Let's walk through this image so it will be helpful to you in each chapter.

You will see a *depiction of the brain* in the background to remind you that all these functions occur within the brain. You will see the four big functions of *cognition, emotion, motor,* and *sensation* distributed on the diagram along with a circle that represents the brain's *internal processes*.

Below the brain image, you will see a depiction of a person, with five lines pointing to various parts of the body.

On the left side of the diagram, you will see:

- **A line pointing to the face**: we have written "make a face, cry, talk, bite and chew" as examples of output that might occur on the face area.
- **A line pointing to the legs and feet**: we have written "dance and walk" as examples of output that might occur in the lower extremities.

On the right side of the diagram, you will see:

- **A line pointing to the head**: we have written "think, plan and wonder" as examples of output that might occur in the brain.
- **A line pointing to the arms**: we have written "point, reach and hold" as examples of output that might occur in the upper extremities.
- **A line pointing to the body**: we have written "sick stomach and heart racing" as examples of internal body actions that might occur.

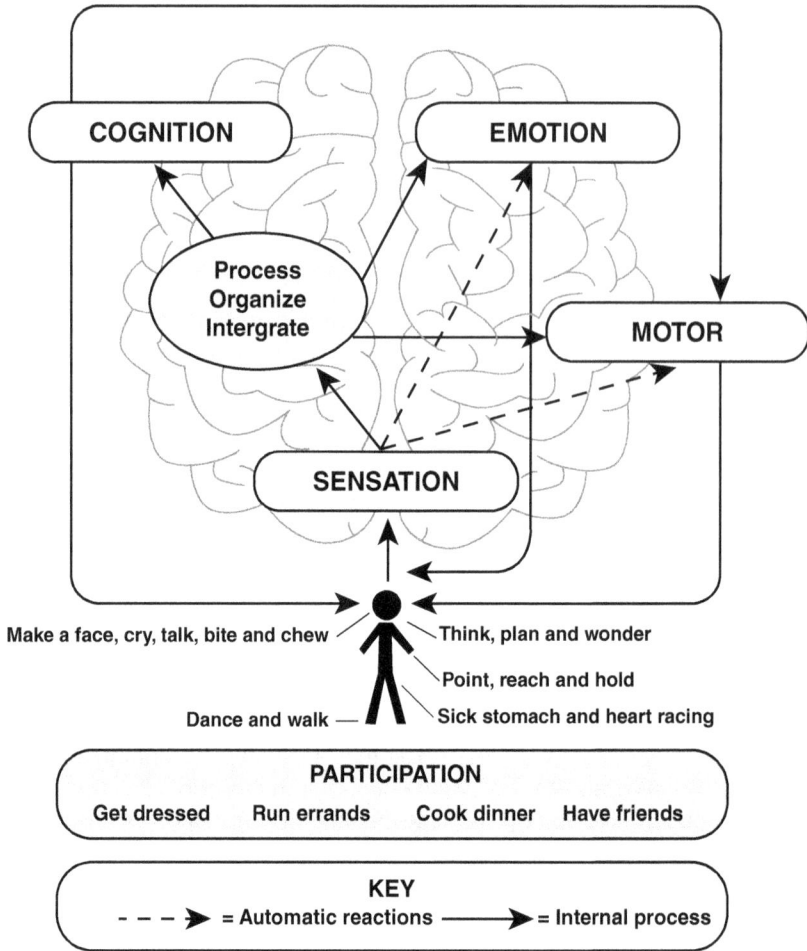

Figure 0.1 Brain figure

Below the person is a PARTICIPATION box. We have written examples of areas of participation that matter to people in their everyday lives.

The KEY tells you about the internal actions and processes that are depicted with arrows in the diagram. A dotted line represents automatic reactions, while the solid arrow shows internal processes. You will learn about these actions as you study the people in this book.

You will find a specific version of this figure at the beginning of each chapter. The bold arrows show you what functions we are emphasizing in that chapter. In class you can talk about how each person's brain processing happens, and you can compare and contrast across chapters to see how all the operations might fit together.

Remember: all the brain functions are working together to support your life every day. The highlighted arrows show what matters in each chapter. As you move through the book, you will see all the different ways that cognition, motor, and emotional outputs happen from a neuroscience point of view.

Have fun with this learning tool; it will get easier as you learn more about the nervous system, and will create an image in your mind that you can use when you are in practice.

Further reading

MedicineNet. (n.d.). What are the 4 main functions of the nervous system? www.medicinenet. com/4_main_functions_of_the_nervous_system/article.htm (accessed September 14, 2022)

Reference.com. (2015). What are the four functions of the nervous system? www.reference.com/ science/four-functions-nervous-system-78ef29631e4be78b (accessed September, 15, 2022)

References

Goldenberg, S. (2022). *Radical curiosity: Challenging commonly held beliefs to imagine a flourishing future*. New York: Crown Publishing.

Illich, I. (1971). Deschooling society. Retrieved from www.davidtinapple.com/illich/1970_ deschooling.html

Kandel, E., Schwartz, J., Jessell, T, Siegelbaum, S. & Hudspeth, A. (2013). *Principles of neural science*, 5th edition. New York: McGraw-Hill Publishing.

Unit I
Sensorimotor systems

1 Alex wants to put on make-up and has Bell's palsy

Neuroscience facilitates our understanding of self-care routines

Andrea L. Garcia and Jacqueline Daniel

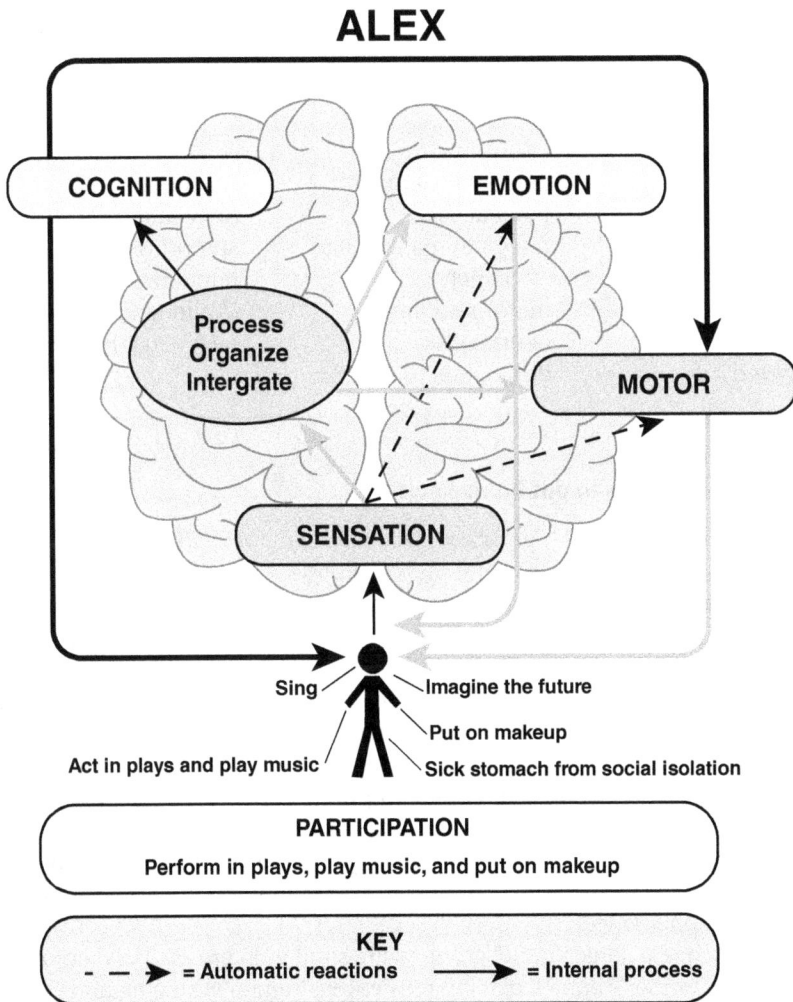

Figure 1.1 Alex brain figure

DOI: 10.4324/9781003524380-3

Purpose of this chapter

The purpose of this chapter is to explore how Alex, a 17-year-old, non-binary high-school senior who wants to put on make-up might be affected by Bell's palsy, a condition that impacts the functioning of cranial nerve VII (facial nerve). People with Bell's palsy have full lives with their daily routines, relationships and learning, but may require modifications for function.

The key neuroscience concepts that will be explored in this chapter include structure and function of cranial nerve VII (facial nerve), principles of peripheral nervous system regeneration, and the neuromuscular junction, acetylcholine transmission, and reflex arcs. As with all the chapters, these components of the nervous system work with other systems to support overall human function.

Keywords for this chapter are listed in the box below. Be sure you learn what these key features are so you can get the most out of the chapter.

Keywords for this chapter

acetylcholine (ACh)	geniculate ganglion	regenerative sprouting
Bell's palsy	hyperacusis	Schwann cells
buccal branch	marginal mandibular	sprouting
cervical branch	branch	temporal branch
collateral sprouting	motor synkinesis	Wallerian degeneration
corneal reflex	neuropathy	zygomatic branch
facial nerve	ophthalmic division	

Alex, a person who wants to put on makeup

Alex is a 17-year-old senior in high school. Alex lives at home with their younger sibling, parents, and two dogs. Alex is enjoying their senior year of high school but is excited to attend college next year. They have been visiting colleges with their parents that have strong academic programs in the performing arts. Alex plans to major in vocal arts, and dreams of performing on Broadway in New York City someday. Alex has participated in community and school-based theater companies and performances since they were in first grade and has been a voice student since middle school. Alex's parents have encouraged Alex to explore all of their dreams and aspirations of performing.

Alex has relied heavily on their parents' support in the last 5 years. At the age of 14, Alex came out to their family as a non-binary individual after several years of socially isolating, experiencing negative self-perception, and periods of painful body self-image. With support, Alex now feels more confident expressing themself in their interests as well as their outward appearance.

Socially, Alex has a large friend group with similar interests. They enjoy spending afternoons in each other's homes playing musical instruments, singing and dancing, and practicing new make-up applications that they have seen demonstrated online. They spend hours trying new cosmetics and matching them to costumes and outfits they have crafted from their closets.

Recently, Alex woke up one morning and discovered, upon looking in the mirror, that their right eye was not blinking or closing properly, and the right side of their mouth seemed to be frowning. Looking closer at themself, Alex attempted to raise their eyebrows, but only the left one lifted. Concerned, Alex sought their mom's help. Alex's mom began to touch their face lightly, to which Alex said that they felt Mom's light touch around their right ear, but remarked that the area around their ear felt painful. Alex's mom took them to the local emergency room, as she feared Alex was experiencing a stroke.

In the hospital, Alex received many tests to attempt to give Alex a diagnosis. The team of doctors and nurses explained to Alex and their family that facial paralysis can be due to several reasons, and it is important to uncover the underlying cause to determine the course of treatment. Some of the diagnoses that were ruled out for Alex prior to finding the root of the facial paralysis were Ramsay-Hunt syndrome, trauma, Lyme's disease and/or other bacterial infections, cysts and/or other tumors, myasthenia gravis, multiple sclerosis, and stroke (Balakrishnan, 2015; Lundy-Ekman, 2022). It appeared as if there was no identifiable cause for Alex's symptoms and thus they received a diagnosis of Bell's palsy (BP).

Box 1.1   Learning activity

Having read the narrative, what sparks your curiosity? Discuss with your peers.

What will you need to know more about? Prior to reading the chapter, work with your small group to talk about what you already know.

Box 1.2   Learning activity

1. How can scientific reasoning about neuroscience expand your insights?
2. What neurological structures are involved with Bell's palsy?

After taking some time to discuss all of this, let's consider the functions of the nervous system and how impairments result in physical presentations.

What is Bell's palsy?

BP is the most common cause of facial nerve palsy (Chung et al., 2022; Portelinha et al., 2015), and scientists have yet to find its definitive prognosis (Ahn et al., 2023; Patel & Levin, 2015; Singh & Deshmukh, 2022; Somasundara & Sullivan, 2017). However, empirical findings gained from research and exploring the connections between neuroscience and clinical presentations can help us understand BP more broadly, despite its unknown etiology. BP is characterized by a sudden onset of one-sided facial paralysis or muscle weakness, with common signs and symptoms including one-sided facial droop, facial tingling, vestibular dysfunction, pain around the ear on the affected side, headache, neck pain, decreased salivation or taste, and motor synkinesis (Chung et al., 2022; Balakrishnan,

2015; Eviston et al., 2015; Patel & Levin, 2015; Somasundara & Sullivan, 2017). The severity of symptoms varies, from mild weakness or dysfunction to complete one-sided facial paralysis, and usually last for a few weeks or months in some cases (Ahn et al., 2023; Eviston et al., 2015; Patel & Levin, 2015; Singh & Deshmukh; Somasundara & Sullivan, 2017).

Neuroscience information to guide your thinking about Alex

Cranial nerves

Our brain communicates with the rest of our body through neural pathways to initiate various functions and voluntary or involuntary actions. There are 12 cranial nerves (CN) that arise from the brain (the majority from the brain stem) and branch out to innervate different parts of the head, neck, and trunk, enabling movement and discrimination of sensory input. Although CNs originate from the brain, they are mainly considered to be part of the peripheral nervous system, with the exception of the olfactory and optic nerves (cranial nerves I and II). Please see Table 1.1 for a reference table of all 12 cranial nerves and their associated functions. The olfactory and optic nerves reside in the central nervous system and are myelinated by oligodendrocytes. The remaining CNs, or peripheral nerves, are myelinated by Schwann cells, glial cells that support rapid propagation of action potentials. Unlike oligodendrocytes, Schwann cells can regenerate and repair damaged nerves. This ability of peripheral nerve regeneration is especially important in promoting recovery from BP.

Each CN has distinct functions and are categorized as either sensory or motor nerves. Some CNs carry both sensory and motor fibers, including the facial nerve (CN VII), and the trigeminal (CN V), glossopharyngeal (CN IX) and vagus (X) nerves. Also, the facial nerve, along with the oculomotor (CN III), the glossopharyngeal and vagus nerves are considered part of the parasympathetic nervous system. Although the exact etiology of BP remains unclear, studies suggest that viral infections may cause acute exacerbation, with inflammation, edema, and/or ischemia of the facial nerve being the most common underlying causes presented in the literature (Balakrishnan, 2015; Somasundara & Sullivan, 2017; Zhang et al., 2020).

Table 1.1 Cranial nerve and function

Cranial nerve	Associated function
I Olfactory	Smell
II Optic	Vision
III Oculomotor	Somatic skeletal motor and autonomic
IV Trochlear	Somatic skeletal motor
V Trigeminal	Somatic sensory and branchiomeric motor
VI Abducens	Somatic skeletal motor
VII Facial	Branchiomeric motor, taste, somatic sensory, and autonomic
VIII Vestibulocochlear	Hearing and balance
IX Glossopharyngeal	Somatic sensory, viscerosensory, taste, autonomic, and branchiomeric motor
X Vagus	Somatic sensory, viscerosensory, taste, autonomic, and branchiomeric motor
XI Spinal Accessory	Branchiomeric motor
XII Hypoglossal	Somatic skeletal motor

Source: Martin (2021)

Box 1.3   Learning activity

Find a picture online of the facial nerve pathway illustrating the five exterior branches that emerge from the skull, so you have a visual reference as you read the next section.

Keywords: facial nerve anatomy, branches, pathway, intracranial course, distribution, innervations

Facial nerve

The clinical presentation of BP reflects the anatomical course of the facial nerve. To understand how dysfunction along the facial nerve contributes to the myriad of symptoms, it is important to explore the related neuroanatomy. The facial nerve originates from the pons-medullary junction of the brainstem and enters the internal acoustic meatus (opening) of the temporal bone, then travels into a long osseous canal known as the facial or fallopian canal. Within the facial canal is where you will find the facial nerve's primary sensory neurons (called the geniculate ganglion), that receive input for taste sensation. The motor branch exits the skull through the stylomastoid foramen, and passes through (but doesn't supply) the parotid gland which is responsible for salivary production. The facial nerve then divides into two trunks, the temporofacial and cervicofacial. These trunks then divide to form five terminal branches that innervate facial musculature:

- The **temporal branch** innervates muscles of the forehead (frontalis) and superior aspect of orbicularis oculi
- The **zygomatic branch** innervates middle part of face (nasalis and zygomaticus), inferior part of orbicularis oculi
- The **buccal branch** innervates cheek muscles (buccinator) and muscles of the mouth
- The **marginal mandibular** branch innervates muscles of the lower part of face and mouth depressors (depressor anguli oris and mentalis)
- The **cervical branch** innervates superficial muscle of the neck (platysma)

Box 1.4   Learning activity

1. Having read the neuroanatomy, think about what would occur as a result of a lesion anywhere along the course of the facial nerve.
2. Draw a quick sketch of a face. Identify on your sketch which facial structures are impacted.
3. What might the physical presentation look like if the person has BP?
4. Create two sketches of faces with this physical presentation: one sketch of a smiling face, and another sketch of a face with their eyes closed.
5. Discuss your sketches with a partner. How has Bell's palsy impacted facial movements?

Somatic, motor, and sensory features

Functions of the facial nerve include blinking and closing eyes, smiling or frowning, lacrimation, salivation, raising the eyebrows, and taste sensations from the anterior aspect of the tongue (Balakrishnan, 2015; Eviston et al., 2015; Singh & Deshmukh, 2022). Injury to the facial nerve may result in paralysis or weakness of facial muscles on the affected side, limiting movement of the face. Motor deficits in BP are almost always ipsilateral (occurring on the same side as the injured nerve), and physical presentations may include drooping of the corner of the mouth and eyebrow, incomplete eye closure when a person attempts to close the eyes, and loss of nasolabial fold or facial creases that normally form with facial expressions (Singh & Deshmukh, 2022). People with BP may also lose taste sensation in the anterior two-thirds of the tongue, most likely due to injury of the facial nerve proximal to the geniculate ganglion (Balakrishnan, 2015; Patel & Levin, 2015). Another clinical feature includes pain around the ear on the affected side, and numbness of the face, tongue, and ear (Balakrishnan, 2015; Eviston et al., 2015; Kim et al., 2018; Patel & Levin, 2015). Prolonged pain has been associated with worse outcomes (Eviston et al., 2015).

Facial neuropathy

People with BP present with a number of symptoms that reflect peripheral neuropathy, which is characterized by damage of one or more nerves due to trauma or disease, and can result in sensory loss, motor dysfunction, and pain (Ginsberg, 2020). Remember, nerves send signals to different body structures in order to initiate muscle contractions or movement and send signals to the brain to make sense of sensations. When there is damage to a motor nerve, muscles no longer receive signals, affecting the ability to move parts of the body. Additionally, when there is damage to a sensory nerve, sensations that are normally felt are no longer processed and numbness may result. Within the extended pathway of the facial canal, the facial nerve has been found to be more vulnerable to trauma and compression (Patel & Levin, 2015). Nerve swelling or inflammation and compression within the facial canal can temporarily inhibit neural communication, disrupt blood supply, and can lead to permanent nerve damage with continuous and increased compression (Balakrishnan, 2015; Lundy-Ekman, 2022). Nerve compression, or ischemia, can impair Schwann cells, interfering with the transmission of electrical signals that are essential for motor and sensory functions (Weyer & Lundy-Ekman, 2022). The following section introduces the microscopic anatomy and physiology of neurotransmission for voluntary movement, to provide background knowledge on typical functions before motor impairment.

Acetylcholine transmission at the neuromuscular junction

Muscle contractions are initiated by the neurotransmitter Acetylcholine (ACh), a chemical messenger that binds onto receptors of a postsynaptic membrane or muscle fiber. Binding occurs at the neuromuscular junction, the site of communication between a nerve ending and a muscle fiber, also known as the synaptic cleft. Before ACh transmission occurs within the synaptic cleft, an electrical signal (called action potential) needs to travel down the axon of a motor neuron to trigger the release of ACh. Once ACh is released into the neuromuscular junction, it diffuses across the synaptic cleft and binds onto the ACh receptors (AChRs) that line a muscle fiber. While binding on AChRs, a fast-acting chemical response is initiated within the muscle membrane, enabling contraction of a skeletal muscle to promote movement. ACh is also responsible for autonomic nervous system function (e.g., slowing heart rate, increasing bodily secretions, dilates blood vessels) and regulating brain activity (e.g., feelings of reward or pleasure). The remaining ACh in the synaptic cleft is broken down into acetyl and choline by acetylcholinesterase (AChE), preventing further muscle contractions.

Although the exact pathogenesis of BP remains unclear (Evitson et al., 2015), some signs and symptoms closely resemble the diagnosis of Myasthenia Gravis (MG) (Elnazeir et al., 2020). Unlike BP, MG is an autoimmune neurological disorder that is characterized by muscle weakness during voluntary movement (see Chapter 2). Presentation of symptoms in people diagnosed with MG vary (see Chapter 2), including asymmetrical or ipsilateral muscle weakness of the eye, mouth, limb, or respiratory muscles that worsen with prolonged movement (Elnazeir et al., 2020). Presentation of ipsilateral facial symptoms such as of the eyes and mouth can make differentiation of BP and MG challenging (see Chapter 2).

Box 1.5   Learning activity

Prior to reading the next section find an image on the internet that shows a typical reflex with the afferent (sensory) and efferent (motor) limbs of the reflex clearly identified so that you have it available as a reference.

Keywords: corneal reflex arc diagram; schematic representation of corneal reflex; blink reflex; corneal reflex pathway

---

Reflex arc

When a foreign substance or object comes into contact with the cornea of the eye, an automatic and protective response (called the corneal reflex) is initiated causing both eyes to blink. This blink reflex occurs bilaterally when one eye is touched, which can be explained by the anatomical loop between the trigeminal sensory nerves and the facial motor nerves that innervate the orbicularis oculi (muscle that closes the eye) (Peterson & Hame, 2022). When the cornea is touched, sensory and motor information travel along a reflex arc. First, touch activates sensory fibers from the eyeball through the trigeminal nerve (the ophthalmic division), and sensory signals travel toward the brainstem where they synapse with neurons in the spinal trigeminal nucleus. Nerves from the spinal trigeminal nucleus then project to the facial motor nuclei, where the motor fibers of the facial nerves on both sides of the head originate. The motor fibers synapse with the orbicularis oculi, resulting in muscle contraction for bilateral eye closure. In people with BP, the absence or delay of the corneal reflex due to a lesion along the facial nerve can be identified by stimulating the cornea with a wisp of cotton (Patel & Levin, 2015). The eyelid of the affected side may exhibit slow closure or may not close at all indicating interruption of signal transmission along the reflex arc.

Nerve regrowth principles

If an axon in the peripheral nervous system is severed, the distal or end segment that becomes separated from the cell body will undergo the process of Wallerian degeneration, which involves the morphologic and biochemical deterioration of axons and myelin sheath (Lee, 2016; Siengsukon, 2022; Zhang et al., 2021). Luckily, peripheral nerves have the capacity to regrow and restore connectivity and function of muscles (Siengsukon, 2022). Schwann cells are capable of nerve regeneration and can form tracks that guide regenerating axons back to their anatomical targets (Jessen et al., 2015; Lee, 2016). The regrowth of axons following nerve damage is known as sprouting and can be classified as collateral or regenerative. Collateral sprouting occurs when an intact axon sends branches to denervated muscles to restore function. Regenerative sprouting occurs when both an axon and its target are damaged, and the axon of the injured neuron sends branches to a new target.

It is important to note, however, that the nervous system has limited ability to repair itself and nerve fibers may regenerate aberrantly (through different pathways than expected) (Siengsukon, 2022). Thus, in BP, motor neurons may improperly innervate another muscle during the process of regeneration (regenerative sprouting), resulting in abnormal facial movements. For example, an individual may experience involuntary mouth movements while voluntarily closing their eyes. This is formally known as motor synkinesis, or involuntary contraction of muscles that occur simultaneously with deliberate movements (Evitson et al., 2015; Somasundara & Sullivan, 2017). Another complication that can arise from inappropriate nerve regeneration is production of tears while eating, known as crocodile tears (Somasundara & Sullivan, 2017). Nerve (gustatory) fibers that originally innervated salivary glands now innervate the lacrimal gland, resulting in this abnormal response while eating. Although a high percentage of people do functionally recover after some time (Somasundara & Sullivan, 2017), there is a potential for incomplete recovery resulting in chronic facial palsy (Evitson et al., 2015). Successful axonal regeneration requires a comprehensive and well-regulated orchestration of molecular and cellular functions to ensure accurate projection and innervation of nerves to its intended target (Zhang et al., 2021). The next section will describe the impact of Bell's palsy on sensory functions. Consider the consequential implications of sensory impairment on daily life.

Box 1.6   Learning activity

In small groups discuss the regenerative properties of a peripheral nerve. Find a YouTube video that explains peripheral nerve regeneration. (Be sure to get guidance from your instructor about how to find quality YouTube videos for this activity.) View it together, and then answer these questions:

1. What parts of the nerve are involved in recovery?
2. What can prevent or delay nerve regeneration?
3. What complications can occur during recovery?

Keywords: peripheral nerve regeneration, neuroregeneration, peripheral nerve repair

---

Living with changes in sensation patterns in Bell's palsy

Peripheral nerves follow a distinct pathway of sensation loss. Similar to how nerves supply information to specific muscles, they also innervate specific regions in the body with sensation information. When experiencing facial paralysis such as BP, sensation around the ears and tongue can be affected (Balakrishnan, 2015; Hotton et al., 2020; Kim et al., 2018; Libreros-Jimenez et al., 2024). As discussed, the facial nerve is primarily a motor nerve, but supplies sensation around the ear and taste sensation to the tongue which can result in pain and numbness in specific areas if sensory nerve fibers are affected (Balakrishnan, 2015; Eviston et al., 2015; Kim et al., 2018; Libreros-Jimenez et al., 2024; Patel & Levin, 2015; Vargo et al., 2023). The facial nerve also innervates the stapedius muscle in the ear, which is responsible for regulating sounds, and disruption of its nerve fibers can result in hyperacusis (sensitivity to sounds) on the affected side, or decreased tolerance to loud sounds (Chung et al., 2022; Libreros-Jimenez et al., 2024; Patel & Levin, 2015; Somasundara & Sullivan, 2017). Sensation patterns also include the tongue due to autonomic innervation by the facial nerve, impairing taste to the anterior two-thirds of the tongue (Balakrishnan, 2015; Eviston et al., 2015; Homer & Fay, 2018; Kim et al., 2018; Libreros-Jimenez et al., 2024; Patel & Levin, 2015). There are five basic tastes of the tongue, including sweet, bitter, salty, sour, and umami (also known as *savory*), and all five can be affected with BP because there are no specific regions of the tongue that are responsible for specific tastes (Yeung & Hummel, 2020).

It is important to note that with BP, light touch and pinprick sensation remain intact because the trigeminal nerve innervates the skin of the face (Lundy-Ekman, 2022). It is possible for people to feel numb in areas of their face when diagnosed with BP, but this is typically a result of lack of proprioception (position sense) in the muscles that are experiencing paralysis (Lundy-Ekman, 2022). Individuals may report dryness in the eye, but this is due to motor loss impairing lacrimal gland secretion, not somatosensation disruption (Balakrishnan, 2015; Eviston et al., 2015; Libreros-Jimenez et al., 2024). With changes to sensation, participation in functional activity can shift.

Box 1.7   Learning activity

Think about a time when you experienced loss of feeling in part of your body, particularly your face.

1. Have you ever felt numbness after leaving the dentist, for example?
2. Take 1–2 minutes and jot down how you think it might feel to drink from a straw, eat soup from a spoon, brush your teeth, apply lip balm, brush hair off your face, and lick your lips if you are experiencing numbness in or around your mouth.

Psychosocial aspects of living with facial palsy

After completing this exercise, you may be deepening your understanding of how the effects of BP related to changes in sensation affect individuals' participation in functional activities. Combine this understanding of changes in sensation with what you know about changes in movement and BP, and let's think about it from a more holistic perspective.

We know that with BP, the ability to smile and frown symmetrically, raise both eyebrows, and wink (and blink) the affected eye can look different from those who are not experiencing facial paralysis. We also know that taste and sound might feel different, as well as a possible new presence of pain, and/or numbness, in certain areas of the face.

What might that mean for the mental health and wellness for individuals with BP? Let's now consider the psychosocial aspects of living with BP.

Box 1.8   Learning activity

1. Think for a moment about what smiling means to you. Consider the act of smiling in different contexts: when you are with family, friends, peers or colleagues, and strangers.
2. Pair up with a peer and share your thoughts. Do you share a similar meaning of smiling? What is different?
3. Together, go to an online search engine and explore the meaning of a smile across cultures. Discuss your findings with your partner.
4. Share what it might look like for you as an individual if your smile was asymmetrical. Discuss: How might this affect you (or not) in different contexts, related to your mental health and wellness? How might you adapt (or not) to this change?

Keywords: smiling across cultures, function of smiling across cultures, cross-cultural meaning of a smile, cultural perceptions of a smile

---

The evidence suggests that, overall, changes in the ability to smile are directly correlated with higher levels of anxiety, a withdrawal from social interaction, and short-term periods of depressed mood (Hotton et al., 2020; Kim et al., 2018; Vargo et al., 2023). Does this ring true for your think, pair, share exercise?

Our ability to express our emotions is heavily reliant not just on smiling, but on our other facial expressions such as frowning, winking, and raising our eyebrows. Expressing emotions through facial expressions changes for those with facial paralysis, and this is important to pay attention to, because the expression—and perception—of emotions is essential for social interaction.

There is a plethora of research available that dives into the neuroscience and psychology of human emotions and emotional processing (de Jongh et al., 2021; Vargo et al., 2023) (Chapter 7 provides an example). Comprehending someone's emotions, particularly in response to your own, is a crucial component of social interaction and interpreting social cues (Hotton et al., 2020; Vargo et al., 2023). For example, mimicking others' expressions such as winking and reciprocating smiles provide cues during social interactions that help us relate to each other (Hotton et al., 2020). Research has found that people who have altered facial expressions due to facial palsy experience more social isolation, avoidance of social encounters, and require more support for their psychological quality of life (Hotton et al., 2020; Vargo et al., 2023). Sometimes people living with BP will cover their face, which in turn affects the social exchange of facial expression (Hotton et al., 2020).

One's health-related quality of life, including their social interaction and social activities, self-esteem, mood, and self-expression, may be affected or changed while living with BP (Hotton et al., 2020; Kim et al., 2018; Vargo et al., 2023). The literature suggests that it is important to pay attention to individual's mental health and wellness history, including anxiety, distress related to body image and appearance, depression and depressed mood, and low self-confidence, as this can correlate to how the individual copes while living with BP (Hotton et al., 2020; Kim et al., 2018; Vargo et al., 2023).

Box 1.9   Learning activity

1. In a small workgroup, jot down some quick notes about what you know about Alex, including their gender identity, age, social participation, hobbies, and interests.
2. Together, answer this question through the use of an online word cloud platform such as www.wordclouds.com: How might Alex's mental health and wellness be affected–or not–by their experience with Bell's palsy?
3. What words stand out the most? Share with the larger group.

Daily life routine: putting on makeup

Typically, the occupation of applying cosmetics begins in adolescence (Mafra et al., 2022). This is a time period in which social and emotional changes occur, and the development of one's own sexuality (Vroman, 2015; Jaworska & MacQueen, 2015; Kaestle et al., 2021). However, an interest in the occupation itself may emerge earlier in life as play or leisure exploration. During adolescence, the development of self and identity occurs in a social context (Kaestle et al., 2021; Vargo et al., 2023; Vroman, 2015). Through engagement in social activities, adolescents are able to acquire hobbies and shared interests, resulting in the formation of friendships (Sundqvist & Hemberg, 2021). Additionally, social interactions tend to elicit concerns of the perception of others, inadvertently impacting perception of self (Vroman, 2015). As teens navigate and explore the more complex social world, makeup can serve as an outlet for self-expression. Makeup can be used on a daily basis as a part of one's self-care routine, and/or can serve as an artistic medium for creative expression.

Back to the person's life: Alex putting on makeup

So now that you know more about BP in the context of neuroscience, signs and symptoms, and its psychosocial impact, how can we use this information to support Alex and their hobbies? After reading this chapter, a more holistic understanding of BP as it relates to Alex can assist in intervention planning.

Box 1.10   Learning activity

In class or small group, discuss intervention approaches that can support Alex and their involvement in daily activities and hobbies. Consider their understanding of BP, its prognosis, and the psychosocial implications to guide your thinking.

What do we know about ourselves and the population at large from this brain condition and this family story?

Although we learned a lot about Alex as an individual and their experience with BP, we also discussed how symptoms might vary, such as heightened sensitivity to loud sounds, or feeling numbness around the ear. We also explored how Alex's experiences with their relationship to self—both physically and psychosocially—may have impacted their experience with BP. Just like with Alex, not everyone will feel and experience occurrences in their lives the same way. There are some common threads that we can generalize to the population at large.

Think about the impact of facial expressions on people in the general population as it relates to expressing our emotions, social participation, and how we engage in meaningful activities. During the COVID-19 pandemic when most people were covering their faces with masks, people found that the way they communicated interpersonally had changed, as they were not able to see each other's facial expressions (Dragomir et al., 2021). We changed the way we interacted with each other so that our brains could interpret the social situation. This included using hands and upper limbs to gesture excitement, happiness, and other emotions. It also included signals from our voices, head orientation, and body posture (Dragomir et al., 2021). These might be suggestions for Alex and others as they navigate their social interactions with BP.

We also talked about experiences with changes in sensation to the face. Many people in the general population have experienced some form of numbness in the face, often from trips to the dentist. This might change the way we eat from a spoon, for example. Individuals with BP may experience changes in the way they engage in hobbies and self-care activities, so it is important to consider the activity analysis of each meaningful occupation, in order to better support these individuals in their participation.

Overall, although we can generalize experiences between Alex and the general population, it is important to consider the individual when working with people who have BP. Their individual backgrounds, social supports, culture, and interests can change the support and interventions that you might offer to folks like Alex and their family. If you're interested in exploring more about BP, there are resources listed under "Further reading" below.

Box 1.11   Learning activity

With your small group, complete the table in the Appendix about the integration of Alex's body functions and social participation demands to successfully complete the task of makeup application with friends.

Further reading

If you're interested in further reading about Bell's palsy and what it is like to live with BP, check out these resources.

Carola. (n.d.). My Bell's palsy story: What it is, treatment, and recovery. *Lili and Bella*. https://liliand-bella.com/my-bells-palsy-story/

Dingman, M. (n.d.). *2-minute neuroscience: Bell's palsy*. Neuroscientifically challenged: Neuroscience made simpler. https://neuroscientificallychallenged.com/posts/2-minute-neuroscience-bells-palsy

Listen Notes. (n.d.). Top podcast episodes. Retrieved January 6, 2023. www.listennotes.com/top-podcasts/bells-palsy/

Mayo Clinic. (n.d.). *Bell's palsy*. www.mayoclinic.org/diseases-conditions/bells-palsy/symptoms-causes/syc-20370028

Moore, L. L. (2016). *Bell's palsy: Facing all odds*. CreateSpace Publishing.

National Institute of Health. (n.d.). *Bell's palsy*. National Institute of Neurological Disorders and Stroke. www.ninds.nih.gov/health-information/disorders/bells-palsy

References

Ahn, H., Jung, W. J., Lee, S. Y., & Lee, K. H. (2023). Recovery from Bell's palsy after treatment using uncultured umbilical cord-derived mesenchymal stem cells: A case report. *World Journal of Clinical Cases, 11*(12), 2817–2824. https://doi.org/10.12998/wjcc.v11.i12.2817

Balakrishnan, A. (2015). Bell's palsy: Causes, symptoms, diagnosis and treatment. *Journal of Pharmaceutical Sciences and Research, 7*(11), 1004–1006.

Balakrishnan, A., Belfiore, L., Chu, T. H., Fleming, T., Midha, R., Biernaskie, J., & Schuurmans, C. (2021). Insights into the role and potential of Schwann cells for peripheral nerve repair from studies of development and injury. *Frontiers in Molecular Neuroscience, 13*, 608442. https://doi.org/10.3389/fnmol.2020.608442

Chung, E. J., Matic, D., Fung, K., MacNeil, S. D., Nichols, A. C., Kiwan, R., Tay, K., & Yoo, J. (2022). Bell's palsy misdiagnosis: Characteristics of occult tumors causing facial paralysis. *Journal of Otolaryngology—Head & Neck Surgery, 51*(1), 39. https://doi.org/10.1186/s40463-022-00591-9

de Jongh, F. W., Sanches, E. E., Luijmes, R., Pouwels, S., Ramnarain, D., Beurskens, C. H. G., Monstrey, S. J., Marres, H. A. M., & Ingles, K. J. A. O. (2021). Cosmetic appreciation and emotional processing in patients with a peripheral facial palsy: A systematic review. *Neuropsychologia, 158*, 107894. https://doi.org/10.1016/j.neuropsychologia.2021.107894

Dragomir, G. M., Fărcașiu, M. A., & Şimon, S. (2021). Students' perceptions of verbal and non-verbal communication behaviors during and after the COVID-19 pandemic. *Applied Sciences, 11*(18), 8282. https://doi.org/10.3390/app11188282

Dresser, L., Wlodarski, R., Rezania, K., & Soliven, B. (2021). Myasthenia gravis: Epidemiology, pathophysiology and clinical manifestations. *Journal of Clinical Medicine, 10*(11), 2235. https://doi.org/10.3390/jcm10112235

Elnazeir, M., Narayanan, S., Badugu, P., Hussain, A., Tareen, T., Hernandez, A. R., Liu, W., Palade, A. E., & Brown, M. E. (2020). Myasthenia gravis masquerading as an idiopathic unilateral facial paralysis (Bell's palsy): A very rare and unique clinical find. *Frontiers in Neurology, 11*, 709. https://doi.org/10.3389/fneur.2020.00709

Eviston, T. J., Croxson, G. R., Kennedy, P. G., Hadlock, T., & Krishnan, A. V. (2015). Bell's palsy: Aetiology, clinical features and multidisciplinary care. *Journal of Neurology, Neurosurgery, and Psychiatry, 86*(12), 1356–1361. https://doi.org/10.1136/jnnp-2014-309563

Ginsberg L. (2020). Acute and chronic neuropathies. *Medicine, 48*(9), 612–618. https://doi.org/10.1016/j.mpmed.2020.06.009

Homer, N., & Fay, A. (2018). Facial paralysis: Diagnosis and management. *Advances in Ophthalmology and Optometry, 3*(1), 357–373. https://doi.org/10.1016/j.yaoo.2018.05.004

Hotton, M., Huggons, E., Hamlet, C., Shore, D., Johnson, D., Norris, J. H., Kilcoyne, S., & Dalton, L. (2020). The psychosocial impact of facial palsy: A systematic review. *British Journal of Health Psychology, 25*, 695–727. https://doi.org/10.1111/bjhp.12440

Jaworska, N., & MacQueen, G. (2015). Adolescence as a unique developmental period. *Journal of Psychiatry & Neuroscience, 40*(5), 291–293. https://doi.org/10.1503/jpn.150268

Jessen, K. R., Mirsky, R., & Lloyd, A. C. (2015). Schwann cells: Development and role in nerve repair. *Cold Spring Harbor Perspectives in Biology, 7*(7), a020487. https://doi.org/10.1101/cshperspect.a020487

Kaestle, C. E., Allen, K. R., Wesche, R., & Grafsky, E. L. (2021). Adolescent sexual development: A family perspective. *The Journal of Sex Research, 58*(7), 874–890. https://doi.org/10.1080/00224499.2021.1924605

Kafle, D. R., & Thakur, S. K. (2021). Evaluation of prognostic factors in patients with Bell's palsy. *Brain and Behavior, 11*(11), e2385. https://doi.org/10.1002/brb3.2385

Kim, S., Lee, H., Kim, N., Yook, T. H., Seo, E., & Kim, J. U. (2018). The association between paralytic side and health-related quality of life in facial palsy: A cross-sectional study of the Korea National Health and Nutrition Examination survey (2008–2012). *Health and Quality of Life Outcomes, 16*, 213–218. https://doi.org/10.1186/s12955-018-1038-0

Lee D. H. (2016). Clinical efficacy of electroneurography in acute facial paralysis. *Journal of Audiology & Otology*, *20*(1), 8–12. https://doi.org/10.7874/jao.2016.20.1.8

Libreros-Jimenez, H. M., Manzo, J., Rojas-Duran, F., Aranda-Abreu, G. E., Garcia-Hernandez, L. I., Coria-Avila, G. A., Herrera-Covarrubias, D., Perez-Estudillo, C. A., Toledo-Cardenas, M. R., & Hernandez-Aguilar, M. E. (2024). On the cranial nerves. *NeuroSci*, *5*(1), 8–38. https://doi.org/10.3390/neurosci5010002

Lundy-Ekman, L. (2022). Cranial nerves. In L. Lundy-Ekman & A. Weyer (Eds.), *Neuroscience: fundamentals for rehabilitation* (6th ed.). Elsevier Inc.

Mafra, A. L., Silva, C. S. A., Varella, M. A. C., & Valentova, J. V. (2022). The contrasting effects of body image and self-esteem in the makeup usage. *PloS One*, *17*(3), e0265197. https://doi.org/10.1371/journal.pone.0265197

Martin, J. H. (2021). Somatic sensation: Trigeminal and viscerosensory systems. In J. H. Martin (Ed.), *Neuroanatomy: Text and atlas* (5th ed., pp. 119–137). McGraw Hill.

Patel, D. K., & Levin, K. H. (2015). Bell palsy: Clinical examination and management. *Cleveland Clinic Journal of Medicine*, *82*(7), 419–426. https://doi.org/10.3949/ccjm.82a.14101

Peterson, D. C., & Hamel, R. N. (2022, July 25). Corneal reflex. In *StatPearls* [Internet]. StatPearls Publishing. www.ncbi.nlm.nih.gov/books/NBK534247/

Portelinha, J., Passarinho, M. P., & Costa, J. M. (2015). Neuro-ophthalmological approach to facial nerve palsy. *Saudi Journal of Ophthalmology*, *29*(1), 39–47. https://doi.org/10.1016/j.sjopt.2014.09.009

Siengsukon, C. (2022). Neuroplasticity. In L. Lundy-Ekman & A. Weyer (Eds.), *Neuroscience: Fundamentals for rehabilitation* (6th ed.). Elsevier Inc.

Singh, A., & Deshmukh, P. (2022). Bell's palsy: A review. *Cureus*, *14*(10), e30186. https://doi.org/10.7759/cureus.30186

Somasundara, D., & Sullivan, F. (2017). Management of Bell's palsy. *Australian Prescriber*, 40(3), 94–97. https://doi.org/10.18773/austprescr.2017.030

Sundqvist, A., & Hemberg, J. (2021). Adolescents' and young adults' experiences of loneliness and their thoughts about its alleviation. *International Journal of Adolescence and Youth*, 26(1), 238–255, https://doi.org/10.1080/02673843.2021.1908903

Vargo, M., Ding, P., Sacco, M., Duggal, R., Genther, D. J., Ciolek, P. J., & Byrne, P. J. (2023). The psychological and psychosocial effects of facial paralysis: A review. *Journal of Plastic, Reconstructive, & Aesthetic Surgery*, *83*, 423–430. https://doi.org/10.1016/j.bjps.2023.05.027

Vroman, K. (2015). Adolescent development: Transitioning from child to adult. In J. Case-Smith & J. C. O'Brien (Eds.), *Occupational therapy for children and adolescence* (pp. 107–112). Mosby Elsevier.

Weyer, A., & Lundy-Ekman, L. (2022). Physical and electrical properties of cells in the nervous system. In L. Lundy-Ekman & A. Weyer (Eds.), *Neuroscience: Fundamentals for rehabilitation* (6th ed.). Elsevier Inc.

Yeung, A. W. K. & Hummel, T. (2020). Literature analysis in relation to research on the five basic tastes. *Nutrition & Food Science*, *50*(1), 34–46.

Zhang, K., Jiang, M., & Fang, Y. (2021). The drama of Wallerian degeneration: The cast, crew, and script. *Annual Review of Genetics*, 55, 93–113. https://doi.org/10.1146/annurev-genet-071819-103917

Zhang, W., Xu, L., Luo, T., Wu, F., Zhao, B., & Li, X. (2020). The etiology of Bell's palsy: A review. *Journal of Neurology*, *267*(7), 1896–1905. https://doi.org/10.1007/s00415-019-09282-4

2 Omar wants to cook meals for his children and has myasthenia gravis

Neuroscience facilitates our understanding of self-care routines

Lauren Winterbottom and Dawn M. Nilsen

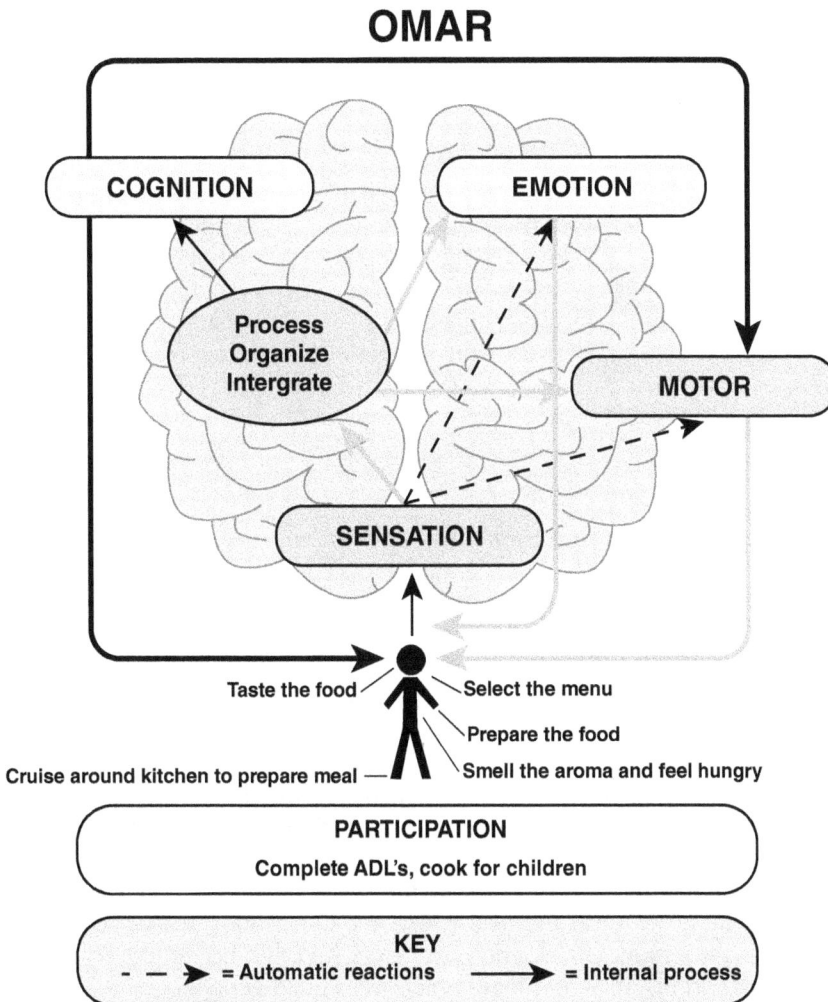

Figure 2.1 Omar brain figure

DOI: 10.4324/9781003524380-4

Purpose of this chapter

The purpose of this chapter is to explore how Omar a 45-year-old, cisgender male who wants to cook dinner for his children might be affected by myasthenia gravis (MG), a condition that disrupts the functioning of the neuromuscular junction (NMJ) impacting muscle functions. People with MG have full lives with their daily routines, relationships and learning, but may require modifications for function.

The key neuroscience concepts that will be explored in this chapter include: the role of upper and lower motor neurons in the production of movement, the motor tracts that influence the functioning of the muscles of the head, neck, and body, neuronal communication, and the neuromuscular junction. As with all the chapters, these components of the nervous system work with other systems to support overall human function.

Keywords for this chapter are listed in the box below. Be sure you learn what these key features are so you can get the most out of the chapter.

Keywords for this chapter

acetylcholine (ACh)
acetylcholinesterase
   (AChE)
action potential
chemical synaptic
   transmission
endplate potential
equilibrium potential
excitatory post-synaptic
   potential

graded potentials
inhibitory post-synaptic
   potential
lower motor neurons
   (LMNs)
myasthenia crisis
myasthenia gravis (MG)
neuromuscular junction
nicotinic acetylcholine
   receptors (AChR)

post-synaptic neuron
pre-synaptic neuron
pyridostigmine
resting membrane
   potential
synapses
upper motor neurons
   (UMNs)

Omar, a man who wants to cook dinner for his children

Omar is a 45-year-old man who lives in a three-bedroom condo in Edgewater, New Jersey. He is recently divorced from his wife with whom he has three children, Elena (aged 12), Hugo (aged 10), and Anna (aged 7). He has joint custody of his children with his wife and highly values his role as a father. Although the divorce was stressful for the whole family, he has found time to connect with his children and loves cooking family dinners. His specialty is chicken parmesan over pasta and garden salad. Omar works from home as a free-lance graphic designer and enjoys his work, although he has recently been overwhelmed with keeping up with both his job and his responsibilities as a father. Omar was diagnosed with ocular MG at age 40 when he noticed that his right eyelid was drooping, and his vision was blurry. He found out that those symptoms were caused by weakness in his eye muscles. His doctors prescribed pyridostigmine initially, which helped improve his symptoms right away. Over the next two years, Omar noticed that he had more difficulty getting up from low chairs, and his doctors said that his condition progressed to affect the strength in his arms and legs, which was called generalized MG. Because the pyridostigmine was no longer effective in improving his muscle strength, Omar now takes prednisone daily to help manage his symptoms. Omar has had difficulty keeping up with his work due to double vision and fatigue when working at the computer. He feels concerned with the need to provide for his kids by maintaining steady freelance work but has had difficulty keeping up with his normal work hours.

More recently Omar has noticed increasing weakness in his hands and difficulty keeping a good grip on objects while cooking. He has been limited by overwhelming fatigue, particularly in the evenings around dinnertime. Omar has noticed that his symptoms come and go unpredictably, adding to his stress because he never knows which days will be "bad days." Omar has found that he always needs to have a back-up plan in case his symptoms are so great that he is unable to meet his responsibilities for the day. This uncertainty has contributed to anxiety, frustration, and sense of isolation. Omar has put a lot of pressure on himself to keep things as normal for his kids as possible, and he feels a great deal of guilt when he is unable to keep up. Although Omar loves cooking dinner for his kids, he has found that he always needs to have a frozen dinner in the freezer as back-up in case his weakness and fatigue make it too difficult for him to cook.

Box 2.1   Learning activity

Discuss with your peers:

1. Having read the narrative, what are you curious about?
2. What will you need to know more about?

What is myasthenia gravis?

Myasthenia gravis is an autoimmune disease in which antibodies block receptors at the neuromuscular junction. This leads to reduced synaptic transmission between lower motor neurons and muscle fibers. This results primarily in muscle weakness and fatigue (Dresser et al., 2021). Weakness can occur in eye muscles, bulbar muscles, axial muscles, limb muscles, and respiratory muscles. Around 15 to 20% of individuals with this disease may experience a myasthenia crisis requiring mechanical ventilation (Dresser et al., 2021). Weakness can fluctuate and may worsen with heat and stress. In addition to fluctuating muscle weakness, individuals with MG also report generalized fatigue, exhaustion, and poor sleep (Law et al., 2021). Non-motor symptoms of the disease may also include cognitive, psychosocial, sensory, and autonomic dysfunction along with reports of pain and headache. Long-term use of steroids may have a negative impact on memory. In addition, those with MG report higher levels of cognitive fatigue when compared with healthy controls. However, the relationship between MG and cognitive dysfunction is not well understood (Tong et al., 2018).

Box 2.2   Learning activity

1. What structures of the nervous system are impaired in MG? Locate pictures of these structures.
2. What motor impairments are associated with MG? Which are most common? Create a list of clinical symptoms you may observe and include definitions of clinical terms.
3. For individuals living with MG, how might each of these symptoms impact their ability to participate in daily activities?

Keywords: myasthenia gravis (MG), myasthenia crisis, pathophysiology, neuromuscular junction, clinical symptoms

MG Subtypes

MG is caused by antibodies that target different molecules in the neuromuscular junction, leading to reduced neuromuscular transmission that results in muscle weakness. Most commonly, antibodies target nicotinic acetylcholine receptors (AChR). While there are other subtypes of the disease in which antibodies target different molecules, this chapter will focus on AChR MG, which affects about 85% of individuals with the disease (Koneczny & Herbst, 2019). Typically, weakness initially presents in the muscles of the eyes. Within two years, most individuals with the disease then progress to generalized MG, in which other muscles become affected. Individuals with ocular MG only have eye muscle weakness. Myasthenia gravis can occur any age. Early onset MG occurs before the age of 50 and is more common in women. Late onset MG occurs after age 50 with a slightly higher prevalence in men (Dresser et al., 2021; Jayam Trouth et al., 2012; Koneczny & Herbst, 2019). For a more detailed discussion of MG subtypes, see Koneczny and Herbst (2019).

Neuroscience information to guide your thinking about Omar

Introduction

To engage in an activity such as cooking, we often rely on postural stability in our trunk, coordinated movements in our arms and hands to grasp and manipulate task objects, and eye movements to locate items in the kitchen. Multiple structures in the nervous system are needed to produce voluntary movements, such as motor neurons that are located within the nervous system (see Chapters 4–6).

Motor neurons

Voluntary movement is produced by a two-neuron pathway comprised of upper motor neurons (UMNs) and lower motor neurons (LMNs). UMNs integrate signals from the cortex and translate them into signals that either initiate or inhibit voluntary movement or modify reflexive movements (Emos & Agarwal, 2023). The axons of UMNs form the pyramidal tract, which then divides into two nerve tracks carrying motor information to the brainstem and spinal cord (Lohia & McKenzie, 2023). UMNs communicate with LMNs, and LMNs communicate with muscles using different neurotransmitters (Zayia & Tadi, 2023).

Box 2.3   Learning activity

1. Find an image that shows the relationship between UMNs and LMNs. Where are UMNs and LMNs located?
2. The pyramidal tract divides into two main tracts. What are the names of those two tracts? They project to the LMNs in which locations?
3. The axons of these LMNs innervate muscles in which locations?
4. What are the clinical signs associated with UMN lesions? LMN lesions? (See Chapters 1–6.)
5. How do these signs differ from MG symptoms?

Keywords: motor neurons, upper motor neurons, lower motor neurons, pyramidal tract

Neuronal communication

Neurons are the "communicators" of the nervous system. These important cells have three basic functions: (1) they receive information (signals); (2) they integrate information to determine whether or not the information should be passed along; and (3) they send information to target cells (i.e. other neurons or effector target, such as muscle or glands) (Mihailoff & Haines, 2018).

Neurons communicate with one another at junctions called synapses. At a synapse, one neuron (pre-synaptic neuron) sends a message to a target neuron (post-synaptic neuron) or an effector target cell (e.g., muscle cell) (Mihailoff & Haines, 2018).

Box 2.4   Learning activity

1. What are the two basic types of synapses? What is the difference between them? Which is the most common?
2. Which is involved in MG?

Keywords: electrical synapse, chemical synapse, pre-synaptic neuron, post-synaptic neuron, neuromuscular junction

---

Chemical synaptic transmission occurs when a neurotransmitter is released from a pre-synaptic neuron. This neurotransmitter then transfers information by binding to a receptor on the post-synaptic neuron or target tissue. We will explore this type of transmission a bit later in this section, but first you need to have a basic understanding of how neurons generate electrical signals (Dwyer, 2018a).

Box 2.5   Learning activity

1. Find an image that clearly labels the pre-synaptic neuron (sending cell), the post-synaptic neuron (receiving cell) and the synapse.
2. Search the National Institutes of Health or Open Access Neuroscience Textbooks from Medical Universities (e.g., UTHealth McGovern Medical School: https://nba.uth.tmc.edu/neuroscience/index.htm) to find a definition of a neurotransmitter and a receptor.
3. What are the major neurotransmitters of the brain and spinal cord?
4. Which neurotransmitter is considered the chief excitatory neurotransmitter of the brain?
5. Which neurotransmitter is considered the chief inhibitory neurotransmitter of the brain?
6. What is the name of the neurotransmitter that allows UMNs to communicate with LMNs?
7. What is the name of the neurotransmitter that allows LMNs to communicate with muscle fibers?
8. Which receptor is important for skeletal muscle contraction?

Keywords: chemical synaptic transmission, neurotransmitter, glutamate, gamma-aminobutyric acid (GABA), acetylcholine (ACh), nicotinic acetylcholine receptors (AChR)

In order to communicate, neurons generate electrical signals to encode and transfer information from one location to another. These electrical signals arise from ion fluxes across the cell membrane resulting in changes in the neuronal membrane potential. Membrane potentials arise from the separation of cations (positively charged ions, such as sodium, potassium, and calcium) and anions (negatively charged ions such as chloride and organic anions) across the neuronal membrane. This separation of charges is due to the concentration gradients (chemical gradient) of the ions and the cell membrane's permeability (the ease with which ions can cross the membrane) to those ions. It is also important to note that ions are subject to both chemical (related to ion concentration gradients and the principle of diffusion) and electrical forces (related to ion charges and the principle of electrostatic pressure). These forces cause ions to either move into the cell or out of the cell, and each ion has what is known as an equilibrium potential. This represents the electrical potential necessary to prevent an ion from diffusing down its chemical gradient (Dwyer, 2018b).

There are three important types of membrane potentials: (1) the resting membrane potential; (2) graded potentials (receptor and post-synaptic); (3) the action potential. Each of these potentials play important roles in neuronal communication (Dwyer, 2018b). Let's explore the differences between them now.

Box 2.6   Learning activity

Access the Kahn Academy website: www.khanacademy.org. Once at the site, in the search bar type in Neuronal Membrane Potentials and access the videos that describe the neuron resting potential, graded potential, and action potential.

1. Why is the resting potential of a typical neuron negative?
2. What causes a graded potential?
3. Describe the differences between an excitatory post-synaptic potential and an inhibitory post-synaptic potential.
4. Reflecting on the neurotransmitters you identified in the learning activity in Box 2.5, which ones are most likely to generate excitatory post-synaptic potentials, and which are most likely to generate inhibitory post synaptic potentials?
5. Which type of potential is caused by the opening of voltage-gated ion channels that are selective for sodium?
6. What is meant by the "all or none" principle of action potentials?

Keywords: resting potential, graded potential, action potential, equilibrium potential, excitatory post-synaptic potential, inhibitory post-synaptic potential

---

Now that you have a better understanding of how neurons generate electrical signals and the functions of the different types of signals, let's return to chemical synaptic transmission. As previously discussed, information transfer between neurons or a neuron and an effector target (e.g., muscle) typically occurs when a pre-synaptic neuron releases a neurotransmitter that binds a receptor on a post-synaptic neuron or the effector target cell. The process of this information transfer involves several important steps. Let's explore the steps involved with chemical synaptic transmission now.

Box 2.7   Learning activity

1. Find a YouTube video or an image on the internet that depicts a chemical synapse and the steps involved with chemical synaptic transmission and list the steps so that you can refer back to them later when we explore a unique chemical synapse the neuromuscular junction. (Be sure to get guidance from your instructor about how to find quality YouTube videos for this activity. A suggestion for a video to help get you started: "2-Minute Neuroscience: Synaptic Transmission.")
2. How is the information transfer at a chemical synapse initiated?
3. How is the information transfer at a chemical synapse terminated?
4. Thinking about how information transfer is initiated and terminated at a chemical synapse, how might drugs act to facilitate or inhibit chemical synaptic transmission?
5. How does understanding chemical synaptic transmission inform your understanding of MG?

Structure and function of the neuromuscular junction

The neuromuscular junction (NMJ) consists of the presynaptic terminal at the end of the lower motor neuron axon where a synaptic bouton is filled with synaptic vesicles. These synaptic vesicles contain the NMJ's neurotransmitter. Here, an action potential from the LMN elicits a muscle contraction through the release of acetylcholine (ACh) into the synaptic cleft, which is the space between the presynaptic terminal and the postsynaptic muscle membrane. ACh crosses the synapse and binds to nicotinic acetylcholine receptors (AChR) that are in the postsynaptic muscle membrane. This membrane contains densely clustered AChRs and numerous junctional folds that increase the membrane surface area. Voltage-gated sodium channels are located within the junctional folds to increase excitability of the membrane. When ACh binds to the AChR, depolarization of the postsynaptic membrane occurs through activation of the voltage-gated sodium channels. This triggers an endplate potential, which then leads to an action potential in the muscle fiber, resulting in a muscle contraction. An enzyme called acetylcholinesterase (AChE), which is part of the extracellular matrix within the synaptic cleft, breaks down remaining ACh to prevent further action (Rodríguez Cruz et al., 2020).

Box 2.8   Learning activity

1. Find an image that depicts the NMJ and clearly labels the presynaptic neuron; junctional folds; postsynaptic muscle fiber and the nicotinic acetylcholine receptors.
2. Now find a video on YouTube that shows chemical synaptic transmission in the NMJ. (You may find the Kahn Academy video "Neuromuscular junction, motor end-plate" helpful.)
3. Why is the NMJ considered a unique chemical synapse?
4. Given what you know about MG, how might this condition lead to weakness and fatigue?

Keywords: neuromuscular junction, acetylcholinesterase (AChE), endplate potential

The NMJ and MG

As we previously discussed, most people with MG have muscle weakness because their neuromuscular junction is impaired. They have antibodies against the AChR. These antibodies can cause the disease in different ways. Antibodies can block AChR or prevent ACh from binding to the receptors by binding to them first. These antibodies can crosslink between AChRs and pull them into the cell in a process called endocytosis. This results in AChR destruction. Antibodies can also activate the complement cascade, which is an immune system response that can damage structures in the postsynaptic muscle membrane, such as the junctional folds. This leads to further loss of AChRs and voltage-gated sodium channels. A reduction in AChRs and other important structures in the postsynaptic membrane can lead to decreased sensitivity to ACh over time (Koneczny & Herbst, 2019). Remember that AChE is an enzyme that breaks down ACh in the NMJ to prevent it from constantly inducing muscle contractions. For people with MG, drugs that inhibit AChE, such as pyridostigmine, can increase the action of ACh in the NMJ, causing an increase in strength. However, as the disease progresses, these drugs may no longer be effective due to structural damage at the postsynaptic membrane. For later stages of the disease, steroids such as prednisone and other therapies that directly target the immune system are often prescribed (Farrugia & Goodfellow, 2020).

Box 2.9   Learning activity

Find an image that shows the difference between normal NMJ function and NMJ dysfunction in MG. How might this dysfunction lead to challenges with daily participation for people with MG?

Keywords: neuromuscular junction, myasthenia gravis, pyridostigmine

---

Daily life routine: cooking chicken parmesan over pasta and garden salad

The activity of cooking a complex meal requires numerous motor skills. Other cognitive and visual skills are also needed for successful meal preparation.

Box 2.10   Learning activity

1. Complete an activity analysis of a meal of your choice using the performance skills listed in the Occupational Therapy Practice Framework (OTPF). Create a list of all the motor skills and process skills in the OTPF and give one example of how each skill could be used during your cooking activity.
2. How might motor skill performance be affected by the symptoms of MG when cooking a meal? Make sure to consider oculomotor symptoms in your discussion.

Back to the person's life: Omar cooking a meal for his children

Although Omar loves to cook, the symptoms caused by MG have made it very challenging for him to prepare meals for his family the way that he used to. The double vision that he experiences makes it difficult to see what he is doing, making him nervous that he will cut himself when chopping vegetables. Additionally, the weakness in his hands has made it challenging to keep a good grip on the knife. He also finds that he fatigues very quickly with the repeated chopping motion. Omar finds it is exceptionally difficult to strain pasta due to weakness in his arms and is worried that he could burn himself. He also feels unsteady when taking pans in and out of the oven due to proximal weakness in his extremities. On top of all this, Omar experiences cognitive fatigue and has difficulty maintaining his endurance while cooking dinner. Omar has learned to adapt by prepping dinner ahead of time and using adaptive recipes that make it easier to manage making dinner for his children. For instance, he will make chicken parmesan subs using frozen pre-breaded chicken cutlets and salad with pre-chopped vegetables. He also keeps a backup option for dinner in the freezer in case his symptoms flair up (or orders a pizza). With his children getting older, he has considered having them help with prep activities the evening before so he can still assemble foods for dinner the next day.

Box 2.11   Learning activity

1. Using your knowledge of the Occupational Therapy Practice Framework, what are the best intervention strategies for Omar?
2. List some interventions that you think might help Omar with cooking meals.

What do we know about ourselves and the population at large from this neurological condition and this family story?

Individuals with MG have expressed that one challenge of living with MG is that symptoms fluctuate and can be unpredictable, causing the need for constant adaptation and tradeoffs in order to make it through the day (Law et al., 2021). They have also expressed feeling disconnected with their healthcare providers as their medical management may not adequately address the effect the disease has on their day-to-day lives. Individuals with MG may experience anxiety, depression, guilt, and loneliness as a result of their symptoms and may lack social support. Due to the unpredictable nature of their symptoms and generalized fatigue, they may have difficulty making plans with friends and maintaining employment (Law et al., 2021). While many aspects of MG can often be managed medically, prolonged use of medications and disease progression over time can limit meaningful participation and engagement. Even though we may understand the symptoms and mechanisms of the disease, each person has a different lived experience and story. This condition also demonstrates the importance of the motor system to our daily lives, how our environments are built for well-functioning motor systems, and how much our daily life can be disrupted when there is dysfunction in this system. As occupational therapists, we can lessen the impact of such conditions by modifying environments and tasks to circumvent motor challenges. It is important to listen to each person's story and learn about their unique challenges and strengths to create the best environmental and task matches to maximize daily participation and occupational engagement.

Box 2.12   Learning activity

With your small group, complete the table in the Appendix about how to facilitate Omar in his desire to cook dinner for his children.

Further reading

If you're interested in further reading about MG and the lived experience of those with MG, please see these resources:

Dresser, L., Wlodarski, R., Rezania, K., & Soliven, B. (2021). Myasthenia gravis: Epidemiology, pathophysiology and clinical manifestations. *Journal of Clinical Medicine*, *10*(11), 2235. https://doi.org/10.3390/jcm10112235

Farrugia, M. E., & Goodfellow, J. A. (2020). A practical approach to managing patients with myasthenia gravis—Opinions and a review of the literature. *Frontiers in Neurology*, *11*. https://doi.org/10.3389/fneur.2020.00604

Jayam Trouth, A., Dabi, A., Solieman, N., Kurukumbi, M., & Kalyanam, J. (2012). Myasthenia gravis: A review. *Autoimmune Diseases*, *2012*(1), 1–10. https://doi.org/10.1155/2012/874680

Koneczny, I., & Herbst, R. (2019). Myasthenia gravis: Pathogenic effects of autoantibodies on neuromuscular architecture. *Cells*, *8*(7), 671. https://doi.org/10.3390/cells8070671

Law, N., Davio, K., Blunck, M., Lobban, D., & Seddik, K. (2021). The lived experience of myasthenia gravis: A patient-led analysis. *Neurology and Therapy*, *10*(2), 1103–1125. https://doi.org/10.1007/s40120-021-00285-w

Rodríguez Cruz, P. M., Cossins, J., Beeson, D., & Vincent, A. (2020). The neuromuscular junction in health and disease: Molecular mechanisms governing synaptic formation and homeostasis. *Frontiers in Molecular Neuroscience*, *13*, 610964. https://doi.org/10.3389/fnmol.2020.610964

References

Dresser, L., Wlodarski, R., Rezania, K., & Soliven, B. (2021). Myasthenia gravis: Epidemiology, pathophysiology and clinical manifestations. *Journal of Clinical Medicine*, *10*(11), 2235. https://doi.org/10.3390/jcm10112235

Dwyer, T. M. (2018a). Chemical signaling in the nervous system. In D. E. Haines & G. A. Mihailoff (Eds.), *Fundamental Neuroscience for Basic and Clinical Applications* (5th ed., pp. 54–71). Elsevier.

Dwyer, T. M. (2018b). The electrochemical basis of nerve function. In D. E. Haines & G. A. Mihailoff (Eds.), *Fundamental Neuroscience for Basic and Clinical Applications* (5th ed., pp. 34–53). Elsevier.

Emos, M. C., & Agarwal, S. (2023). Neuroanatomy, upper motor neuron lesion. In *StatPearls* [Internet]. StatPearls Publishing.

Farrugia, M. E., & Goodfellow, J. A. (2020). A practical approach to managing patients with myasthenia gravis—Opinions and a review of the literature. *Frontiers in Neurology*, *11*. https://doi.org/10.3389/fneur.2020.00604

Jayam Trouth, A., Dabi, A., Solieman, N., Kurukumbi, M., & Kalyanam, J. (2012). Myasthenia gravis: A Review. *Autoimmune Diseases*, *2012*(1), 1–10. https://doi.org/10.1155/2012/874680

Khan, Y. S., & Lui, F. (2023). Neuroanatomy, spinal cord. In *StatPearls* [Internet]. StatPearls Publishing.

Koneczny, I., & Herbst, R. (2019). Myasthenia gravis: Pathogenic effects of autoantibodies on neuromuscular architecture. *Cells*, *8*(7), 671. https://doi.org/10.3390/cells807067

Law, N., Davio, K., Blunck, M., Lobban, D., & Seddik, K. (2021). The lived experience of myasthenia gravis: A patient-led analysis. *Neurology and Therapy*, *10*(2), 1103–1125. https://doi.org/10.1007/s40120-021-00285-w

Lohia, A., & McKenzie, J. (2023). Neuroanatomy, pyramidal tract lesions. In *StatPearls* [Internet]. StatPearls Publishing.

Mihailoff, G. A., & Haines, D. E. (2018). The cell biology of neurons and glia. In D. E. Haines & G. A. Mihailoff (Eds.), *Fundamental neuroscience for basic and clinical applications* (5th ed., pp. 15–33). Elsevier.

Rodríguez Cruz, P. M., Cossins, J., Beeson, D., & Vincent, A. (2020). The neuromuscular junction in health and disease: Molecular mechanisms governing synaptic formation and homeostasis. *Frontiers in Molecular Neuroscience*, *13*, 610964. https://doi.org/10.3389/fnmol.2020.610964

Tong, O., Delfiner, L., & Herskovitz, S. (2018). Pain, headache, and other non-motor symptoms in myasthenia gravis. *Current Pain and Headache Reports*, *22*(6), 39. https://doi.org/10.1007/s11916-018-0687-3

Zayia, L. C., & Tadi, P. (2023). Neuroanatomy, Motor neuron. In *StatPearls* [Internet]. StatPearls Publishing.

3 Danea wants to complete personal hygiene to go out with friends and has a spinal cord injury

Neuroscience facilitates our understanding of personal hygiene

Alison Bell and M. J. Mulcahey

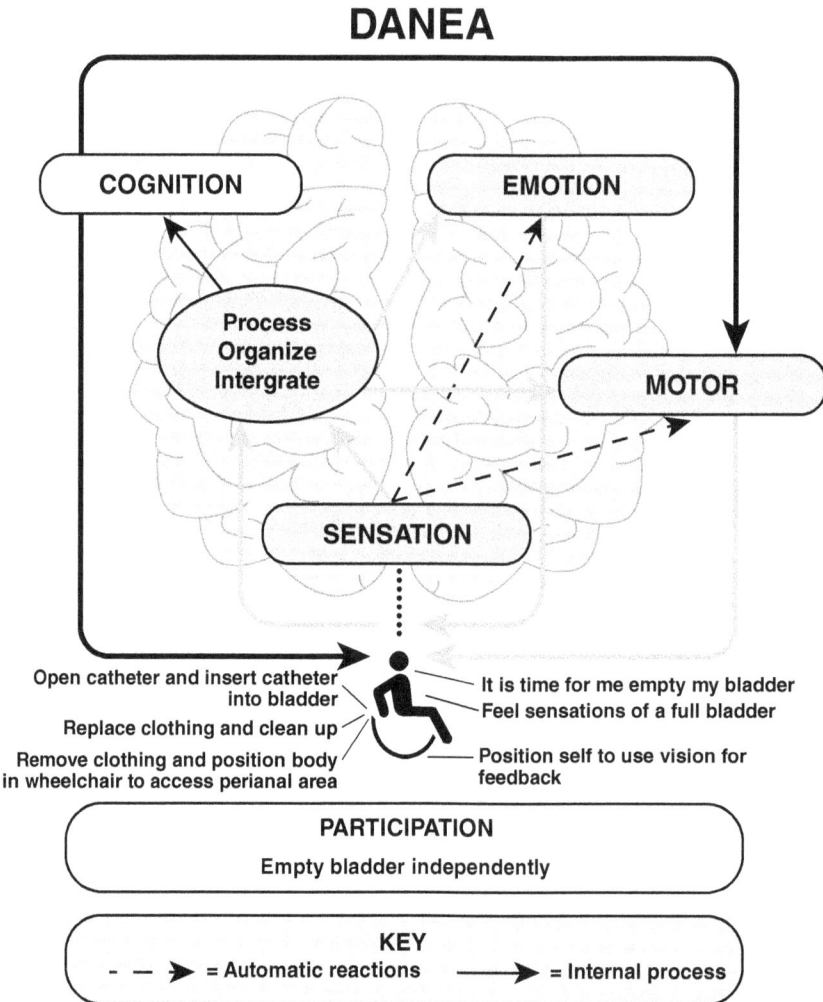

Figure 3.1 Danea brain figure

DOI: 10.4324/9781003524380-5

Purpose of this chapter

The purpose of this chapter is to explore how Danea, a 23-year-old who wants to complete personal hygiene to go out with friends might be affected by a spinal cord injury (SCI), a condition caused by traumatic or non-traumatic events that disrupts the functioning of the spinal cord impacting autonomic, cognitive, motor and sensory functions. People with SCI participate in daily routines, relationships, and vocational and avocational pursuits, but often require modifications for function.

The key neuroscience concepts explored in this chapter are the structure and function of the spinal cord, including upper and lower motor neurons, ascending (sensory) and descending (motor) tracts and their connections to and communication with central and peripheral targets, and the autonomic nervous system. As with all the chapters, these components of the nervous system work with other systems to support overall human function.

Keywords for this chapter are listed in the box below. Be sure you learn these key features to get the most out of the chapter.

Keywords for this chapter

anterior cord syndrome	central cord syndrome	dermatomes
autonomic dysreflexia (AD)	corticospinal tract (CST)	Lissauer's tract
autonomic nervous system	deep tendon reflex (DTR)	spinal thalamic tract
Brown-Sequard syndrome	dorsal-column medial lemniscus	posterior cord syndrome

---

Danea, who uses "they," "their," and "them" pronouns, is a 23-year-old who wants to be more independent in personal hygiene without relying on their mother so that they can go out with friends, including weekend trips. Danea graduated from cosmetology school and briefly worked as an apprentice in a hair salon near home. They live with their mother and younger sibling in a one-story home. Danea loves to sing, particularly at venues with open-microphone karaoke, and gets great pleasure in dressing up, applying make-up, and fixing their hair for photo shoots with friends. Danea has a small tight-knit group of friends who spend several evenings a week and most weekends together, usually on the beach or at a beach club.

Danea sustained a C6 motor and sensory complete SCI one year ago. After the injury, Danea spent eight weeks in an acute rehabilitation hospital to begin to learn basic activities of daily living (ADL) and to be evaluated for adaptive equipment and wheelchair mobility. Since discharge from rehabilitation, the strength of Danea's shoulder muscles has greatly improved, and elbow flexion and wrist extension are strong in both arms. They have not regained function in muscle groups supplied by lower spinal cord levels and do not have active hand grasp, elbow extension, or movement in the trunk and legs. They have some (not typical) feeling in their fingers and thumb, but do not have feeling in their trunk and lower body. Danea continues to work with occupational and physical therapy on goals of physical functioning, ADL, and instrumental ADL (IADL).

Danea can move around the house in a power-assist chair and uses adaptive equipment to apply make-up, brush teeth, and use utensils for meals. Danea uses their smart phone for music, communicating with friends through text and social media and for internet access. They use SMART devices to activate music and turn computers on and off. Using their knuckles, Danea easily uses keyboards and swipes the phone to open and close applications; they send most text messages using voice assistance.

Danea's mother helps with morning and evening routines such as getting in and out of bed, showering, dressing, and undressing. As a result of the injury, Danea needs assistance to ensure that their bowel and bladder are empty. Their mother performs a bowel program every other night using a combination of an enema, oral medications and digital stimulation to ensure they fully empty their bowels as to prevent bowel impaction as well as bowel incontinence. Danea's bladder is emptied every four hours using intermittent catheterization, performed by their mother or sister. Danea would like to be more independent in performing these personal hygiene tasks so they can stay out with friends for extended periods, including overnight.

Danea tells the occupational therapist that they have incredible pain, especially burning painful sensations in their legs despite being unable to feel them. Danea cannot actively move their legs but has figured out how to make them "spasm" and "stiffen up," especially in bed. Danea wonders why they can make their paralyzed legs spasm but cannot make their paralyzed fingers spasm. Danea also shared that they tried singing again but feels winded with frequent episodes of low blood pressure, and time spent with friends is limited because of their catheterization schedule, occasional urinary incontinence, and inability to stay outside in the heat for long periods.

Before you continue reading the chapter, work in your small group to discuss what you already know.

Box 3.1   Learning activity

1. How can knowledge of neuroscience help you understand the clinical presentation of SCI?
2. What regions of the spinal cord supply motor and sensory function to the arms? To the trunk? To the legs?
3. How many vertebrae are in the cervical, thoracic, lumbar and sacral spinal column, and what is the structural relationship between them and the spinal nerves emanating from the spinal cord?
4. What else are you curious about?

What is spinal cord injury?

Despite its small size in the nervous system, the spinal cord significantly influences how we move, our body sensations and automatic behaviors like breathing, blood pressure control, and bowel, bladder, and sexual functions (just to name a few!). While it may be easier to think of the spinal cord as only communication between the brain and peripheral body, it would be a mistake and underestimate the neurologic activity occurring in the spinal cord. After a SCI, most people expect sensory and motor loss due to understanding the spinal cord as a communication system between the brain and body. However, changes in bowel, bladder, sexual function, respiration, pain, and other autonomic functions (cardiac, digestion, temperature control, as examples) are among the additional challenges after SCI, and the unique presentations (you will explore these later) are reflective of the organization and function of the spinal cord.

Neuroscience information to guide your thinking about Danea

Structure of the spinal cord

The spinal cord extends from the medulla to the lumbar segments of the spinal column, where it terminates as a structure known as the conus medullaris. The spinal cord does not extend the full length of the spinal column due to different processes during embryonic development. At the caudal (bottom) end, the spinal cord is anchored to the coccyx by an extension of the pia mater (a membrane that is the innermost part of the layers that cover the brain and spinal cord) called the filum terminale. At the base of the spinal cord is a structure known as the cauda equina. It is called this because the collection of spinal nerves looks like a horse's tail (Ganapathy et al., 2023). The cauda equina is not part of the true spinal cord and is a transitional area between the central and peripheral nervous systems. Despite this transitional zone, damage to this area is classified as a type of SCI.

Box 3.2   Learning activity

The spinal cord is highly organized. This organization can be appreciated by examining cross-sections (slices) of the spinal cord. Find figures or images depicting cross-sections of the spinal cord that clearly label the following structures: gray matter; white matter; dorsal columns central canal; dorsal, ventral and lateral horns; dorsal and ventral roots, dorsal root ganglion and a spinal nerve.

Look for drawings showing all these parts, and then find an actual image of the cross section of the spinal cord and look for the color changes that show the parts.

1. What is contained in the gray matter?
2. What type of information is contained in the ventral, dorsal and lateral horns, respectively?
3. What is contained in the white matter?

   a. Which of these tracts are considered ascending (sensory) tracts?
   b. Which of these tracts are considered descending (motor) tracts?

Keywords: cross section, spinal cord, labeled

The spinal cord contains 31 segments. Each segment has a pair of spinal nerves that exit to supply peripheral structures. There are eight cervical segments, twelve thoracic segments, five lumbar segments, five sacral segments, and one coccygeal segment. The gray matter of each spinal segment is dedicated to specific regions in the body. For sensory information, these regions are called dermatomes. For muscles, they are called myotomes. In practice we use dermatomes to guide our sensory evaluation, but we do not use myotomes to guide our motor testing. This is because multiple segments of the spinal cord innervate most muscles, clinicians must think about the spinal cord levels of motor innervation for the muscle strength testing as opposed to relying entirely on myotome distribution.

Box 3.3   Learning activity

1. What is the definition of a dermatome?
2. What is the definition of a myotome?
3. Find an image of a dermatome chart and answer the following questions:

   a. Which dermatomes supply the upper limb?
   b. Which dermatomes supply the lower limb?
   c. Which dermatomes supply the trunk?
   d. Which dermatomes supply the buttocks?

4. Find an image showing myotomes for the upper and lower limb muscles, and muscles in the trunk.

   a. Which spinal cord levels innervate (supply motor function to) the upper limb?
   b. Which spinal cord levels innervate the lower limb?
   c. Which spinal cord levels innervate the trunk

Keywords: myotome; image search

5. How does knowledge of dermatomes, myotomes and segmental innervation help occupational therapists identify motor and sensory levels of SCI?
6. Why is it important for an occupational therapist to know the motor and sensory level of someone's SCI?

The cervical segments contain neurons that control neck and arm areas and are also crucial for breathing. The diaphragm is the primary muscle of breathing and is supplied by neurons in the upper cervical spine. Accessory muscles of breathing are supplied by neurons in the cervical and thoracic spine. These muscles include the scalene (innervated by the cervical spinal cord), sternocleidomastoid (innervated by the upper cervical spinal cord and cranial nerve XI) and intercostal muscles (innervated by the thoracic spinal cord). The thoracic segments support the trunk, lumbar segments the hips and legs, and sacral segments the hips, legs and bowel, bladder, and sexual functions. Due to the arrangement of the spinal cord, after a SCI, there is dysfunction that corresponds to the level that was damaged as well as the areas below that level of injury. This is because the white matter carrying information to and from the brain can no longer ascend or descend through the damaged spinal cord segment.

Box 3.4   Learning activity

1. Based on Danea's case description, what segment in the spinal cord is Danea's injury?
2. Consider what you know about Danea's abilities in ADLs, specifically personal hygiene and discuss them relevant to what you know about Danea's motor level of injury and motor function.

3. View a short video to learn more about intermittent catheterization. View a video about independent self-catheterization after spinal cord injury. (Be sure to get guidance from your instructor about how to find quality YouTube videos for this activity.) Continue your discussion about Danea's motor function relevant to their goal for self-catheterization.

Keywords: intermittent catheterization, spinal cord injury, bladder management, demo, demonstration

4. Based on your understanding of the structure of the spinal cord, consider what you know about Danea's respiratory function and discuss the implications on singing and open-microphone karaoke nights.

Somatosensory pathways

Sensory information is transmitted through several pathways from the periphery to the central nervous system. The two major pathways for conscious body sensations are the dorsal-column medial lemniscus and spinal thalamic tract. Other body sensory pathways provide unconscious sensory information to influence motor behaviors and even pain control. These pathways are functionally important, however, rarely talked about in clinical practice as clinicians cannot measure their function or integrity.

Dorsal-column medial lemniscus

The dorsal-column medial lemniscus (DCML) transmits information about conscious awareness of light touch and proprioception. When sensory mechanoreceptors in the skin, muscles, or joints are stimulated, axons will carry that information into the spinal cord. Axons that transmit somatosensory information have cell bodies in the dorsal root ganglion and the axon extends into the dorsal horn of the spinal cord and ascend in the spinal cord through the ipsilateral (on the same side) white matter. Like the rest of the nervous system, the spinal cord is organized. The conscious light touch and proprioception information carried by the DCML is somatotopically (specific part of the body is associated with a distinct location) organized within the spinal cord. Moving from caudal (bottom) to rostral (top), each new entering axon will layer lateral to each other and ascend in the dorsal columns (Augustine et al., 2023).

The dorsal columns are named for their appearance (column) and location in the spinal cord (dorsal aspect). Within the dorsal columns, lower extremity and lower trunk information travel in the gracile fasciculus (or gracile tract) and upper extremity and upper trunk information travel in the cuneate fasciculus (or cuneate tract). Axons in the dorsal columns synapse on neurons in the caudal medulla. The axons that ascend in the dorsal columns are known as the first-order neurons. These *first-order neurons* synapse on *second-order neurons* in the caudal medulla. Second-order neurons cross the midline of the medulla. The second order neurons that have crossed travel in a white matter pathway called the medial lemniscus and ascend through the contralateral (opposite side in respect to sensory input) brainstem and travel to the thalamus where they synapse on *third-order neurons*. The thalamus is a large egg-shaped nucleus where almost all sensory information is received, processed and relayed to other areas of the brain. Third-order neurons then travel through a white matter pathway called the internal capsule to arrive at the primary somatosensory cortex. The primary somatosensory cortex is located in the anterior aspect of the parietal lobe and is the cortical area that is important for the conscious perception of sensory stimuli. Like the spinal cord the primary somatosensory cortex is also somatotopically organized (Augustine et al., 2023).

Box 3.5   Learning activity

1. Take a moment and view a short video on the DCML, taking note of the 1st, 2nd and 3rd order neurons. Be sure to get guidance from your instructor about how to find quality YouTube videos for this activity. (keyword: dorsal column medial lemniscus)
2. What are some of the clinical signs of damage to the DCML?
3. Using your knowledge about the DCML and Danea's level of spinal cord injury, what might you expect in terms of sensation in the hand, fingers and thumb?
4. How may these sensory impairments impact functional use of the hand, especially for activities associated with personal hygiene such as self-catheterization.
5. Consider the impact of sensory loss on motor control. Discuss the importance of stereognosis and proprioception on everyday functioning. In the absence of stereognosis and sense of position, such as in Danea's situation, what other sensory system may be useful for object manipulation and personal hygiene activities?

Spinal thalamic tract

The spinal thalamic tract (STT) is part of a larger system known as the anterolateral system. The STT provides information on conscious awareness of pain and temperature sensations. The other tracts in the anterolateral system provide information to the brain stem to influence arousal and emotional responses to pain (Mosconi & Graham, 2017).

Box 3.6   Learning activity

1. Take a moment and view a short video on the STT, and notice that impairment of the STT causes loss of appreciation to pain and temperature. *Be sure to get guidance from your instructor about how to find quality YouTube videos for this activity.*

Keyword: spinal thalamic tract

2. Localization of pain is not as accurate as localization to light touch. Consider the differences in the DCML and STT and offer a reason why.
3. When testing for pinprick sensation, an occupational therapist will alternate between sharp stimuli and light touch stimuli and record accuracy rather than only using a sharp object and asking for when the client feels the stimuli. Why do you think this is?
4. Consider the implications of loss of protective sensations (ability to detect stimuli that can be harmful) in everyday activities. Think about usual activities, such as cooking and risk for burns, but also think about how activities may be adapted

---

such as placing a hot dish on lap while propelling wheelchair from stove to table. What other activities or adaptations pose risk due to loss of sensory input? What is the role of occupational therapy?
5. View a quick video on the risk for pressure injuries after spinal cord injury. What is the relationship between risk for pressure injury and sensory pathways?

Keywords: pressure injury ("pressure ulcer" is an older term for pressure injury and you may find this during your searches), spinal cord

Axons that transmit information about noxious (painful) stimuli (mechanical, chemical, thermal) as well as itch and crude touch from the body have cell bodies in the dorsal root ganglia. The axons transmit pain, itch and crude touch information into the dorsal horn of the spinal cord. Most axons will enter the spinal cord through a small pathway known as Lissauer's tract. This tract extends up and down and a few segments before the first-order neuron synapse on the second-order neuron in the dorsal horn. The second-order neuron crosses in the spinal cord. The crossing will happen immediately in the spinal cord through a white matter pathway called the anterior white commissure (Ku & Morrison, 2022). This is anterior (or ventral) to the gray matter. These second-order neurons now travel contralaterally (on the opposite side from where they entered) in the white matter of the spinal cord. The pathway is called the anterior lateral pathway because the second-order neurons are located in an anterior and lateral position in the spinal cord. Like the DCML, the second-order neuron ascends through the brainstem and eventually synapses with neurons in the thalamus. These neurons travel through the internal capsule to reach the primary somatosensory cortex (Al-Chalabi et al., 2023).

Box 3.7   Learning activity

Danea has a cervical level SCI and cannot feel their legs, however, reports burning and painful sensations in their legs. The STT has been damaged and does not transmit conscious pain sensation, so why does Danea have pain?

Danea has neuropathic pain. Neuropathic pain refers to any pain that is caused by damage to the nerve or nervous system. Neuropathic or neurogenic pain is not specific to SCI, though it is extremely common in SCI. People with spinal cord injuries can have neuropathic pain at the level of the injury or below the level of injury.

It may seem impossible to have pain below the level of injury, where Danea cannot feel; however, this happens due to a complex cascade that occurs after the injury. The injury creates an environment where the neurons become easily excited and can transmit pain signals in the absence of activation of sensory/nociceptor receptors (Lee et al., 2013). Neuropathic pain is more common in cervical level injuries (Burke et al., 2017).

1. What do you know about chronic neuropathic pain following SCI, and its association with sleep, function and quality of life?
2. How can occupational therapy support clients who experience neuropathic pain?

Motor pathways

Motor commands are transmitted from the central nervous system to the periphery through several descending pathways. The motor pathway clinicians test during a motor/muscle examination is the corticospinal tract (CST). This is the pathway for most conscious motor commands. Several other pathways are important for automatic responses to maintain balance and posture, and while functionally very important, clinicians do not have good measures, and these are rarely addressed in SCI medicine.

Located in the frontal lobe, the primary motor cortex executes motor commands for muscles in our body. CST neurons begin in the primary motor cortex and descend through the internal capsule to the brain stem. The CST descends through the medulla and will create a protruding and distinct landmark on the ventral aspect, known as the medullary pyramids (Augustine et al., 2023). The CST is often called a pyramidal tract. There are many other motor tracts that do not travel through the pyramids are often called extrapyramidal tracts. Extrapyramidal tracts are most often associated with automatic movements and postural reactions.

At the level of the pyramids, about 90% of the neurons will cross midline (Lohia & McKenzie, 2023). Where these neurons cross is called the pyramidal decussation. The fibers that cross (decussate) are known as the lateral cortical spinal tract and contain motor information from the contralateral (opposite side) cortex. These fibers descend through the spinal cord in the lateral white matter and enter the spinal cord gray matter in the ventral horn. Neurons in the lateral CST primarily support distal movements and fine motor control. The fibers that do not cross represent the ventral corticospinal tract. These fibers descend in the ipsilateral (on the same side) white matter. When entering the spinal cord gray matter, they may cross so the ventral corticospinal tract does offer some bilateral innervation. The ventral corticospinal tract supply proximal and axial muscles and only extends through the thoracic spinal cord. In the ventral horn, the CST will synapse on motor neurons that will synapse on muscle (Augustine et al., 2023).

Box 3.8   Learning activity

Clinical note: Intact pinprick sensation at 24 hours after SCI is a strong predictor of motor recovery after SCI (Poynton et al., 1997). This is due to the location of the STT as it ascends in the white matter. The STT is anatomically very close to the lateral CST in the spinal cord.

1. Locate a figure/diagram of the corticospinal tract (keyword: lateral corticospinal tract, ventral corticospinal tract). While examining the figure, reread the previous two paragraphs, or view a short video on the CST. Appreciate the lateral and ventral corticospinal tracts below the pyramidal decussation.

   a. What muscle groups are supplied by the lateral CST?
   b. What muscle groups are supplied by the ventral corticospinal tract?
   c. Imagine a spinal cord lesion on the right side of the CST above the pyramidal decussation. What clinical features would you anticipate?
   d. Imagine a spinal cord lesion on the right side of the CST below the pyramidal decussation. What clinical features would you anticipate?

2. To further appreciation SCI and lesions to the CST, take a moment to review the paper by Van Wittenberghe, I.C., & Peterson, D.C. (2023). Corticospinal tract lesion. In: *StatPearls* [Internet]. Treasure Island, FL: StatPearls Publishing. Retrieved from: www.ncbi.nlm.nih.gov/books/NBK542201/

Motor neurons

Motor neurons influence the motor systems. There are two types of motor neurons: upper motor neurons (UMN) and lower motor neurons (LMN).

Upper motor neurons act on other upper motor neurons in the brain or directly on an LMN in the ventral horn. LMNs act directly on muscles (or glands in the case of the autonomic nervous system) (Augustine et al., 2023). It is a mistake to classify LMNs as part of the peripheral nervous system (PNS) because while the majority of a somatic LMN is in the PNS, the cell bodies of somatic LMNs are in the ventral horn of the spinal cord. Injury to the LMN or UMN will both result in loss of communication to the muscle and cause weakness or paralysis, however, UMN and LMN function differently and injuries have different clinical presentations.

Box 3.9   Learning activity

1. Find an image/diagram of the CST that clearly label the primary motor cortex, the medullary pyramids, the pyramidal decussation, lateral and ventral (anterior) CSTs, the spinal cord ventral (anterior) horns, and the communication between UMNs and LMNs and LMNs and muscle

Keywords: corticospinal tract, labeled

   a. What clinical signs are associated with damage to UMNs?
   b. What clinical signs are associated with damage to LMNs?
   c. Why do you think these clinical signs differ?

2. Consider Danea's examination.

   a. They have strong voluntary elbow flexion and wrist extension. What spinal cord level innervates (supplies) the elbow flexors? The wrist extensors?
   b. They cannot extend the elbow nor do they have any motor function of the fingers and thumbs. What spinal cord level innervates the elbow extensors? Extrinsic finger and thumb flexors? Extensors finger and thumb extensors? Intrinsic muscles of the thumb and fingers?
   c. Recall that occupational therapists do not rely entirely on myotome distribution for motor testing. Appreciate the multi-segmental innervation of the muscles of the hand and thumb.
   d. Danea's injury likely resulted in both UMN and LMN injury.

     (i)   Where would you likely see LMN injury?
     (ii)   Where would you likely see UMN injury?

(iii) Offer a hypothesis for the pattern of UMN and LMN injury based on your understanding of neuroscience concepts.

(iv) Why is it important for occupational therapists to assess if weakness if due to an upper versus lower motor neuron injury? How will that impact occupational therapy treatment?

Sensory-motor integration

Only in a neuroscience textbook can we fully separate the sensory and motor systems. Our writing presents the motor and sensory systems as linear and unidirectional, however, the nervous system is complex with vast communication and integration happening even in the spinal cord. One of the easiest ways to understand this sensory-motor connection in the spinal cord is to talk about reflexes.

Reflexes are automatic responses from a sensory stimulus. They are not driven by higher-level cortical centers (though cortical centers will be informed about the activity and can modify it if necessary). Reflexes are necessary for everyday function. Imagine if you needed to consciously send motor commands for every postural reaction or eye movement. It would take too long, and you would fall and have delayed visual responses.

An important reflex in the spinal cord is the stretch reflex (also called monosynaptic stretch reflex). The basis of this reflex is that the sensory receptors in the muscles detect a stretch (of the muscle) which is communicated to the LMN in the ventral horn in the spinal cord, which then responds by contracting the stretched muscle. This sensory-motor communication is the basis for resting muscle tone. In the stretch reflex, receptors in the muscle, called muscle spindle, are specialized to detect change in length in the muscle. Information about muscle length is communicated by the muscle spindle via axons that enter the dorsal horn of the spinal cord where they will synapse with the LMN in the ventral horn stimulating a contraction. This constant communication allows the muscle to have a resting level of tone that is necessary for skilled motor control (Augustine et al., 2023).

Now let's consider this stretch reflex in the context of SCI which is a lower and upper motor neuron injury. In an UMN injury there is no damage to the muscle spindle (receptor), the sensory nerve bringing information to the spinal cord or to the LMN. In an UMN injury resting muscle tone is still possible. That doesn't not mean that the tone is "normal" because in the absence of input from the CST it tends to be overactive resulting in increased muscle tone and spasticity (see Chapter 5). In an LMN injury, the muscle spindle may be able to communicate through the sensory nerve, however, the damaged LMN cannot facilitate muscle contraction. In this case, there is no circuitry for resting muscle tone, and we see a flaccid paralysis.

Box 3.10   Learning activity

1. View a short video on the monosynaptic stretch reflex to further your understanding of the sensory-motor communication that is constantly occurring in the central nervous system. Be sure to get guidance from your instructor about how to find quality YouTube videos for this activity.

Keywords: stretch reflex, monosynaptic

2. Danea does not have movement in their legs but has figured out how to make them stiff to help with moving in bed. How is Danea able to facilitate muscle contractions below the level of their spinal cord injury?
3. Spasticity is a common phenomenon in neurological conditions, such as spinal cord injury. Provide an explanation for the clinical presentation of spasticity after spinal cord injury, and offer a clinical rationale for the statement: "spasticity is a sign of a working nervous system below the level of injury."
4. Spasticity does not appear immediately after injury. After injury to the spinal cord, there is significantly impaired reflex activity in the spinal cord. This phenomenon is known as spinal shock. Use resource to identify how long spinal shock lasts and when spasticity begins to develop.
5. Are you still curious about the spinal cord circuitry underlying muscle stretch reflexes? Consider Purves, D., Augustine, G.J., Fitzpatrick. D., et al. (Eds.). (2001). The spinal cord circuitry underlying muscle stretch reflexes. In *Neuroscience* (2nd ed.). Sunderland, MA: Sinauer Associates.

The deep tendon reflex (DTR) is another important spinal reflex you are likely very familiar with. When a doctor tests your reflexes by hitting a reflex hammer against the patellar tendon, they are testing a DTR and using that information to evaluate the integrity of the sensory and motor systems. As a clinician, you can use DTR to assess the integrity of the sensory and motor system at specific segments in the spinal cord. The loss of DTR suggests an LMN injury. An overactive DTR suggests an UMN. This knowledge should guide your goal setting and intervention planning.

Let us now consider the DTR in the context of SCI. The patellar tendon reflex specifically tests the integrity of the L4–5 spinal segments (appreciate that muscles are typically supplied by more than one level of the cord, aka multi-segmental innervation). If a client had a spinal cord injury at L4, tapping the patellar tendon would cause a stretch on the quadriceps muscles which the muscle spindle would detect. The sensory information from the muscle spindle would travel in an axon into the dorsal horn. However, when it reached the damaged spinal cord, injury to the spinal cord would prevent any further communication to the LMN in the ventral horn. In this case, we would see absent reflexes. If the clinician tested reflexes above the level of injury, for example at the triceps (supplied by the C7 spinal cord), the sensory-motor pathway would be intact, and reflexes would be normal, as would be volitional movement. Now consider if reflexes were tested below the level of injury, the clinical picture will be different. If the clinician tested the S1 reflex (at the Achilles tendon) the sensory information would be transmitted to the dorsal horn of the spinal cord and eventually synapse at the LMN in the ventral horn which would stimulate a contraction of the gastrocnemius muscle. The intact sensory-motor communication allows for the reflex to occur, however, without descending control from the CST the DTR is overactive. Typical DTR are small movements or even just small observable contractions of the muscle. In the presence of a UMN injury, these reflexes are overactive meaning you can see observable large movements during the clinical exam (Zimmerman & Hubbard, 2023).

Box 3.11   Learning activity

1. Find a resource that can guide occupational therapists on how to test reflexes in the clinical practice.

Keywords: reflex testing, clinical exam, deep tendon reflex

2. Consider Danea's motor examination and clinical presentation to fill in this chart. Describe what you would expect to see during a clinical exam at different motor and dermatome levels.

	C5	C7	L1
Muscle activity (normal, weakness, paralysis)			
Resting muscle tone (flaccid, normal, high)			
Spasticity Present (Yes/No)			
Sensation (normal, impaired absent)			

Autonomic nervous system

The autonomic nervous system (ANS) is part of the nervous system that regulates automatic physiologic processes (Gibbons, 2019). The targets of the ANS neurons are most commonly organs like the heart or glands, like the salivary glands. The ANS regulates involuntary reactions necessary for essential functions such as pupillary dilation, blood pressure control, sexual arousal, and breathing. The ANS can be divided into three parts: sympathetic, parasympathetic, and enteric. The enteric nervous system is primarily responsible for the digestive process. The sympathetic nervous system (SNS) is often called our "fight or flight" system because when activated it can increase heart rate, and blood pressure and focus the body's resources to prepare for stressors. The parasympathetic nervous system is known as the "rest and digest" system. Parasympathetic activation will lower blood pressure and heart rate and promote digestion. These are just a few examples of the parasympathetic and sympathetic nervous system functions. Both systems are necessary to carry out the automatic physiologic process and work together to promote homeostasis. It is important to understand that while the SNS is called the flight or fight system, it is active even when fight or flight stresses are absent (Augustine et al., 2023).

Cell bodies of neurons of the ANS can be found in the brainstem and spinal cord, therefore, autonomic dysfunction is common in spinal cord injury. Spinal cord injury is not just a sensory and motor system injury. Spinal cord injury also significantly impacts the ANS and as a result impacts breathing, blood pressure control, digestion, bowel and bladder continence, bowel motility, digestion, body temperature control, and sexual functions (Augustine et al., 2023).

Autonomic dysreflexia (AD) is a life-threatening consequence of autonomic dysfunction in SCI. It is a medical emergency that can occur in people with injuries at the T6 level and above (Lakra et al., 2021). AD causes a rapid rise in blood pressure that can lead to a stroke or death. It is caused by any noxious stimuli below the level of the injury such as a sock that is too tight, an overfilled bladder (most common), ingrown toenail, pressure from an ill-fitting wheelchair or anything that has the potential to cause tissue damage (Allen & Leslie, 2023).

AD results in increased blood pressure with a decrease in heart rate. This occurs due to abnormal autonomic nervous system activity. SCI disrupts some but not all parts of the ANS. Any increase in blood pressure should be offset by parasympathetic activity driven by neurons in the brainstem, but in SCI, the pathways are interrupted so the rise in blood pressure goes largely unchecked, and continues to increase to dangerous levels. The vagus nerve, a cranial nerve (see Chapter 1) and part of the parasympathetic nervous system is not part of the spinal cord and acts to reduce heart rate to counter the high blood pressure accounting for the lower heart rate seen in AD (Allen & Leslie, 2023). Most people with SCI who experience AD know the signs, which can include pounding headache, facial flushing, and nausea, and irritability in babies (Hickey et al., 2004; Karlsson, 2006).

Types of spinal cord injury

As we presented the anatomy and function of the spinal cord, we have assumed complete injuries to the spinal cord. In reality, very few injuries result in complete *transection* of the spinal cord. The majority of SCIs are incomplete injuries meaning some sensory or motor information can pass to and from the brain (National Spinal Cord Injury Statistical Center, 2024). While neuroimaging is available, no clinical measure used by occupational therapists has the capability to determine if the cord is completely transected. However, clinicians, including occupational therapists use standardized assessments to describe the clinical presentation and categorize the injury as *clinically* complete or incomplete.

Box 3.12   Learning activity

1. While the inability to walk and/or use arms due to paralysis is often implicated for loss of independence in ADLs after SCI (and rightfully so!), disruption of the autonomic nervous system due to SCI can create tremendous challenges to functioning and participation in everyday life. Take a moment and view a video or read a short explanation about the autonomic nervous system, and how SCI impacts it.
2. Consider bladder and bowel function.

   a. How would your everyday routines be interrupted by the need for someone to catheterize you to empty your bladder every four hours? How would you fit a one-hour bowel program every day or every other day into your routine?
   b. An over-extended bladder (too much urine in the bladder) is a frequent cause of **AD**, which can be life-threatening. How can occupational therapy work with Danea and their mother to address Danea's desire to spend extended periods of time with friends, with the understanding that the bladder must be emptied every four hours to mitigate risk of AD?

3. Consider temperature control.

   a. Do you know that when you sweat, it is your body's way to cool itself? Do you know that "goosebumps" can mean that your body is trying to warm itself?
   b. The autonomic nervous system is responsible for the body's ability to control its temperature. View a short video on body temperature control and how SCI can interfere with it?

c. One of Danea's favorite leisure activities is to spend time at the beach. Using your knowledge of the autonomic nervous system, discuss the risks faced by Danea if they spend extended periods of time in very hot temperatures.
d. How can occupational therapy support Danea's desire to spend time at the beach, with the understanding about risks due to temperature dysregulation.

The gold standard assessment for evaluating and classifying the neurological consequence of SCI is called International Standards for Neurological Classification of Spinal Cord Injury (ISNCSCI), which was developed by the American Spinal Injury Association (ASIA) and International Spinal Cord Society (ISCoS) (ASIA and ISCoS International Standards Committee) (Kirshblum et al., 2020). The ISNCSCI classifies injuries into five categories: "A" =motor and sensory complete; "B" = preserved sensation below the level of injury; "C" and "D" = preserved sensation and motor function below the level of injury ("D" has stronger and more motor function than "C") and "E" = normal sensation and motor function.

Box 3.13   Learning activity

Visit the American Spinal Injury Association Website and download the ISNCSCI form.

1. What spinal tracts are being tested in the ISNCSCI motor and sensory examinations?
2. What are some of the limitations of the ISNCSCI relevant to understanding the impact of SCI on the central and autonomic nervous systems?

Some incomplete injuries are given specific names that describe a particular type of injury. These injury patterns occur due to the organization of the spinal cord. The work you have done to understand the structure and function of the spinal cord will help you to understand the presentation of these particular types of incomplete injuries.

Box 3.14   Learning activity

1. Find a figure of a cross-section of the spinal cord that has all structures clearly labeled, including blood supply.

Keywords: cross section, spinal cord, labeled

2. Find a description of Brown-Sequard syndrome.

   a. Use the above figure and shade the area in the cord that would be damaged in Brown-Sequard syndrome.
   b. What would you expect to see in clinical presentation? Provide a rationale based on your understanding of spinal cord structure/organization.

3. Find a description of central cord syndrome.

   a. Use the above figure and shade the area of the cord that would be damaged in Central Cord Syndrome.

b. What would you expect to see in clinical presentation? Provide a rationale based on your understanding of spinal cord structure/organization.

c. Simulate an extension of the injury away from the center. As the injury expands, how would the clinical presentation change? Provide a rationale based on your understanding of spinal cord structure/organization.

4. View a short video of the blood supply to the spinal cord. Find a description of anterior cord syndrome and posterior cord syndrome.

Keywords: spinal cord, blood supply, anterior cord syndrome, posterior cord syndrome

a. Use the above figure, shade the area of the cord that would be damaged in anterior cord syndrome.

b. What would you expect to see in clinical presentation? Provide a rationale based on your understanding of spinal cord structure/organization.

c. Repeat this for posterior cord syndrome.

Box 3.15   Learning activity

Clinic note: Although it is not new (Sherwood et al., 1992) nor has it been adopted widespread, the term "discomplete SCI" is used with increasing frequency to describe people who have "clinically complete" SCI but evidence of spinal cord connectivity via neurophysiological methods (Lütolf et al., 2021; Whalgren et al., 2021).

With advancements in innovative methods to facilitate neuroplasticity for recovery of neurological function after SCI, it becomes increasingly important to consider neurophysiological evidence of preserved connectivity in the spinal cord (discomplete SCI) in otherwise "clinically complete" SCI.

Occupational therapists working in the field of SCI will hear the term "discomplete injury."

Back to the person's life: Danea wants to complete personal hygiene to go out with friends for extended periods of time

Although Danea has multiple impairments in sensorimotor and autonomic functions, dependence on their mother and sister for intermittent catheterization is one of the greatest obstacles to going out with friends for extended periods of time, and spending weekends away from home. Danea has been adamant about not letting anyone else other than their mother and sister catheterize them, but their tolerance for not being able to hang out and take weekend trips with friends is waning.

The influence of participation in valued life roles and occupations aligns well with occupational therapy practice and should guide treatment. Providing assistive technology and SMART devices and working with Danea to find alternative ways to complete activities, occupational therapists can support them in resuming the home and community roles they value. The ability to maintain continence and not have accidents is an important predictor of quality of life (Akkoç et al., 2012; Elmelund et al., 2018) and must be considered by occupational therapists. With a C6 SCI, Danea can actively extend their wrist resulting in passive finger and thumb flexion (aka tenodesis grasp) (Jung et al., 2018) and use gravity-assisted wrist flexion to passively extend the fingers and thumb. Tenodesis grasp provides a mechanism to grasp and hold objects, such as a catheter, but is typically not strong enough to insert the catheter into the urethra (Jung et al., 2018; Zlatev et al., 2016). For some, a wrist-driven-flexor hinge orthosis increases the strength of tenodesis grasp (Kang et al., 2013). However, even if Danea had sufficient pinch strength, Danea's greatest challenges may be around managing clothing and positioning themselves in the wheelchair to be able to insert the catheter.

Box 3.16   Learning activity

1. Occupational therapists can use activity analysis to understand the components of the activity "catheterization while sitting in the wheelchair," and to problem solve with Danea on strategies to accomplish the activity. In your small group brainstorm on potential strategies that Danea can use to complete each component of the activity, while keeping in mind the sensorimotor impairments. Think creatively on ways an occupational therapist could coach Danea to reframe their current habits and perspectives about bladder management that get in the way of spending times with their friends.

Activity analysis: Catheterization while sitting in wheelchair	
Component	Potential Strategies
Find Accessible bathroom	
Wash hands	
Remove supplies for catheterization from bag on wheelchair	
Remove clothing enough to access urethra	
Open the sterile package and remove catheter with drainage bag	
Apply lubricant to catheter	
Position body in wheelchair to access urethra and to visually see to insert catheter	
Insert catheter into urethra until urine begins to drain	
Hold catheter in place until urine drainage stops	
Remove catheter from urethra	
Empty drainage bag into toilet	
Dispose catheter and drainage bag	
Pull up clothing	
Reposition self in wheelchair	
Wash hands	

2. While the components for catheterization while sitting in a wheelchair are the same for both biological sexes, some components may be easier for an individual assigned male at birth, even with the same injury level and impairments as Danea. Use your knowledge of the **central nervous system** and the impact of SCI, identify which components may be easier for individuals assigned male at birth with a C6 clinically complete SCI, and provide a rationale based on your understanding of neuroscience concepts.

Box 3.17   Learning activity

Occupational therapists work collaboratively with nurses, physicians and clients with SCI in pursuit of strategies to manage the bladder as independently as possible and in ways that are efficient, safe and acceptable. Individuals assigned male at birth typically can elicit a reflex erection, which reduces the amount of clothing to manage and eliminates the need for special positioning in the wheelchair; the reflex erection also makes it easier to insert the catheter. An individual assigned male at birth with the same level of injury as Danea may be able to achieve independent self-catheterization without any innovative and advanced interventions.

Use your knowledge of neuroscience concepts to describe the underlying neuro-physiological mechanism that allows for a reflex erection.

1. Recall that Danea uses spasms to help with bed mobility. What other ways may spasticity help facilitate function?
2. Understand that spasticity is sometimes problematic (Mills et al., 2020) As an example, spasticity can be strong enough to throw someone out of a wheelchair, or lose balance during body transfers or walking. In these cases, non-pharmacological (Khan et al., 2019) and pharmacological (de Sousa et al., 2022) treatments are considered to reduce spasticity. Using neuroscience concepts, offer a hypothesis for why spasticity fluctuates, and is not static.
3. Spasticity is also not always predictable, meaning it can change in frequency, intensity and duration. Discuss the implication of relying on spasticity for function with the understanding that it can change from day to day, and overtime.

What do we know about ourselves and the population at large?

In the United States, the average age of SCI has increased from 29 years of age in the 1970s to 43 years today (National Spinal Cord Injury Statistical Center, 2024), driven in large part due to falls in older adults who may have age-related delays in protective reactions and degenerative changes in the vertebral column that create a narrowing, making them more vulnerable to SCI due to falls (Ikpeze et al., 2017). There is some evidence that suggests an association between age at injury, and morbidity and functional outcomes, with those injured at an older age having more complications and poorer functional outcomes (Ahn et al., 2015; Keusen et al., 2023).

Box 3.18   Learning activity

Clinical note: Traumatic etiologies of SCI vary as a function of age and region. In the United States motor vehicle crashes, falls, violence (gunshot) and sports are leading causes of SCI in adults (National Spinal Cord Injury Statistical Center, 2024). Although motor vehicle accidents and falls are most common cause of SCI in most regions, variations exist (Kang et al., 2018).

In children etiology of traumatic SCI varies as a function of age at injury. In the United States, younger children are more prone to SCI due to iatrogenic causes and falls while adolescents are more prone to sports and violence related injury. For both groups, motor vehicle crashes are the leading cause of traumatic SCI (Parent et al., 2011; New et al., 2019).

Non-traumatic etiologies of SCI (also called spinal cord dysfunction) include vascular ruptures, tuberculosis, tumors, transverse myelitis, and acute flaccid myelitis. These etiologies occur in both adults and children and tend to be associated with more diffuse LMN involvement. Degenerative cervical myelopathy is a common etiology of non-traumatic SCI in older adults (David et al., 2019).

Efforts to better understand etiology and outcome of SCI from a global scale is under way. These understandings are important for developing SCI prevention programs that are tailored to regional needs.

Box 3.19   Learning activity

With your small group, complete the table in the Appendix about the integration of Danea's central and autonomic nervous system functions to successfully complete the task of emptying their bladder.

Further reading

If interested in further reading about surgical interventions for bladder management:

Banakhar, M. A., Elkilini, M., & Hassouna, M. (2021). Spinal cord injury patients: Effect of urinary intervention therapy type on quality of life, questionnaire-based study. *Turkish Journal of Urology*, 47(3), 205–209.

Chen, S. F., Lee, Y. K, & Kuo, H. C. (2022). Satisfaction with urinary incontinence treatments in patients with chronic spinal cord injury. *Journal of Clinical Medicine*, 11 (19), 5864. https://doi.org/10.3390/jcm11195864

Martens, F. M. J., den Hollander, P. P., Snoek, G. J., Koldewijn, E. L., van Kerrebroeck, P. E. V. A., & Heesakkers, J. P. F. A. (2011). Quality of life in complete spinal cord injury patients with a Brindley bladder stimulator compared to a matched control group. *Neurourology and Urodynamics*, 30: 551–555. https://doi.org/10.1002/nau.21012

If interested in further reading about the lived experience of spinal cord injury, see www.elearnsci.org.

References

Ahn, H., Bailey, C. S., Rivers, C. S., Noonan, V. K., Tsai, E. C., Fourney, D. R., Attabib, N., Kwon, B. K., Christie, S. D., Fehlings, M. G., Finkelstein, J., Hurlbert, R. J., Townson, A., Parent, S., Drew, B., Chen, J., & Dvorak, M. F. (2015). Rick Hansen Spinal Cord Injury Registry Network. (2015). Effect of older age on treatment decisions and outcomes among patients with traumatic spinal cord injury. *Canadian Medical Association Journal*, 187(12), 873–880. https://doi.org/10.1503/cmaj.150085

Akkoç, Y., Ersöz, M., Yıldız, N., Erhan, B., Alaca, R., Zinnuroglu, M., Ozcete, Z. A., Tunc, H., Kaya, K., Alemdaroglu, E., Sarigul, M., Konukcu, S., Gunduz, B., Bardak, A. N., Ozcan, S., Demir, Y., Gunes, S., & Uygunol, K. (2012). Effects of different bladder management methods on the quality of life in patients with traumatic spinal cord injury. *Spinal Cord*, 51(3), 226–231. https://doi.org/10.1038/sc.2012.131

Al-Chalabi, M., Reddy, V., & Alsalman, I. (2023) Neuroanatomy, Posterior Column (Dorsal Column). In: *StatPearls* [Internet]. StatPearls Publishing. Retrieved from: www.ncbi.nlm.nih.gov/books/NBK507888/

Allen K. J., & Leslie, S. W. (2023) Autonomic Dysreflexia. In: *StatPearls* [Internet]. StatPearls Publishing. Retrieved from: www.ncbi.nlm.nih.gov/books/NBK482434/

Al-Shaikh, R. H., Czervionke, L., Eidelman, B., & Dredla, B. K. (2022). Spinal Cord Infarction. In *StatPearls [Internet]*. StatPearls Publishing. Retrieved from: www.ncbi.nlm.nih.gov/books/NBK545185/

ASIA and ISCoS International Standards Committee. (2019). The 2019 revision of the International Standards for Neurological Classification of Spinal Cord Injury (ISNCSCI)—What's new? *Spinal Cord*, 57, 815–817. https://doi.org/10.1038/s41393-019-0350-9

Augustine, G. J., Groh, J. M., Huettel, S. A., LaMantia, A. S., White, L. E., & Purves, D. (2023). *Neuroscience*, 7th Edition. Sinaauer Associates. https://global.oup.com/academic/product/neuroscience-9780197616253?cc=us&lang=en&#

Bryden, A. M., Hoyen, H. A., Keith, M. W., Mejia, M, Kilgore, K. L., & Nemunaitis, G. A. (2016). Upper extremity assessment in tetraplegia: The importance of differentiating between upper and lower motor neuron paralysis. *Archives of Physical Medicine and Rehabilitation*, 97(6 Suppl), S97-S104. https://doi.org/10.1016/j.apmr.2015.11.021

Bryden, A., Kilgore, K. L., & Nemunaitis, G. A. (2018). Advanced assessment of the upper limb in tetraplegia: A three-tiered approach to characterizing paralysis. *Topics in Spinal Cord Injury Rehabilitation*, 24(3), 206–216. https://doi.org/10.1310/sci2403-206

Burke, D., Fullen, B. M., Stokes, D., & Lennon, O. (2017). Neuropathic pain prevalence following spinal cord injury: A systematic review and meta-analysis. *European Journal of Pain*, 21(1), 29–44. https://doi.org/10.1002/ejp.905

David, G., Mohammadi, S., Martin, A. R., Cohen-Adad, J., Weiskopf, N., Thompson, A., & Freund, P. (2019). Traumatic and nontraumatic spinal cord injury: pathological insights from neuroimaging. *Nature Reviews Neurology*, 15, 718–731. https://doi.org/10.1038/s41582-019-0270-5

de Sousa, N., Santos, D., Monteiro, S., Silva, N., Barreiro-Iglesias, A., & Salgado, A. J. (2022). Role of baclofen in modulating spasticity and neuroprotection in spinal cord injury. *Journal of Neurotrauma*, 39(3–4), 249–258. https://doi.org/10.1089/neu.2020.7591

Dijkers, M. (1997). Quality of life after spinal cord injury: a meta analysis of the effects of disablement components. *Spinal Cord*, 35(12), 829–840. https://doi.org/10.1038/sj.sc.3100571

Dijkers, M. P. J. M. (2005). Quality of life of individuals with spinal cord injury: a review of conceptualization, measurement, and research findings. *Journal of Rehabilitation Research and Development*, 42(3), 87–110. https://doi.org/10.1682/jrrd.2004.08.0100

Doherty, J. G., Burns, A. S., O'Ferrall, D. M., & Ditunno, J. F. Jr. (2002). Prevalence of upper motor neuron vs lower motor neuron lesions in complete lower thoracic and lumbar spinal cord injuries. *The Journal of Spinal Cord Medicine*, 25(4), 289–292. https://doi.org/10.1080/10790268.2002.11753630

Elmelund, M., Klarskov, N., & Biering-Sørensen, F. (2018). Prevalence of urinary incontinence in women with spinal cord injury. *Spinal Cord*, 56, 1124–1133. https://doi.org/10.1038/s41393-018-0157-0

Engel-Haber, E., Botticello, A., Snider, B., & Kirshblum, S. (2022). Incomplete spinal cord syndromes: Current incidence and quantifiable criteria for classification. *Journal of Neurotrauma*, 39(23–24), 1687–1696. https://doi.org/10.1089/neu.2022.0196

Ganapathy, M. K., Reddy, V., & Tadi, P. (2023). Neuroanatomy, Spinal Cord Morphology. In: *StatPearls* [Internet]. Treasure Island, FL: StatPearls Publishing. Retrieved from: www.ncbi.nlm.nih.gov/books/NBK545206/

Gibbons, C. H. (2019). Basics of autonomic nervous system function. *Handb Clin Neurol.*, 160, 407–418. doi:10.1016/B978-0-444-64032-1.00027-8.

Hickey, K. J., Vogel, L. C., Willis, K. M., & Anderson, C. J. (2004). Prevalence and etiology of autonomic dysreflexia in children with spinal cord injuries. *J Spinal Cord Med.*, 27 Suppl 1, S54–60. doi:10.1080/10790268.2004.11753786.

Ikpeze, T. C., & Mesfin, A. (2017). Spinal cord injury in the geriatric population: Risk factors, treatment options, and long-term management. *Geriatric Orthopedic Surgery and Rehabilitation*, 8(2), 115–118. https://doi.org/10.1177/2151458517696680

Jung, H. Y., Lee. J., & Shin, H.I. (2018). The natural course of passive tenodesis grip in individuals with spinal cord injury with preserved wrist extension power but paralyzed fingers and thumbs. *Spinal Cord*, 56(9), 900–906. https://doi.org/10.1038/s41393-018-0137-4

Kang, Y., Ding, H., Zhou, H. X., Wei, Z. J., Liu, L., Pan, D. Y., & Feng, S. Q. (2018). Epidemiology of worldwide spinal cord injury: a literature review. *Journal of Neurorestoratology*, 6, 1–9. https://doi.org/10.2147/JN.S143236

Kang, Y. S., Park, Y. G., Lee, B. S., & Park, H. S. (2013). Biomechanical evaluation of wrist-driven flexor hinge orthosis in persons with spinal cord injury. *Journal of Rehabilitation Research and Development*, 50(8), 1129–1138. https://doi.org/10.1682/JRRD.2012.10.0189

Karlsson, A. K. (2006). Autonomic dysfunction in spinal cord injury: clinical presentation of symptoms and signs. *Prog Brain Res.*, 152, 1–8. doi:10.1016/S0079–6123(05)52034-X.

Kirshblum, S., Snider, B., Rupp, R., & Read, M. S. (2020). International Standards Committee of ASIA and ISCoS. Updates of the International Standards for Neurologic Classification of Spinal Cord Injury: 2015 and 2019. *Phys Med Rehabil Clin N Am.*, 31(3), 319–330. doi:10.1016/j.pmr.2020.03.005.

Keusen, P., Vuilliomenet, T., Friedli, M., Widmer, M. (2023). Age at onset of spinal cord injury is associated with increased inpatient care needs, reduced independence at discharge and a higher risk of institutionalization after primary inpatient rehabilitation. *Journal of Rehabilitation Medicine*, 55, jrm00353. https://doi.org/10.2340/jrm.v54.4468

Khan, F., Amatya, B., Bensmail, D., & Yelnik, A. (2019). Non-pharmacological interventions for spasticity in adults: An overview of systematic reviews. *Annals of Physical Rehabilitation Medicine*, 62(4), 265–273. https://doi.org/10.1016/j.rehab.2017.10.001

Ku, J., & Morrison, E. H. (2023). Neuroanatomy, anterior white commissure. www.ncbi.nlm.nih.gov/books/NBK546614/

Lakra, C., Swayne, O., Christofi, G., & Desai, M. (2021). Autonomic dysreflexia in spinal cord injury. *Pract Neurol.*, 21(6), 532–538. doi: 10.1136/practneurol-2021-002956. PMID: 34353860.

Lee, J., & Thumbikat, P. (2015). Pathophysiology, presentation and management of SCI. *Surgery*, 33(6), 238–939. https://doi.org/10.1016/j.mpsur.2015.04.003.

Lee, S., Zhao, X., Hatch, M., Chun, S., & Chang, E. Y. (2013). Central neuropathic pain in spinal cord injury. *Critical Reviews in Physical and Rehabilitation Medicine*, 25(3–4), 159–172. https://doi.org/10.1615/CritRevPhysRehabilMed.2013007944

Lohia, A., & McKenzie, J. (2023). Neuroanatomy, pyramidal tract lesions. www.ncbi.nlm.nih.gov/books/NBK540976/

Lütolf, R., Rosner, J., Curt, A., & Hubli, M. (2021). Identifying discomplete spinal lesions: New evidence from pain-autonomic interaction in spinal cord injury. *Journal of Neurotrauma*, 38(24), 3456–3466. http://doi.org/10.1089/neu.2021.0280

Mills, P. B., Holtz, K. A., Szefer, E., Noonan, V. K., & Kwon, B. K. (2020). Early predictors of developing problematic spasticity following traumatic spinal cord injury: A prospective cohort study. *The Journal of Spinal Cord Medicine*, 43(3), 315–330. https://doi.org/10.1080/10790268.2018.1527082

Mosconi, T., & Graham, V. (Eds.), (2017). The spinal cord. *Neuroscience for Rehabilitation*. McGraw Hill. https://accessphysiotherapy.mhmedical.com/content.aspx?bookid=2258&sectionid=175151376

National Spinal Cord Injury Statistical Center. (2024). *Traumatic spinal cord injury facts and figures at a glance*. Birmingham, AL: University of Alabama at Birmingham, 2024.

New, P. W., Lee, B. B., Cripps, R., Vogel, L. C., Scheinberg, A., & Waugh, M. C. (2019). Global mapping for the epidemiology of paediatric spinal cord damage: towards a living data repository. *Spinal Cord*, *57*(3), 183–197. https://doi.org/10.1038/s41393-018-0209-5

Parent, S., Mac-Thiong, J. M., Roy-Beaudry, M., Sosa, J. F., & Labelle, H. (2011). Spinal cord injury in the pediatric population: a systematic review of the literature. *Journal of Neurotrauma*, *28*(8), 1515–1524. https://doi.org/10.1089/neu.2009.1153

Poynton AR, O'Farrell DA, Shannon F, Murray P, McManus F, Walsh MG. (1997). An evaluation of the factors affecting neurological recovery following spinal cord injury. *Injury*, 28(8), 545–548. doi: 10.1016/s0020-1383(97)00090-9. PMID: 9616393.

Purves, D., Augustine, G.J., Fitzpatrick. D., et al. (Eds.). (2001). The spinal cord circuitry underlying muscle stretch reflex*es*. In *Neuroscience* (2nd ed.). Sunderland, MA: Sinauer Associates. Retrieved from: www.ncbi.nlm.nih.gov/books/NBK10809/.

Sherwood, A. M., Dimitrijevic, M. R., & McKay, W.B. (1992). Evidence of subclinical brain influence in clinically complete spinal cord injury: discomplete SCI. *Journal of the Neurology Sciences*, 110(1–2), 90–98. https://doi.org/10.1016/0022-510x(92)90014-c

Van Wittenberghe, I.C., & Peterson, D.C. (2023). Corticospinal Tract Lesion. In: *StatPearls* [Internet]. Treasure Island, FL: StatPearls Publishing. Retrieved from: www.ncbi.nlm.nih.gov/books/NBK542201/

Wahlgren, C., Levi, R., Amezcua, S., Thorell, O., & Thordstein, M. (2021). Prevalence of discomplete sensorimotor spinal cord injury as evidenced by neurophysiological methods: A cross-sectional study. *J Rehabil Med.*, 53(2), jrm00156. doi:10.2340/16501977-2774.

Zimmerman, B., & Hubbard, J. B. (2023). Deep Tendon Reflexes. In: *StatPearls* [Internet]. Treasure Island, FL: StatPearls Publishing. Retrieved from: www.ncbi.nlm.nih.gov/books/NBK531502/

Zlatev, D., Shem, K., & Elliott, C. (2016). How many spinal cord injury patients can catheterize their own bladder? The epidemiology of upper extremity function as it affects bladder management. *Spinal Cord*, 54, 287–291. https://doi.org/10.1038/sc.2015.169.

4 Thomas wants to stay connected using a computer and has amyotrophic lateral sclerosis

Neuroscience facilitates our understanding of computer use

Meghan Doherty and Sarah Schuman

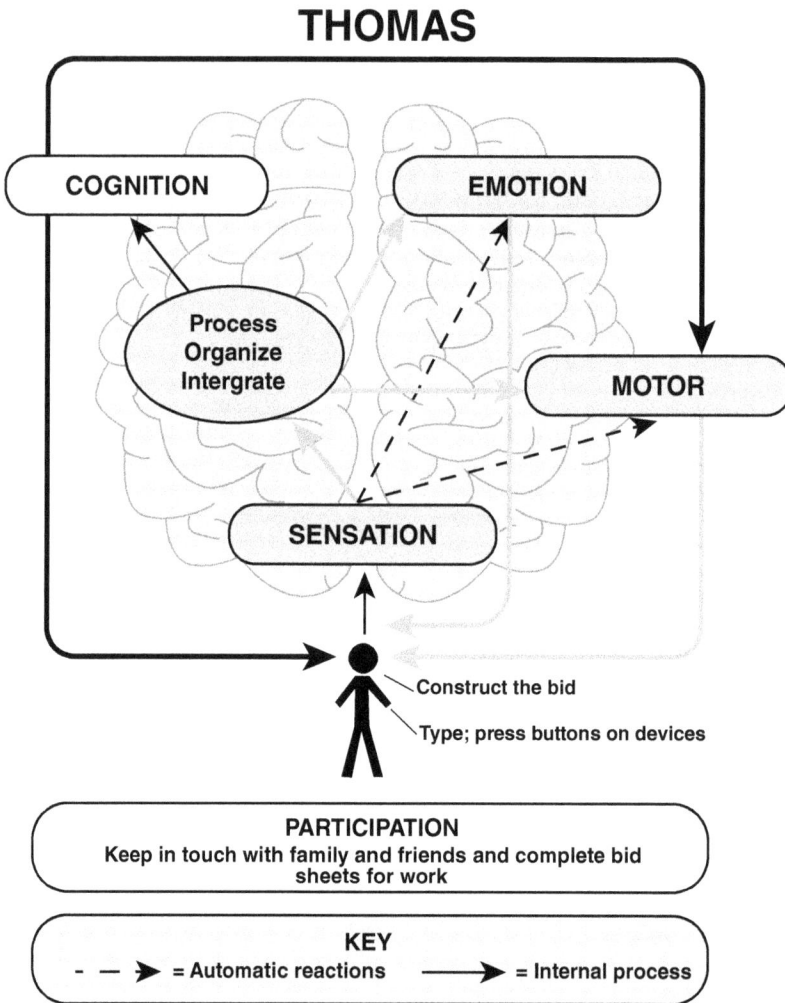

Figure 4.1 Thomas brain figure

DOI: 10.4324/9781003524380-6

Purpose of this chapter

The purpose of this chapter is to discover the neuroscience underpinnings of computer use. As with all chapters in this text, we consider technology use from the lens of an individual with neurological impairment. We will focus on a person, Thomas, with amyotrophic lateral sclerosis (ALS). People experiencing changes in function from ALS or other neurodegenerative conditions, such as multiple sclerosis (MS), alter their use of computers to engage socially with friends and family. While ALS and MS are distinct diseases, it will be helpful to consider them together in this chapter as they involve similar structures. Let's find out more about Thomas so we can have a context for understanding the impact of changes in his nervous system on his life.

Keywords for this chapter are listed in the box below. Be sure to learn what these key features are so you can get the most out of the chapter.

Keywords for this chapter

anterior corticospinal tract	corticospinal tracts	middle pons
anterior horn	internal capsule	motor neurons
basal ganglia	lateral corticospinal tract	myelin sheath
central sulcus	lesions	nodes of Ranvier
cerebellum	lower motor neuron	primary motor cortex
	medulla	upper motor neuron

Thomas, a 45-year-old, wants to keep in touch with friends and family using his computer

Thomas is a father, plumber, Jewish community member, and friend to many. He lives alone, but his daughter recently graduated from college and began her first job as a teacher in the same city; he and his wife divorced eleven years ago. He works with his childhood best friend at their family business. Since his ALS diagnosis six months ago, Thomas has shifted his job as a plumber to traveling and bidding for jobs and some office work, rather than fielding calls. Thomas enjoys live music, staying connected to friends and family through social media, and walking his dog, Munch.

Thomas first noticed clumsiness in his left hand a year ago during plumbing tasks as well as changes in his handwriting and typing accuracy. After being diagnosed with ALS by a neurologist, he now is re-evaluated by an interdisciplinary team every three months. At his most recent appointment, the occupational therapist (OT) noted his grip strength decreased to 32 pounds in his dominant left hand, which is below the 10th percentile for men his age. The physical therapist (PT) shared that his left ankle strength decreased enough that she is recommending a brace called an ankle foot orthosis (AFO) to stabilize it. Thomas feels he can still complete his daily one mile walk with his dog, but needs to sit and rest after he gets home. He has noticed he has lower energy the past month, but doesn't know the cause. He also sometimes laughs even when he doesn't think something is funny which has created some awkward situations; the neurologist says this is called pseudobulbar affect (PBA) and gave him a new medicine to help.

Thomas gets frustrated when he struggles to complete phone and computer tasks with the same efficiency as before ALS. He is slower and makes more mistakes in his typing and clicking. He also gets cramps and fatigued muscles; taking breaks helps. He texts daily with his daughter and enjoys commenting on his friends' social media posts and photos. He sends emails throughout his day at work with bids for plumbing jobs that he types up after taking handwritten notes on site. He spends about two hours a day on his smartphone and another four at his work or personal computer; using these devices is essential both to stay employed at a company he loves and to be connected to his social network.

You are the occupational therapist in an outpatient clinic seeing Thomas, who is looking for strategies, features, and assistive technology options to continue participating in smartphone and computer occupations and improve his efficiency.

Box 4.1   Learning activity

Discuss with your peers:

1. Having read the narrative, what are you curious about?
2. What do you need to know more about?

Before you continue reading the chapter, work with your small group to discuss what you already know.

Box 4.2   Learning activity

1. How do Thomas's work and virtual contexts present a challenge to his nervous system?
2. What parts of the brain and nervous system affect strength in ALS?
3. Why might Thomas be feeling fatigued?

Now that you have had some time to think about this, let's consider what computer and smartphone users require from the brain and nervous system. You already have some great ideas to build on.

Neuroscience information to guide your thinking about Thomas

Neural communication among nerve cells/systems

Healthy communication between the brain, spinal cord, and the rest of the nervous system occurs in specialty cells called neurons (Bear et al., 2020). There is a central portion of these cells called the soma, and extensions called axons that transfer information over distances throughout the nervous system to various parts of the body. These axons reach dendrites on other cells which serve as receptors of information from axons; this is how nerve cells communicate to each other, by transmitting electrical synapses. Surrounding each long axon is a protective coating called the myelin sheath—think of it like insulation around an electrical cord you'd find in your home. The myelin sheath has gaps, called the nodes of Ranvier, which speed up the electrical synapse by increasing voltage (energy) as it travels across the axon. Our body has motor neurons responsible for communicating brain information along the axon to muscles to tell them to contract for movement (Bear et al., 2020). Our body also has sensory neurons which send information from the skin, muscles, and peripheral body parts back to the brain. When a person has a disease such as ALS or MS, this healthy communication becomes disrupted.

Box 4.3   Learning activity

1. Locate a picture of a neuron. Label the following structures: soma, axon, dendrites, node of Ranvier.
2. Where is the connection, or synapse, between a motor and sensory neuron found?
3. What cells are responsible for forming the myelin sheath?

Keywords: neuron, soma, axon, dendrite, node of Ranvier, synapse

---

Basic knowledge of ALS and MS

ALS is characterized as a motor neuron disease and results in the destruction of motor neurons in the central nervous system (i.e. spinal cord, brain, and brainstem). While the specific cause of ALS is not well-understood, the damage to motor neurons is caused by a combination of damage to the myelin sheath (demyelination) and subsequent production of a fibrous "scar" (Allen, 2019). Ultimately, the destruction and loss of motor neurons causes progressive loss of the ability to use muscles, or paralysis, and will result in death within an average of three to five years of symptom onset (Allen, 2019). All people with ALS will have loss of muscle strength, but the first area of the body affected varies. Some individuals will have a limb onset, while others will have a bulbar onset. In individuals with limb onset, weakness will begin in one arm or leg and develop in remaining limbs as disease progresses. However, for those with bulbar onset, symptoms will be associated with damage to cranial nerves, resulting in difficulty swallowing, loss/decreased ability to produce speech, increased saliva production, or even involuntary emotional outbursts (i.e. pseudobulbar affect) (Dal Bello-Haas, 2019, p. 774). We do not have a cure for ALS, and the medications available have limited ability to slow the disease.

Box 4.4   Learning activity

1. What are the different patterns of progression for limb-onset ALS?
2. Identify at least two signs/symptoms of pseudobulbar affect (PBA).
3. How might PBA impact an individual's social interactions/relationships?

Keywords: Limb-onset ALS, bulbar-onset ALS, pseudobulbar affect

---

MS is a progressive neurological condition involving the myelin sheath, it is distinct in that it is a chronic inflammatory condition which results in damage to the central nervous system. In an individual with MS, their immune system mistakenly activates and destroys the myelin sheath. This attack from the immune system will ultimately cause damage, or lesions, to the brain and spinal cord (Ghasemi et al., 2017). The loss of and damage to the myelin sheath disrupts the important connection between nerves and can result in a variety of symptoms. Symptoms that are a direct result of the damage to the myelin sheath, or primary symptoms, are the following: numbness/tingling, trouble walking, vision problems, changes in bladder or bowel function, and cognitive impairments. Additionally, individuals with MS may have changes in emotional regulation such as pseudobulbar affect (Ahmed & Simmons, 2013). Secondary symptoms of MS, or those that are not a direct result of the disease, can include infections, decreased mobility, fatigue, depression/anxiety, and decreased ability to participate in daily activities (Ghasemi et al., 2017).

It is important to keep in mind that MS impacts every individual in a different way. For example, some may use a wheelchair for mobility and have trouble using their hands, while others may use a cane for mobility and require assistance to urinate. The way in which symptoms present and progress can vary widely based upon where the lesions occur. We can look to the subtypes of the disease to better understand the onset and progression of symptoms. The subtypes are relapsing remitting MS (RRMS), primary progressive MS (PPMS), secondary progressive MS (SPMS), and progressive relapsing MS (PRMS). We do not have a cure for MS, but medications and immunotherapies can help manage symptoms and slow disease progression.

Box 4.5   Learning activity

1. What do you already know about the neurological condition MS? Discuss with your peers.
2. Create a list of at least five symptoms specific to MS that would impact someone's ability to use their phone or computer. Use the following topics to guide your work: sensory changes, changes in mobility, vision problems, changes in bowel/bladder function, and cognitive/emotional impairment.
3. Consider how the following could be impacted by various symptoms of MS. Discuss with your peers:

    • Mobility and movement
    • Vision
    • Bowel and bladder
    • Sensation
    • Cognition

4. How would these changes impact one's ability to engage in self-care tasks? Social participation? Work?
5. Find information depicting the progression of symptoms in each MS subtype. Discuss similarities/differences with a partner.

    • Relapsing remitting
    • Primary progressive
    • Secondary progressive
    • Progressive relapsing

While MS is similar to ALS in that they are both progressive conditions and affect the nervous system, they are distinct. Namely, ALS results in death to motor neurons, whereas MS causes damage to motor neurons. This key difference contributes to many of the distinctions between the two conditions, such as life expectancy and symptom presentation. In this chapter we will detail the ways in which each affects participation and bodily functions.

Anatomy of brain and spinal cord regions

The roles of the primary motor cortex and corticospinal tracts are key to understanding the disease processes of ALS and MS. The primary motor cortex is located in the frontal lobe of the brain, just anterior to the central sulcus. To produce movement with the body, the signal must start here. For example, if Thomas wants to depress the spacebar on his keyboard using his index finger, this process will begin in the primary motor cortex. This is also where upper motor neurons originate, the first neuron forming the circuit responsible for connection between the brain and our muscles.

Once the signal has been received by the primary motor cortex, it will travel along the upper motor neuron via the corticospinal tract. The corticospinal tract travels through the white matter of the brain and to the brainstem (i.e. internal capsule, midbrain, middle pons, and medulla). Once the upper motor neuron reaches the posterior aspect of the medulla two paths emerge: the lateral corticospinal tract and anterior corticospinal tract. The upper motor neuron will cross the midpoint (i.e. midline) of the medulla to form the lateral corticospinal tract and continue to the spinal cord. The upper motor neurons that do not cross the midline and descend to the spinal cord form the anterior corticospinal tract. While both tracts do exist, the lateral corticospinal tract is larger and used by the majority of upper motor neurons (approximately 90%) (Zayia & Tadi, 2021). Once the upper motor neuron reaches its intended area, or level, of the spinal cord, it will "peel off" the corticospinal tract to enter the spinal cord and terminate in the anterior horn. Here it will synapse, or connect, with the lower motor neuron, the second neuron forming the circuit we previously discussed. The lower motor neuron is then responsible for carrying the signal from the upper motor neuron all the way to the muscle that is to be activated.

Box 4.6 Learning activity

Find a diagram of the brain and corticospinal tract. Label the brainstem and using two different colors trace the paths of the UMN and LMN.

Keywords: upper motor neuron vs. lower motor neuron, brain, spinal cord, muscle, corticospinal tract

---

Given the important roles of the primary motor cortex and corticospinal tracts, damage to either (or both) of these structures can lead to significant problems or symptoms, like we see in ALS and MS. For example, in ALS hardening of the lateral corticospinal tracts disrupts communication, leading to muscles wasting away from non-use; the messages cannot get through to tell them to contract and so they get weaker over time (VanMeter & Hubert, 2022). Additionally, for individuals with MS, the number of lesions, or damage, on the primary motor cortex and corticospinal tracts are correlated with the severity of disability and disease progression (Kerbrat et al., 2020). As it relates to both ALS and MS, PBA is thought to be the result of damage to the cortico-limbic-subcortical-thalamic-pontocerebellar network, which is heavily involved in emotional expression and regulation (King & Reiss, 2013).

In MS, inflammation causes loss of the myelin sheath surrounding axons in the brain and spinal cord; this is akin to gaps in a communication "road." Later in the disease process plaques form, which are large areas of inflammation and demyelination (VanMeter & Hubert, 2022). When we don't have myelin, the electrical signals sent down the corticospinal tract are either unintelligible or move too slowly. Therefore, muscles do not get signals to contract, or have weaker contractions. If the disruption of the message is due to inflammation in MS, and treatment and time reduce that inflammation, function might return for that person (Gutman, 2017). This could look like weakness resolving or sensation returning. However, MS is characterized by relapses, or recurrences of symptoms, and therefore some myelin degradation is permanent and cumulative (VanMeter & Hubert, 2022). The type of MS determines the relapses as discussed above (i.e. RRMS or PPMS). However, relapses do not occur for individuals with ALS, which is another hallmark difference between the two neurological conditions.

While muscle weakness and atrophy are similar among all individuals with ALS, the presentation of this disease can also vary significantly. Symptom onset and manifestation is largely a result of the severity and location of motor neuron loss (Dal Bello-Haas, 2019, p. 772). For example, upper motor neuron involvement is associated with the following symptoms: increased tension in the muscles called spasticity, rhythmic or oscillating reflexes like clonus, and presence of primitive reflexes that should have disappeared at a young age, such as those that are responsible for the development of grasping or ability to feed in infants. Lower motor neuron involvement is reflective of the following symptoms: muscle weakness, decreased reflexes, decreased/loss of muscle tone, muscle cramps, or muscle twitching (i.e. fasciculations) (Dal Bello-Haas, 2019). However, the symptoms for persons with ALS are not just physical.

Let's consider the impact of these symptoms on one's mood and energy levels. Individuals with ALS must utilize significant compensatory strategies in the way that they move to decrease risk of a fall, prevent injury, and to complete daily tasks. For example, a person with ALS may overuse hip and gluteal muscles during walking because of weakness in the muscles of the calf and ankle. The continued use of these strategies, combined with progressive widespread weakness and changes in respiratory function, results in significant fatigue for some individuals with ALS.

Box 4.7   Learning activity

1. Locate a web resource directed at patients with ALS, that discusses the symptom of fatigue.
2. List four strategies to decrease/manage fatigue in ALS. Brainstorm with your partner.

Keywords: fatigue, weakness, energy conservation, adaptive equipment

---

Involvement of cerebellum and basal ganglia

The cerebellum and basal ganglia (BG) are midbrain structures affected by the neuro-degenerative processes of MS and ALS. The cerebellum is a large structure made up of three lobes that works to coordinate movement, maintain posture, and equilibrium but also assists with spatial organization, memory, and attention shifting (Gutman, 2017). The basal ganglia assist with motor control, behavior, and cognition and comprise several subcortical nuclei: the striatum, the globus pallidus, the ventral pallidum, the substantia nigra, and the subthalamic nucleus (Castelnovo et al., 2023). There are many important functions of the basal ganglia and many pathways of information flow that contribute to complex human actions ranging from production of dopamine to cognitive processing (Gutman, 2017).

Box 4.8   Learning activity

1. Locate a diagram of the basal ganglia structures and the cerebellum.
2. Create a table of six or more BG structures and their primary functions.

Keywords: basal ganglia, cerebellum

In ALS, we see widespread involvement of the basal ganglia both with atrophy of structures and degradation of communication networks (Bede et al., 2013). The caudate nucleus, hippocampus, and nucleus accumbens shrink in size, or atrophy; frontostriatal networks contribute to symptoms including executive dysfunction, apathy, and deficits in social cognition (Bede et al., 2013). However, the brain is able to adapt to change, and in ALS increased connectivity between the caudate and cerebellum has been seen to compensate for other functions (Abidi et al., 2020). The cerebellum is recruited to work more for a person with ALS to compensate for functional motor decline (Prell & Grosskreutz, 2013). Atrophy of the cerebellum is also seen and contributes to cognitive and behavioral decline (Gellersen et al., 2017; Prell & Grosskreutz, 2013).

Some people with ALS develop a type of dementia called frontotemporal dementia (FTD) which affects behavior and memory in addition to loss of strength (Castelnovo et al., 2023; Machts et al., 2015). Changes in the size of basal ganglia structures and their communication to other parts of the brain are impaired with this type of dementia in ALS.

In MS, dysfunction of the basal ganglia is tied to symptoms of fatigue and altered cognitive processing. Fatigue is due to connectivity changes between key regions of the basal ganglia and the motor cortex, medial prefrontal cortex, and more (Finke et al., 2015). The basal ganglia also show changes in density of their gray matter, integrity of white matter, and decrease in volume (Finke et al., 2015). While it is best known for its role in coordination, the cerebellum has the largest impact on cognitive behavioral functions of people with MS (Parmar et al., 2018).

Box 4.9   Learning activity

1. List five signs/symptoms of frontotemporal dementia. How does this type of dementia differ from others?
2. What impact might changes in cognition/memory have on one's independence or overall function?

Keywords: dementia, frontotemporal dementia, memory loss

The cerebellum also impacts gross motor and fine motor coordination which makes tasks like unlocking a door with a key, or pouring a hot beverage difficult. Tremors, impairments in balance like ataxia of gait, and difficulty with moving the muscles of the eye (oculomotor control) are seen when the cerebellum becomes damaged as part of MS demyelination (Parmar et al., 2018).

Processes of change in ALS and MS

People with ALS and MS experience changes in their function over time. The amount of time varies with the disease and subtypes; ALS is fatal and people with ALS generally experience a rapid decline after symptoms begin. People with MS on average have 5–10 years shorter life expectancy than those without MS (Marrie et al., 2015). As we discussed previously, there are four MS subtypes which are named after the way the symptoms affect a person over time. Some people may start with relapsing remitting MS (RRMS) where symptoms appear, but then decrease or go away completely, and over time the individual may then progress to another type.

Box 4.10   Learning activity

Create a Venn diagram to highlight the similarities and differences between ALS and MS. Use the information you have learned so far to guide your work.

Keywords: motor neuron, life expectancy, symptoms at onset

The ALS Functional Rating Scale-Revised (ALSFRS-R), is the measure for staging ALS and is completed by a medical professional through conversation with the person with ALS (Gordon et al., 2004). Other rating systems (King's, Milano-Torino) have been proposed but not yet adopted by all. The scales all identify areas of daily life where a person may be independent or need assistance; a numerical score then indicates how severe the stage of disease. For some, loss of movement in their legs and gross motor activity participation may drop and lower their score, whereas another person might have many swallowing and breathing symptoms that would change their ALSFRS-R score.

The most common scale used to characterize MS progression is the Expanded Disability Status Scale (EDSS), but there are also newer outcome measurement tools that have been developed (Inojosa et al., 2020; Kurtzke, 1983). The EDSS rates a person's ability to walk as well as the function of other bodily systems such as memory and the visual and sensory systems. A higher rating indicates the person is less independent, or experiencing more disability (Kurtzke, 1983).

There are many factors that impact not only a person's disease progression and access to care, but also their independence or experience of disability. Factors that may affect how fast their disease progresses include the quality of healthcare they receive based on insurance, where they live, transportation availability to get to appointments, and other factors, many of which are related to their socioeconomic status at the time they are diagnosed with MS or ALS. Additionally, having supportive caregivers or access to paid caregivers, medical equipment (wheelchairs, bath seats, etc.), assistive technology (computer headsets, voice features, etc.) or adaptive equipment (special knife to cut food with one hand, built up handles, etc.) all can vary from person to person. Community non-profit organizations like the MS Society or ALS Association can also play a large role in helping people with access to these resources.

Daily life routine: Using the computer to keep in touch with family

To keep in touch with family, Thomas relies heavily on his smartphone and computer. He likes to text, send emails, and comment on social media. When he is especially fatigued, he attends services and meetings at his temple virtually instead of in person. Thomas sees a licensed counselor for coping skill development and adjustment to disability via telehealth. His outpatient OTP showed him how to use built-in accessibility features on his smartphone such as talk to text, predictive text, and a virtual assistant ("Hey Siri," "OK Google") to complete activities. They recommended he purchase a headset to wear when using his computer so he can use voice to text with special software when he writes emails. They also showed him some alternative ways to use a mouse in the future including head-mounted options.

The major symptoms of ALS that limit individuals like Thomas's participation in valued daily occupations include muscle weakness, dysarthria, anarthria, dysphagia, dyspnea, muscle spasticity, and at times, frontotemporal dementia (FTD) (*Amyotrophic lateral sclerosis (ALS) fact sheet*). The participation restrictions that people with ALS experience over the course of the disease are varied, but areas most reported are decreased participation in recreational activities and work-related activities. Van Groenestijn et al. (2017) reported that more than one third of patients decreased their participation in community activities, hobbies, and recreation. McCabe et al. (2008) similarly found that patients with ALS as well as their caregivers are negatively impacted by the disease, and as a result, both groups experienced decreased participation in social activities and hobbies. McCabe et al. (2008) reported that 83% of patients had ceased their participation in paid work as a result of their diagnosis, by moving from full-time work to unemployment. The result of decreased participation in work is two-fold, as 28% of patients reported a negative impact on their social life as a result (McCabe et al., 2008). With a decrease in participation in meaningful activities, both socially and related to work, individuals with ALS may experience subsequent diminished quality of life.

Box 4.11   Learning activity

With your small group, complete the table in the Appendix about the integration of Thomas's social computer and smartphone use demands and the neuroscience that affects his participation.

Back to the person's life: Thomas using his computer to keep in touch

Now that you know more about brain and nervous system functioning in people with MS and ALS, how can we use this scientific reasoning to help Thomas continue using technology to participate socially? Throughout your education and career you will spend time exploring specific intervention details. However, knowledge of the neuroscience underpinnings provides a solid foundation to select intervention options that will support the intact brain and nervous system functions that Thomas has at his current stage of ALS. Always start with the occupational profile—which activities are valued by the client? How can we problem-solve to preserve their participation in these meaningful social activities?

Occupational therapy practitioners can encourage clients to use built-in technology features that are already available with the devices they own. Downloading or purchasing additional software or assistive technology devices might be beneficial, particularly as the symptoms of MS or ALS progress and a person has to re-adapt how they access them. These features and devices will vary based on the pattern of degeneration the client experiences. For example, someone with a bulbar form of ALS in the mild and moderate stages would not benefit from the same technology as someone like Thomas with limb onset ALS, as they will experience dysarthria (trouble speaking) prior to loss of fine motor control. Many individuals with progressing ALS will opt to use an augmentative and alternative communication (AAC) device to aid communication.

Box 4.12   Learning activity

Now that you know about how Thomas uses built-in features and assistive technology to keep in touch with family and friends, consider how he could use these same ideas for his *work* communication needs. With a partner, use your knowledge of neuroscience and what you know about Thomas and ALS to guide your idea generation about what intervention strategies you may use for Thomas.

What do we know about ourselves and the population at large from this brain condition and this family story?

While we framed technology use for social activities in the case of ALS, we ALL use technology to be social. We perceive technology to be a basic requirement to function in many home, work, and social settings. We also know that sometimes using technology can be frustrating when it doesn't work for us! We maintain a calendar on our smartphone and communicate with healthcare professionals through an electronic medical chart application. As we age and as new technologies rapidly become available, all people experience the need to form new routines and learn new strategies. An example of this is the advent of virtual meeting technology due to the COVID-19 pandemic of 2020–2023 for participation in school, work, and social activities. Adopting new technology or routines is easier for some people than others based on our visual, motor, cognitive, and other abilities. Normal aging brings unique changes to these systems that affects participation further. Lastly, the costs of technology may be out of reach for some clients.

We all have to prioritize the things we need and want to do throughout our day and across the weeks and months. Individuals living with neurodegenerative diseases have additional considerations that affect how they can prioritize and participate in daily activities including fatigue management, changes in strength and thinking abilities, and more. They also need to consider the big picture of how to spend their time when facing choices including end-of-life care. The "Further reading" list below provides additional insights if you are interested.

Further reading

If interested in further reading about ALS and MS, consult the following websites:

- ALS Association—www.als.org
- American Occupational Therapy Association ECHO Series—www.aota.org/practice/practice-essentials/evidencebased-practiceknowledge-translation/ms-echo
- National MS Society—www.nationalmssociety.org
- Roon—www.roon.com
- Your ALS Guide—www.youralsguide.com

References

Abidi, M., de Marco, G., Couillandre, A., Feron, M., Mseddi, E., Termoz, N., Querin, G., Pradat, P. F., & Bede, P. (2020). Adaptive functional reorganization in amyotrophic lateral sclerosis: coexisting degenerative and compensatory changes. *European Journal of Neurology, 27*(1), 121–128. https://doi.org/https://doi.org/10.1111/ene.14042

Ahmed, A., & Simmons, Z. (2013). Pseudobulbar affect: Prevalence and management. *Therapeutics and Clinical Risk Management*, 483–489. https://doi.org/10.2147/TCRM.S53906

Allen, D. D. (2019). Neuromuscular Diseases. In R. T. Lazaro, S. G. Reina-Guerra, & M. Quiben (Eds.), *Umphred's Neurological Rehabilitation-E-Book* (7th ed., pp. 457–458). Elsevier Health Sciences.

National Institute of Neurological Disorders and Stroke (n.d.). *Amyotrophic lateral sclerosis (ALS) fact sheet*. Retrieved May 26 from www.ninds.nih.gov/Disorders/Patient-Caregiver-Education/Fact-Sheets/Amyotrophic-Lateral-Sclerosis-ALS-Fact-Sheet

Bear, M., Connors, B., & Paradiso, M. A. (2020). *Neuroscience: Exploring the brain* (4th ed.). Jones & Bartlett Learning.

Bede, P., Elamin, M., Byrne, S., McLaughlin, R. L., Kenna, K., Vajda, A., Pender, N., Bradley, D. G., & Hardiman, O. (2013). Basal ganglia involvement in amyotrophic lateral sclerosis. *Neurology, 81*(24), 2107–2115.

Castelnovo, V., Canu, E., De Mattei, F., Filippi, M., & Agosta, F. (2023). Basal ganglia alterations in amyotrophic lateral sclerosis. *Frontiers in Neuroscience, 17*.

Dal Bello-Haas, V. (2019). Amyotrophic Lateral Sclerosis. In S. B. O'Sullivan, T. J. Schmitz, & G. Fulk (Eds.), *Physical Rehabilitation, 7e* (11th ed., pp. 769–795). F. A. Davis Company. fadavispt.mhmedical.com/content.aspx?aid=1197010940

Finke, C., Schlichting, J., Papazoglou, S., Scheel, M., Freing, A., Soemmer, C., Pech, L., Pajkert, A., Pfüller, C., & Wuerfel, J. (2015). Altered basal ganglia functional connectivity in multiple sclerosis patients with fatigue. *Multiple Sclerosis Journal, 21*(7), 925–934.

Gellersen, H. M., Guo, C. C., O'Callaghan, C., Tan, R. H., Sami, S., & Hornberger, M. (2017). Cerebellar atrophy in neurodegeneration—a meta-analysis. *Journal of Neurology, Neurosurgery & Psychiatry, 88*(9), 780–788. https://doi.org/10.1136/jnnp-2017-315607

Ghasemi, N., Razavi, S., & Nikzad, E. (2017). Multiple sclerosis: Pathogenesis, symptoms, diagnoses and cell-based therapy. *Cell Journal (Yakhteh), 19*(1), 1. https://doi.org/10.22074/cellj.2016.4867

Gordon, P. H., Miller, R. G., & Moore, D. H. (2004). ALSFRS-R. *Amyotrophic lateral sclerosis and other motor neuron disorders, 5*(1, Suppl.), 90–93. https://doi.org/https://doi.org/10.1080/17434470410019906

Gutman, S. A. (2017). *Quick reference neuroscience for rehabilitation professionals: The essential neurologic principles underlying rehabilitation practice* (3rd ed.). Slack Incorporated.

Inojosa, H., Schriefer, D., & Ziemssen, T. (2020). Clinical outcome measures in multiple sclerosis: A review. *Autoimmunity Reviews, 19*(5), 102512. https://doi.org/https://doi.org/10.1016/j.autrev.2020.102512

Kerbrat, A., Gros, C., Badji, A., Bannier, E., Galassi, F., Combès, B., Chouteau, R., Labauge, P., Ayrignac, X., & Carra-Dalliere, C. (2020). Multiple sclerosis lesions in motor tracts from brain to cervical cord: Spatial distribution and correlation with disability. *Brain, 143*(7), 2089–2105. https://doi.org/doi: 10.1093/brain/awaa162.

King, R. R., & Reiss, J. P. (2013). The epidemiology and pathophysiology of pseudobulbar affect and its association with neurodegeneration. *Degenerative neurological and neuromuscular disease*, 23–31.

Kurtzke, J. F. (1983). Rating neurologic impairment in multiple sclerosis: An expanded disability status scale (EDSS). *Neurology, 33*(11), 1444. https://doi.org/https://doi.org/10.1212/WNL.33.11.1444

Machts, J., Loewe, K., Kaufmann, J., Jakubiczka, S., Abdulla, S., Petri, S., Dengler, R., Heinze, H.-J., Vielhaber, S., & Schoenfeld, M. A. (2015). Basal ganglia pathology in ALS is associated with neuropsychological deficits. *Neurology, 85*(15), 1301–1309.

Marrie, R. A., Elliott, L., Marriott, J., Cossoy, M., Blanchard, J., Leung, S., & Yu, N. (2015). Effect of comorbidity on mortality in multiple sclerosis. *Neurology, 85*(3), 240–247. https://doi.org/https://doi.org/10.1212/WNL.0000000000001718

McCabe, M. P., Roberts, C., & Firth, L. (2008). Work and recreational changes among people with neurological illness and their caregivers. *Disability and Rehabilitation, 30*(8), 600–610. https://doi.org/https://doi.org/10.1080/09638280701400276

Parmar, K., Stadelmann, C., Rocca, M. A., Langdon, D., D'Angelo, E., D'Souza, M., Burggraaff, J., Wegner, C., Sastre-Garriga, J., & Barrantes-Freer, A. (2018). The role of the cerebellum in multiple sclerosis—150 years after Charcot. *Neuroscience & Biobehavioral Reviews, 89*, 85–98.

Prell, T., & Grosskreutz, J. (2013). The involvement of the cerebellum in amyotrophic lateral sclerosis. *Amyotrophic Lateral Sclerosis and Frontotemporal Degeneration, 14*(7–8), 507–515. https://doi.org/https://doi.org/10.3109/21678421.2013.812661

Van Groenestijn, A. C., Schroder, C., Kruitwagen-Van Reenen, E. T., Van Den Berg, L. H., & Visser-Meily, J. M. A. (2017). Participation restrictions in ambulatory amyotrophic lateral sclerosis patients: Physical and psychological factors. *Muscle & Nerve, 56*(5), 912–918. https://doi.org/10.1002/mus.25574

VanMeter, K. C., & Hubert, R. J. (2022). *Pathophysiology for the Health Professions E-Book*. Elsevier Health Sciences.

Zayia, L. C., & Tadi, P. (2021). Neuroanatomy, motor neuron. In *StatPearls [Internet]*. StatPearls Publishing.

5 Erna wants to clean her home and has cerebral palsy

Neuroscience facilitates our understanding of home maintenance

Lorie Gage Richards and Mozhgan Valipour

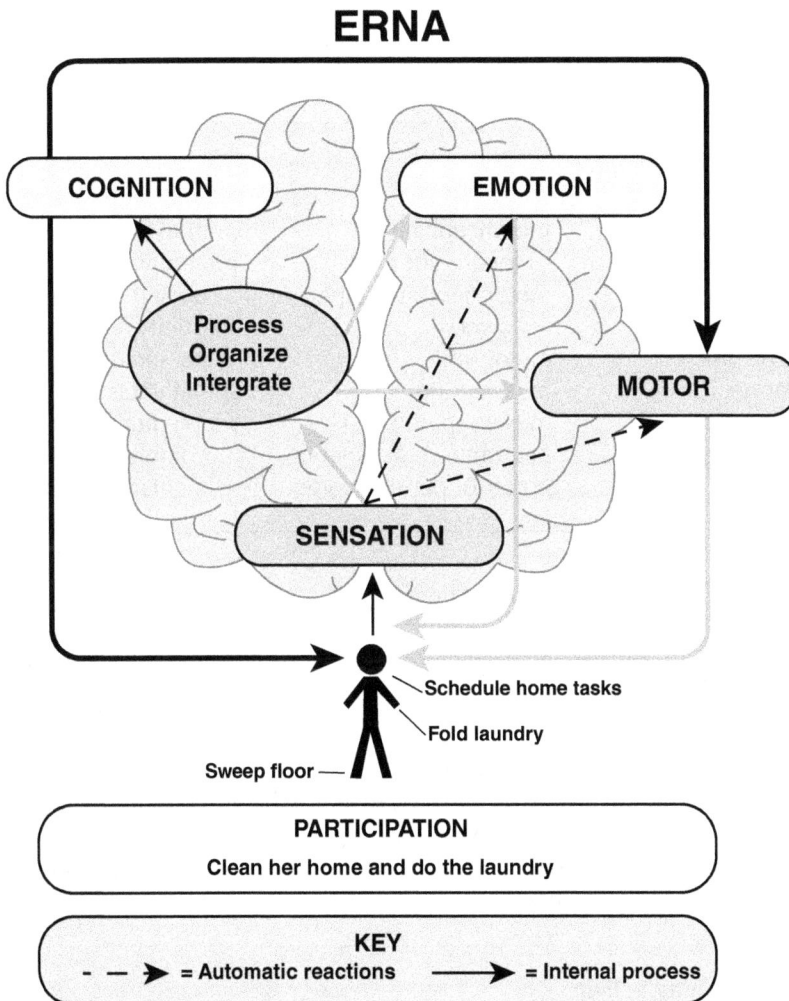

Figure 5.1 Erna brain figure

DOI: 10.4324/9781003524380-7

Purpose of this chapter

The purpose of this chapter is to discover how Erna, a 29-year-old, African American woman who wants her apartment to be spotless, might be affected by having spastic cerebral palsy (CP), a condition affecting her motor skills. People with spastic CP have full lives with their daily routines, relationships, and learning, but may require modifications for function.

The key neuroscience concepts we will explore in this chapter include functions of the motor system, which includes brain cortical and subcortical areas, spinal tracts carrying neural commands from the brain to the spinal cord, peripheral motor nerves that carry motor commands from the spinal cord to muscles, and muscle structures involved in performing motor aspects of activities and occupations. We will discuss voluntary motor acts and motor reflexes and how spastic CP impacts both.

As with all the chapters, these nervous system components work with other systems to support overall human function.

Keywords for this chapter are listed in the box below. Be sure you learn what these key features are so you can get the most out of the chapter.

Keywords for this chapter

alpha motor neurons	mesencephalic	primary motor cortex (M1)
basal ganglia (BG)	locomotor area	premotor cortex (ventral,
cerebellum	motor neurons (upper,	dorsal)
cerebellar tracts	lower)	spasticity (tonic, phasic)
gamma (fusimotor)	motor unit	spinal circuits
motor neurons	muscle tone	spinal tracts
inhibition (1a, 1b,	muscle spindle	supplementary motor
descending)	neuromuscular junction	complex (aka supple-
interneurons	posterior parietal cortex	mentary motor area)

Erna, a person who wants to clean her home

Erna lives alone in a one-story apartment in a small U.S. city. She is an associate professor at a university, teaching and conducting research in public health. Erna likes to keep her apartment spotless because she has friends and family over frequently for dinners, game nights, and other socializing.

At two months of age, she was diagnosed with tetraplegic (aka quadriplegic) spastic CP. This has caused motor control difficulties which impact her ability to tidy her apartment. Due to her budget, hiring a domestic worker would require giving up some of her leisure activities. She has come to Occupational Therapy to help her determine strategies that would allow her to clean her home more easily.

Box 5.1   Learning activity

1. Having read the narrative, what are you curious about?
2. What do you need to know more about?

More about Erna

Erna completes basic housecleaning independently. She can wipe off surfaces, wash dishes, and pick up objects to reduce clutter from surfaces, but her movements are slow and more uncoordinated than a person without CP. At times she knocks objects over or off their surface. Erna often must reach a few times before she grasps an object. Other housework is harder. Heavier objects (e.g., a ceramic casserole dish, heavy books), large and awkward objects (e.g., bed pillow), and small objects (e.g., pens, coins) are difficult to pick up. Erna walks in her home, but if she walks a lot, she becomes fatigued. Erna has trouble with her balance. For example, if she changes directions quickly, or reaches for something that is far away, she easily stumbles or falls.

She has a laundry service as her washer and dryer are in the basement. She can put her clothes away, but this takes time as she often drops clothes trying to hang them up. She sometimes has difficulty maneuvering the vacuum in tight places. When she has to use a lot of effort, her muscles tend to contract more and get stiffer, especially her finger and elbow flexors and her leg extensors. This further interferes with her performing her activities and occupations.

What is cerebral palsy?

Before birth, your neurons formed and migrated to their final places, which was based on their gene expression, mainly determined by their location in the neural tube.[1] The neurons began to connect with each other. At birth, you were able to make movements and had automatic reflexes that helped you perform the infant occupations that kept you alive, such as the rooting reflex that helped you find and latch on to a nipple for feeding. Yet, many oligodendrocytes surrounding neuron axons were not fully formed.[2] Much of your motor system was less efficient than now. This is one reason you were unable to hold your head up or walk. Also, as a newborn, you had little experience moving against gravity or using objects. As your motor axons become myelinated, your movements become more coordinated, and stronger. Most of this happened because connections between motor (and sensory) neurons formed, strengthened, weakened, or were pruned based on your motor experiences. This learning process has continued and will continue throughout your life.[3,4]

With CP, there is damage to the brain, especially the motor system.[5] This damage can occur before, during, or shortly after birth up to three years of age.[6]

The motor problems that result depend on when, where, and how much the motor system is damaged.[7] This damage makes it difficult for individuals with CP to produce movements that match the demands of the activity. Additionally, the more difficulty a child has making movements, the less they interact with objects and move around their environment. Limiting motor experiences interferes with motor network development.[8] Most people with CP learn better motor skills. However, due to the neural damage and limited motor experiences, they usually have motor control problems throughout their lives.

Box 5.2   Learning activity

1. What can cause CP?
2. What are the four kinds of CP?

---

3. What is the characteristic motor pattern seen with each?
4. Find pictures or YouTube videos of a person with spastic CP walking and picking up objects to help you visualize what Erna's movements look like. *Be sure to get guidance from your instructor about how to find quality YouTube videos for this activity.*
5. Describe those movements that you see.

Neuroscience information to guide your thinking about Erna

How does the nervous system control voluntary movement?

There are two basic types of movements: reflexive and voluntary movements. We will focus mostly on voluntary movement but will briefly cover reflexive movements later as they relate to Erna's spastic CP. To perform voluntary movements, you create an action goal—something you need or want to do. You might need to move your leg if your foot falls asleep. Your stomach growls so you need to go find some food. Forming such goals uses parts of the nervous system, like the prefrontal cortex, that are not considered part of the motor system, but might be impaired in people with CP.[9] However, we won't talk more about that area here.

Once you have a goal, your motor system network forms a motor program for it. Your sensory system (see Chapters 7–9) provides information on where your body and limbs are in relation to gravity, each other, and any relevant objects. This data is transformed into a form that can be used for motor actions. Plus, once you have some movement experience, your nervous system has motor memories of similar activities.[10] The motor memories are combined with sensory information and task demands to plan the current motor program.[11] Multiple neural areas contribute to the planning of motor programs. Many of these areas have reciprocal connections to each other and work in parallel (mostly at the same time) to modify the motor program.[12,13] Brain motor areas have more heterogeneous roles than previously thought, but certain areas are more associated with particular planning aspects than others.

The final motor command is sent from the brain's upper motor neurons to the spinal cord through several pathways. For some actions, most of the motor action features are specified in your brain; for others, such as walking, spinal circuits determine the primary motor pattern.[14] At each motor system level the motor program can be modified. At the spinal level, the motor command is sent to the peripheral nerves. The motor command travels over these lower motor neurons to those muscles needed to achieve the goal.

Box 5.3   Learning activity

To help you understand what is meant by a neural network, find some pictures of motor system neural networks.

How a person without CP reaches for the books and pens

To help you understand more deeply, let's focus on a particular housekeeping activity—picking up and putting items away. Erna wants to pick up books and pens that she put on the floor by her couch and then put the books away in her bedroom. First, we'll learn how a person without CP might perform this activity. Then how Erna performs it.

Box 5.4   Learning activity

1. With a partner or group, place some books and pens on the floor. Each of you, one at a time while the other watches, bend over to pick up a book and a pen.
2. Describe the motions of the arm, hand, legs, and trunk as the person reaches for and grasps the book and the pen.
3. Did the arm movement and the bending occur one after the other or at the same time?
4. Was the same type of grasp and strength of grasp used to pick up both objects?
5. Did everyone do the action the same?

As in most activities, you also made movements that were harder to see. In planning the movement, your motor system anticipated how raising your arm and bending/squatting would move your center of mass (COM) towards the edge, or beyond, your base of support (BOS).

Box 5.5   Learning activity

Find a picture of human center of mass and center of pressure.

1. What is meant by "COM" and "BOS"?
2. Stand with your back and heels against a wall.
3. Move your arms up quickly so they are out straight in front of you. Did you feel your back push harder against the wall?
4. Now try to bend over to touch the floor without moving away from the wall? What happened?

When you bend forward or raise your arms, your COM moves forward. If your COM moves out of your BOS, you will fall. Thus, prior to bending or moving your arms, you may have put one foot forward to widen your BOS. You also activated your plantarflexors and other extensor muscles that move the COM backwards to counteract its future forward movement.[15]

How Erna reaches for the books and pens

Due to spastic CP, Erna struggles to make coordinated movements—with muscle patterns matching the task demands. She has trouble reaching with her elbow extended. Her movements are stiff and slow, often jerky. She may over- or undershoot reaches, requiring more small corrective movements than a person without CP. She also has hypertonicity (tightness) in some muscles. During reaches she finds it hard to open her hand all the way (extend/abduct all her digits simultaneously) so she wiggles her fingers on the edge of the book to grab it. She can close her hand, but her grip is too weak to lift heavy books very far or hold them for long. She has difficulty picking up the pens due to their small size and rounded shape. She can move her fingers separately but has difficulty opposing just the index finger and thumb in exactly the right configuration to easily pick them up. Often the other fingers interfere, or the thumb hits the side of the index finger, and the pen rolls out of the pinch. Erna also has trouble with her postural control due to her CP. Her legs are adducted so that her knees touch (aka, "scissors" position). Her hips and knees are slightly flexed; her weight is forward towards her toes. She bends from the hips with only slightly bent knees.

Box 5.6   Self-directed learning activity

Look up a picture of "spastic legs scissors position." Try putting your legs in a scissors position like Erna's. Now try bending to pick up a book or pen. What did you notice about your balance?

Just as you faced, this posture makes Erna unstable; therefore, she grabs furniture for stabilization while bending to pick things up and tends to walk as close as possible to the books and pens before bending to pick them up.

Nervous system control of reaching and grasping movements

Your motor system creates the motor program as a forward internal model of the kinematics and the kinetics necessary for you to perform the action. In this model, limb/body joint angles and the muscle patterns needed to achieve these joint angles of the action are estimated.[16,17] The internal model is formed and refined in the cortex.

Box 5.7   Learning activity

1. Look up pictures of the following cortical motor areas and where they are located: primary motor cortex (M1), ventral premotor cortex (vPMC), dorsal premotor cortex (dPMC), supplementary motor complex (aka, supplementary motor area), posterior parietal cortex intraparietal sulcus.
2. Many motor areas are organized somatotopically. In M1, this organization is called, the homunculus. Find a picture of this. From this picture, can you tell what "somatotopically" means?
3. Which parts of motor planning and/or execution do each of these areas contribute to?

The basal ganglia (BG) can modify the motor program. The exact role in motor control of the BG is debated.

Box 5.8   Learning activity

1. Find a picture of the BG.
2. Find a picture of the three main BG pathways related to motor control.
3. What is the major theory of the role of the BG in motor control?
4. Identify each pathway's effect on the motor cortex.

Kandel, et al.[18] nonetheless, suggest that, in addition to the main role you found above, the BG might also impact stimulus-driven movement (e.g., grabbing a napkin when you spill a drink), as well as self-paced and memory-driven actions. The BG may help to control which sensory inputs should be attended to, directly impacting which motor programs are selected.

In contrast, some authors note that timing of BG activation compared to cortical activity suggests that the BG's role is more about reinforcing the commitment to an action rather than motor selection.[19] The BG may also help determine movement parameters, such as speed, and the probability that a movement will be performed. The neural signals that code options about the movement type and where it is to be performed may be sent via pathways using the neurotransmitter glutamate. Signals using dopamine may modify options about when movement occur. (See Chapter 23 for more on the BG.)

The cerebellum also contributes to making smooth, accurate limb movements.[20] (See Chapter 6 for more on the cerebellum.)

Box 5.9   Learning activity

1. Find a picture of the cerebellum and its location in the brain. What parts of the cerebellum are involved in making movements?
2. Find a picture of the cerebellar tracts to the rest of the motor system. What are the roles of the cerebellum in voluntary motor control?
3. Describe what is meant by "efference copy" and its role in motor control.

Many of the areas already discussed connect to M1. When activated by premotor areas, M1 sends a motor command to the spinal cord. There are direct connections to motor neurons from the premotor and supplementary motor areas (e.g., Maier et al.[21]), but most motor commands come from M1. There are four descending tracts that carry motor information to the body. Each runs from either the cortex or brain stem nuclei to spinal circuits at various levels of the spinal cord.

Descending motor commands synapse on alpha motor neurons, gamma motor neurons (more on these later), or interneurons at various spinal levels associated with limb movement. Here, the motor program can be further modified.

Box 5.10   Learning activity

1. Find pictures of the four descending white matter tracts that carry motor information to the spinal cord. (There is actually a fifth tract, the corticobulbar tract, that
   deals with head and face motor control, but we will not deal with this tract in this
   chapter.) What are the names of the four descending motor white matter tracts?
   Note which tracts have two branches.
2. Describe each tract's path, from its origin, through the brain and into the spinal cord.
   Do this for all the branches of these tracts. Be sure to note brain stem structures that
   these tracts pass through and indicate what these structures do in motor control.
3. Do they control muscles on the same (ipsilateral) or opposite (contralateral) side
   of the body?
4. Do they cross to the other side in the pathway? If so, how many times?
5. Do they control trunk, proximal, or distal limb muscles?
6. What spinal levels are responsible for arm movement?
7. Which is the only tract in primates that control hand and finger movements?

The final motor command is sent to the muscles from the alpha motor neurons. Their
axons exit the spinal cord and traverse large plexi before becoming the final peripheral
nerves. The peripheral nerves synapse onto the muscle at the neuromuscular junction (see
Chapter 2).

Box 5.11   Learning activity

1. Find a picture of the plexus for the arm and hand.
2. What is this plexus called?
3. After you study these pictures for a bit, see if you can draw and label this plexus
   with its spinal roots.
4. List the peripheral nerves that emerge from the plexus, with their spinal root origins and their innervation(s).

Box 5.12   Learning activity

1. What is the difference between an alpha motor neuron and a spinal interneuron?
2. What types of spinal interneurons are there?
3. Where do spinal interneurons project?
4. What does an alpha motor neuron project to?

Box 5.13   Learning activity

1. Find pictures of a motor unit, the neuromuscular junction, and the contractile fibers (extrafusal fibers) in a muscle. Use these pictures to help you with the answers

to the following questions. You will also probably have to investigate websites other than images to answer some of them.
2. What is the definition of a motor unit?
3. What is the principal neurotransmitter used at the neuromuscular junction?
4. What are the three types of extrafusal muscle fibers and their characteristics?
5. What determines the number of motor units in a muscle?
6. Describe the size principle of motor fiber recruitment.
7. What are the contractile molecules in motor fibers? How do they create muscle force?

The motor command has to produce forces sufficient and in the right direction to perform the activity. Force level produced is determined by many aspects of the neural-muscle system, but two principles of this control are the number of motor units activated and the frequency of action potentials arriving at the muscle with a certain amount of time. A larger number of activated motor units and action potentials that arrive close together produce forceful contractions. Most movements require activation patterns across multiple muscles. Also, movements cause movement at unintended joints. Muscles produce movement at each joint they cross. Body movements produce momentum at multiple limb segments that cause movement, even at joints quite distant from an activated muscle. These **joint interaction torques** are larger for fast movements than slow movements. Lastly, movements may cause body parts to be in positions where gravity has a torque at certain joints. If movement there is not wanted, other muscles need to activate to stabilize those joints.

Box 5.14   Learning activity

1. Move your arm slowly out in front of you while standing (flex your shoulder) without contracting any muscles at your elbow. Now do the same thing really fast. What happened at your elbow? This is an example of a joint interaction torque.
2. Hold your arm out in front of you (shoulder flexion). Bend your elbow a little bit. Now relax your elbow muscles. What happened to your elbow? This is an example of gravity's pull on your elbow that has to be opposed by a muscle contraction if you don't want that to happen to your elbow.
3. What is the term used when muscles activate at the same time? What is the role of the agonist muscle(s), antagonist muscle(s), and synergist muscle(s) in making a movement? Your motor system has to coordinate the activation of all of these for any given movement.

Motor programs are created partly based on information about the muscles: their length and tone. Muscles typically have a certain resting length and muscle tone. Muscle tone is regulated to help ready the muscles for action.[22,23] (Think about what happens to your muscles when you are afraid or when you are waiting for the ball in tennis, volleyball, or baseball.) Information about muscle length change, the length change velocity, and muscle tension is communicated by the sensory organs in the muscle spindle and tendon.

Box 5.15   Learning activity

1. Define what is meant by muscle tone.
2. Find a picture of the muscle spindle. There are muscle fibers in the muscle spindle to which sensory nerves are attached. What is the general name for all these fibers?
3. What are the specific fibers called (there are three of them) that provide information about muscle length and velocity of changes in length?

   a. What stimulation do each of these respond to?
   b. What type of sensory nerve are attached to each of these?

4. The muscle spindles receive commands from special motor nerves that innervate muscle spindle muscle fibers What are they called? (There are two basic types with one type having two subtypes.)

   a. Which muscle fibers to they innervate?

5. What sensory organ is in the tendon?

   a. What type of stimulation does it respond to?
   b. What type of sensory nerve is attached to this organ?

The muscle spindle plays an important role in muscle tone. The active part of muscle tone occurs by both dynamic and static stretch reflexes. Reflexes are primarily controlled via spinal cord circuits, although we now know that reflexes can be somewhat modified by descending motor commands.[24,25] The dynamic stretch reflex occurs rapidly (within 1 ms). The static stretch reflex is concerned with continuous muscle tension.[18] (See Chapter 1 for more on stretch reflexes.) Erna has hypertonicity, part of which impacts her stretch reflexes.

Box 5.16   Learning activity

1. Define hypertonicity.
2. What is the difference between hypertonicity and spasticity?
3. What are the causes of spasticity?

Box 5.17   Self-directed learning activity

1. Find a picture of the basic reflex arc.
2. Find pictures of the stretch reflex testing (also known as deep tendon reflex testing). There are also videos of this testing that can be found on the Web.
3. You have probably all had a physician demonstrate such a dynamic or phasic stretch reflex on you, but let's demonstrate it here. With a partner, have that

partner hit your patellar tendon with a reflex hammer or the side of the hand (like a karate chop). What happens to your partner's lower leg when you do that?
4. This reflex can also be tested at the Achilles tendon. Place your partner's foot in your hand with your finger cupped over the heel and their toes over your wrist or forearm. Now tap the tendon briskly. What happened to their foot? Are these dynamic or static stretch reflexes?
5. Describe the dynamic stretch reflex, including whether the synapse involved is excitatory or inhibitory. What are other names for this reflex?
6. Is this monosynaptic or polysynaptic? What do these terms mean?
7. What muscles does the dynamic stretch reflex affect?
8. Describe the static stretch reflex. Is this monosynaptic or polysynaptic? What muscles does the static stretch reflex affect?

Posture and balance

Box 5.18   Learning activity

1. Describe these structures and concepts involved in the stretch reflex and muscle tone:
2. Renshaw cells, recurrent inhibition, 1a inhibition, reciprocal inhibition, non-reciprocal 1b inhibition, and fusimotor drive.
3. What are the descending inputs to the spinal circuit of the stretch reflex? Are they inhibitory or faciliatory?

Part of Erna's difficulty in picking up the books and pens is her unsteady postural control and balance. Posture and balance are controlled by different systems.

Box 5.19   Learning activity

1. Look up the definition of postural stability.
2. Look up the difference between anticipatory postural actions and reactionary postural responses.
3. Why are we continuously having to activate and deactivate muscles around joints to maintain upright, "still" posture? Which muscles are especially important for upright posture?
4. Remember how Erna positions her legs due to her spastic cerebral palsy? Put your legs that way and then try to pick up something from the floor. Was that difficult or easy?

As Erna plans her movements, her nervous system anticipates the pull of gravity on her body parts and what will happen as the book is added to her hand and plans the muscle activations needed to counteract gravity, integrates them with the primary movement plans, and activates those muscles just prior to her bending and arm movements. These are anticipatory postural actions.[26] Her motor system can do this because of stored memories of what happened during previous bending and reaching experiences.

Reactionary postural responses are movements produced to prevent falls once something has disturbed balance. As Erna bends over, her cat unexpectedly bangs his head against her leg, disturbing her balance causing her to hang onto the couch more strongly to prevent falling. To make such responses, the nervous system requires adequate sensory information about immediate risk to posture and balance and to implement a response rapid and large enough to re-establish a safe posture. Because Erna has fallen many times, she is somewhat afraid of falling when she picks items up from the floor. This reduces her ability to make efficient postural reactions.

Box 5.20   Learning activity

1. Look up some videos on anticipatory and reactionary postural actions.
2. What parts of the nervous system are involved in planning anticipatory postural actions.
3. What part of the nervous system is involved in her quick postural reaction to the cat's action?
4. What characteristics of Erna's sensorimotor functioning, because of her CP, make postural activities more challenging for her?
5. What effect does fear of falling have on muscle tone and stiffness?

Walking

Erna walks to her bedroom to put the books in her bookcase. Her gait is slow, in a somewhat scissors and toe walking pattern. This fatiguing gait tires Erna after a few trips. Therefore, straightening up the house takes longer than she would like.

Box 5.21   Learning activity

1. In groups, have one of your group walk slowly across the room. What happened just before they took their first step? Can you describe the pattern that their legs made as they walked?
2. Look up the gait pattern of a person without cerebral palsy (e.g., the step cycle) and see if you got all the pieces.
3. What part of the central nervous system is responsible for controlling the basic, rhythmic pattern of gait? Describe its parts.
4. What part(s) of the central nervous system controls the initiation of gait?
5. What parts of the central nervous system are involved in planning locomotor actions?
6. A unique part of the motor system related to gait is the mesencephalic locomotor area. Locate this on a picture and describe what it does.

---

7. What part is especially involved in vision-guided gait planning?
8. As in the upper limb, the spinal circuits at the lumbar region that control walking send their motor commands through alpha motor neurons that traverse a plexus before separating into various peripheral nerves. Find a picture of this plexus. Name and diagram this plexus, including its spinal roots and resulting peripheral nerves.

Application of the neuroscience to understanding Erna's performance

Erna's motor abilities and challenges can help us determine where the damage to Erna's motor system occurred. The following questions guide us in this endeavor:

1. Can she produce easy, fluid, smooth voluntary arm and move different fingers independently? Can she reach her arm out straight when the shoulder is in flexion?
2. Are her arms and legs weak? Does she have reduced sensation?

   a. If so, is it in a dermatome or innervation pattern for a specific part of her upper or lower limb? Is it on only one or both sides of the body?
   b. Is the weakness more proximal, distal, or similar in both sets of muscles?

3. Does she have problems initiating gait? Is she able to alter the speed of her gait when the task requires changes in speed?
4. Does she show a tremor? If so, is this an intention tremor or resting tremor?
5. Does she consistently overshoot the books or the pens? Or does she both undershoot and overshoot? Does she demonstrate ataxia when she walks?
6. After effort does her hand get tight so that she has trouble opening her hand?
7. When she moves quickly or is startled, does she experience unwanted muscle contractions or clonus? Does she appear stiff as she moves?

Erna makes voluntary movements with her arms and legs, including independent finger movement. She initiates gait and alters speed as needed. Yet, her movements are poorly coordinated and weak, more distally than proximally. She struggles to raise her arm and extend her elbow at the same time, in other words, selectively activate muscles. These answers suggest that she is relying more on motor command signals from spinal tracts other than the corticospinal tract (CST), such as the retriculospinal tract (ReST) and rubrospinal (RST). Her independent, but uncoordinated, finger movements imply that, at least some of her CST is intact. Her gait initiation argues for lack of major damage to her mesencephalic locomotor region. Her limbs have decreased proprioception and tactile sensation, but it and her weakness are not in a dermatome or peripheral nerve distribution. Thus, she does not have a spinal cord injury or peripheral nerve damage. Her sensory loss and motor problems are on both sides. Therefore, there is likely damage to both the right and left hemisphere motor areas.

Erna's hand tightens into a fist with effort. She needs to stretch it before reaching again. Her gait pattern shows leg adduction with toe walking. These motor patterns are indicative of hypertonicity. They might indicate tonic spasticity but could be co-contraction caused by difficulty coordinating opposing muscle activation timing seen with CST damage. Tonic spasticity indicates reduced inhibitory descending commands from the lateral ReST, and potentially some increased facilitation from various sources (more sensory group Ia transmitters release, more alpha motor neuron excitability, more excitable interneurons).[27]

In decluttering, it is unlikely that Erna's phasic spasticity is involved as her slow movement velocity would be unlikely to trigger the phasic spastic stretch reflex. If she moves quickly, as if she tries to catch a slipping book, the phasic spastic stretch reflex might be triggered; her upper limb flexors and her leg extensors would contract quickly, unlike someone without hypertonicity whose spinal circuits are less excitable requiring faster movements to trigger the phasic stretch reflex. We should note there is controversy around whether the increased spinal circuit excitability is a pathology, and thus bad, or whether this is an adaptation to the reduced descending inputs that assist with muscle activation. In the latter, the adaptation allows movement, and task performance at some level, to still occur.[28] One clue this might be an adaptation is that spasticity develops only after some weeks post brain injury.[28,29]

Erna does not have a tremor. She under- or overshoots targets, but not severe enough to indicate intention tremor (tremor seen with movement) or ataxia (uncoordinated, often ballistic movements). She does not have a resting tremor (tremor at rest). These answers tell you that she does not have cerebellar, BG, or vestibulospinal tract damage.

In summary, Erna's difficulties with doing her housekeeping stem mostly from the brain damage to her CST and ReST (or their neurons). This, in turn causes heighted excitation of and insufficient motor commands to her spinal circuits. The resulting hypertonicity and insufficient motor commands have produced stiff muscles that don't get activated in the coordinated patterns needed for efficient motor actions, including less effective postural and balance.

Back to the person's life: Erna cleaning her home to her own satisfaction

---

Box 5.22   Learning activity

In class or small groups, discuss what intervention approaches from the OTPF you might use with Erna. Discuss the pros and cons of each that you think are relevant.

So now that you know more about neural motor system functioning in people with CP, how can we use this scientific reasoning to help Erna more easily do her housekeeping?

Knowing the root cause of the poor motor performance is important. It helps to direct the best intervention for the functional problems. If it is likely that one problem is in generating facilitatory motor commands, then it is possible to improve motor skills through a lot of motor skill practice, especially early after damage when the brain is more plastic.[e.g.30] If the problem is sensory, a person may not learn better motor skills, although there is some emerging evidence that proprioception and tactile perception may be improved with training.[31,32] As Erna is an adult and she has had CP since infancy, it might be unlikely that Erna's motor skills would improve sufficiently. She might not want or have the time to spend the hours of motor practice it would take to improve her motor function. Thus, strategies to decrease the motor coordination demands of her housekeeping tasks can be used to improve her function.

Often, however, motor skills can be improved to a meaningful level in in people with longstanding motor system damage.[33,34] As such, a combination approach might be used. Task modification to make the task motorically easier can occur in conjunction with motor practice if the strategy does not eliminate or reduce the use of the paretic arm and hand.[35] In this way, Erna could obtain the satisfaction of performing her housekeeping more easily with the just-right practice challenge. It might also encourage more motor practice than just setting aside time each day to practice.

Erna's difficulty also stems from hypertonicity. Some interventions for hypertonicity can be provided by occupational therapists. Others need to be provided by a physician.

Box 5.23   Self-directed learning activity

1. What are the most common interventions for hypertonicity? Identify the one that is most often used in children with CP with scissors gait
2. What is the physiology underlying their effectiveness?
3. Are their effects permanent?
4. What are the side effects?

It is unlikely that Erna's walking would be similar to someone without CP even if her hypertonicity were now eliminated for multiple reasons. Current anti-spasticity medicine usually results in various amount of muscle weakness[36,37]; individuals with spasticity have difficulty moving with more common movement patterns post-medication administration. In addition, Erna's brain and spinal cord have learned her current balance and walking patterns over years of practice in interacting with various environments with her current hypertonicity status. She has formed deep habits of moving (strong neural network synaptic connections) that would take many hours of practice to change. Lastly, she also has difficulty producing coordinated motor activation patterns. Thus, she may have difficulty planning and executing a locomotor pattern that is more typical of a person without CP, even without hypertonicity. As a result, people with CP might need therapy to improve motor coordination in addition to hypertonicity intervention.

Another factor that is important to note is that Erna may be using her hypertonicity as a stabilizing force due to her trouble with voluntary motor control. In this case, anti-spasticity medicines could make her less functional, at least until she builds greater ability to voluntarily activate muscles with appropriate patterns and forces. Two examples illustrate this concept. In one of our research studies, we administered botulinum toxin A to the arm and hand muscles of a woman with voluntary arm/hand movement. She reported dissatisfaction after the medicine administration as she was no longer able to push her shopping cart. After the botulinum, she was unable grasp the cart well enough to push it. Another example is that many children with spastic CP, who could run before given anti-spasticity medicine, albeit using a different and awkward-looking pattern, are unable to run after receiving the medicine. This prevents them from engaging in some desired activities, such as playing baseball, for quite some time until they develop sufficient voluntary motor control to run again, if they do.

What do we know about ourselves and the population at large from this brain condition and this family story?

We have learned that people with CP have strengths and weaknesses, as do all humans. We also learned that CP is heterogeneous; people with CP have different types of motor difficulties ranging from very mild to very severe. The CP type and severity depends on the neural damage location and extent and its timing during development. Consequently, we cannot know a person's abilities and challenges from their diagnosis. We must evaluate their abilities to know this. People with CP often learn strategies that allow them to perform their required and desired occupations, just as all humans do. They are often satisfied with how they complete them and do not want therapy to learn how to do those tasks differently. We cannot assume what they want help with, and which approach they'll want to use until we talk with them.

We have learned that completing housekeeping uses the entire motor system. Performing such activities requires effective motor planning that integrates sensory information about the status and location of the body and its parts. The plan is refined over several cortical areas, the BG, and cerebellum. It is then sent to the spinal cord via several motor tracts. Motor program modification can also occur at the spinal circuit before the motor command is sent through the peripheral nerves to the muscles. People with spastic CP have hypertonicity in which loss of descending inhibition, among other neural changes, produces spasticity, a component of hypertonicity. The latter also includes non-neural components, such as muscular stiffness, which also impact motor function. As neural damage is early, people with CP also have alterations in motor development due to more limited motor experiences. Thus, the motor challenges of adults with CP result from both the initial damage, the adaptations of the motor system to the damage, and their altered motor development. Interestingly, the motor system of people with spastic CP is still able to learn in ways similar to an undamaged motor system—through modifying existing neural connections and creating new ones.

People with spastic CP can choose between the Occupational Therapy Practice Framework interventions of establish (remediation, restoration) and modify (compensation, adaptation) for improving their ability to perform daily activities, such as housekeeping. Such choices require weighing the likelihood for sufficient gains in motor skills and the amount of practice needed to achieve those gains with the relative ease and expense of alternative strategies, such as assistive technology and activity modification.

Box 5.24   Learning activity

With your small group, complete the table in the Appendix about how Erna can be assisted to clean her apartment.

Further reading

Two novels that tell the story of a young girl growing to adulthood with CP, as told by her mother:

Killilea, M. *Karen*. Open Road Media, 2016
Killilea, M. *With Love from Karen*. Open Road Media, 2016
CP resources online:

- Information about cerebral palsy: www.ninds.nih.gov/health-information/disorders/cerebral-palsy
- Cerebral Palsy Foundation: https://cpresource.org/
- A site connecting families with children with CP to research about CP: www.canchild.ca/en/research-in-practice/current-studies/childhood-cerebral-palsy-integrated-neuroscience-discovery-network-cp-net
- Center for Parent Information and Resources: www.parentcenterhub.org/cp/
- MedlinePlus resources on CP: https://medlineplus.gov/cerebralpalsy.html
- Information about the neuroscience of motor control: www.physio-pedia.com/Motor_Control_and_Learning

References

1 Alberts B, Johnson A, Lewis J, Raff Ml, Roberts K, Walter P. Neural development. *Molecular Biology of the Cell*. (5th ed.) Garland, 2007.
2 Kessarism N, Fogarty M, Iannarelli P, Grist M, Wegner M, Richardson WD. Competing waves ofl oligodendorcytes in the forebrain and postnatal elimination of an embryonic lineage. *Nat Neurosci*. 2006;*9*:173–179. doi: 10.1038/nn1620
3 Nudo RJ, Milliken GW, Jenkins WM, Merzenich MM. Use-dependent alterations of movement representations in primary motor cortex of adult squirrel monkeys. *J Neurosci*. 1996;*16*(2):785–807. doi: 10.1523/JNEUROSCI.16-02-00785.1996.
4 Monje M. Myelin plasticity and nervous system function. *Annual Rev Neurosci*. 2018;*41*:61–76. https://doi.org/10.1146/annurev-neuro-080317-061853
5 National Center on Birth Defects and Developmental Disabilities, Centers for Disease Control and Prevention. cerebral palsy (CP). (2022, May 2). www.cdc.gov/ncbddd/cp/causes.html
6 Larsen ML, Rackauskaite G, Greisen G, Laursen B, Uldall P, Krebs L, Hoei-Hansen, CE. Continuing decline in the prevalence of cerebral palsy in Denmark for birth years 2008–2013. *Eur J Paediatr Neurol*. 2021;*30*:155–161. doi: 10.1016/j.ejpn.2020.10.003.
7 Hadders-Algra M. Early diagnosis and early intervention in cerebral palsy. *Front Neurol*. 2014;*5*:185. https://doi.org/10.3389/fneur.2014.00185
8 Adolph KE, Franchak JM. The development of motor behavior. *Wiley Interdiscip Rev Cogn Sci*. 2017;*8*(1–2):10.1002/wcs.1430. doi: 10.1002/wcs.1430.
9 Barakat MKA., Elmeniawy GH, Abdelazeim FH. Sensory systems processing in children with spastic cerebral palsy: a pilot study. *Bull Fac Phys Ther*. 2021;26:27. *https://doi.org/10.1186/s43161-021-00044-w*
10 American Psychology Association. *Motor program*. APA Dictionary of Psychology. (2023, February 22). https://dictionary.apa.org/motor-program
11 O'Sullivan SB, McKibben RJ, Portney LG. Examination of motor function: Motor control and motor learning. In O'Sullivan SB, Schmitz TJ, Fulk G. eds. *Physical Rehabilitation*, 7e. McGraw Hill, 2019. Accessed August 18, 2023. https://fadavispt.mhmedical.com/content.aspx?bookid=2603&sectionid=214786051.
12 Burman KJ, Bakola S, Richardson KE, Reser DH, Rosa MGP. Patterns of cortical input to the primary motor area in the marmoset monkey. *J Comp Neurol*. 2014;*522*:811–843. Doi: 10.1002/cne.23447

13 Dea M, Hamadjida A, Elgbeili G, Quessy S, Dancause N. Different patterns of cortical inputs to subregions of the primary motor cortex hand representation in cebus apella. *Cereb Cortex.* 2016;*26*:1747–1761. Doi: 10/1093/cercor/bhv324

14 Minassian K, Hofstoetter US, Dzeladini F, Guertin PA, Ijspeert A. The human central pattern generator for locomotion: Does it exist and contribute to walking? *Neuroscientist.* 2017;*23*(6):649–663. doi: 10.1177/1073858417699790.

15 Massion J. Movement, posture and equilibrium: interaction and coordination. *Prog Neurobiol.* 1992;*38*:35–56. 10.1016/0301–0082(92)90034-c

16 Wolpert DM, Ghahramani Z, Jordan MI. An internal model for sensorimotor integration. *Science.* 1995;*269*:1880–1882. doi: 10.1126/science. 7569931

17 Dogge M, Custers R, Aarts H. Moving forward: on the limits of motor-based forward models. *Trends Cogn Sci.* 2019;*23*;743–753. doi: 10.1016/j.tics. 2019.06.008

18 Kandel ER, Koester JD, Mack SH, Siegelbaum, S.A. *Principles of neural science.* (6th ed.). McGraw Hill, 2021.

19 Hudspeth AJ, Jessell TM, Kandel ER, Schwartz JH, Siegelbaum SA. eds. *Principles of Neural Science.* McGraw-Hill, Health Professions Division, 2013.

20 Manto M, Bower JM, Conforto AB, et al. (2012). Consensus paper: roles of the cerebellum in motor control--the diversity of ideas on cerebellar involvement in movement. *Cerebellum (London, England),* 2012;*11*(2):457–487. https://doi.org/10.1007/s12311-011-0331-9

21 Maier MA, Armand J, Kirkwood PA, et al. Differences in the corticospinal projection from primary motor cortex and supplementary motor area to macaque upper limb motoneurons: An anatomical and electrophysiological study, *Cereb Cortex.* 2002;*12*(3):281–296. https://doi.org/10.1093/cercor/12.3.281

22 Latash ML, & Zatsiorsky VM. Muscle tone. *Biomechanics and Motor Control: Defining Central Concepts. Elsevier, 2016,* 85–98. doi: 10.1016/b978-0-12–800384-8.00005-3.

23 Profeta VL, Turvey MT. Bernstein's levels of movement construction: A contemporary perspective. *Hum Mov Sci. 2018;57*:111–133. doi: 10.1016/j.humov.2017.11.013.

24 Hsu LJ, Zelenin PV, Orlovsky GN, Deliagina TG. (2017). Supraspinal control of spinal reflex responses to body bending during different behaviours in lampreys. *J Physio. 2017;595*:883–900. doi: 10.1113/JP272714.

25 Horslen BC, Zaback M, Inglis JT, Blouin JS, Carpenter MG. Increased human stretch reflex dynamic sensitivity with height-induced postural threat. *J Physiol.* 2018;*596*(21):5251–5265. doi: 10.1113/JP276459.

26 Cavallari P, Bolzoni F, Bruttini C, Esposti R. The organization and control of intra-limb anticipatory postural adjustments and their role in movement performance. *Front Hum Neurosci.* 2016;*10*:525. DOI=10.3389/fnhum.2016.00525

27 Ganguly J, Kulshreshtha D, Almotiri M, Jog M. (2021). Muscle tone physiology and abnormalities. *Toxins.* 2021;*13*(4):282. doi: 10.3390/toxins13040282

28 Burke D. Spasticity as an adaptation to pyramidal tract injury. *Adv Neurol.* 1988;*47*:401–23.

29 Trompetto C, Marinelli L, Mori L, Pelosin E, Currà A, Molfetta L, Abbruzzese G. Pathophysiology of spasticity: implications for neurorehabilitation. *Biomed Res Int. 2014;2014*:354906. doi: 10.1155/2014/354906.

30 Nudo RJ. Recovery after brain injury: mechanisms and principles. *Fron. Hum. Neurosci.* 2013;7. https://.doi.org/10.3389/fnhum.2013.00887

31 Bolognini N, Russo C, Edwards DJ. The sensory side of post-stroke motor rehabilitation. *Restor Neurol Neurosci.* 2016;*34*(4):571–586. https://doi.org/10.3233/RNN-150606

32 Serrada I, Hordacre B, Hillier SL. (2019). Does sensory retraining improve sensation and sensorimotor function following stroke: A systematic review and meta-analysis. *Front Neurosci.* 2019;*13*: 402. doi: 10.3389/fnins.2019.00402.

33 Uswatte G, Taub E, Lum P, Brennan D, Barman J, Bowman MH, Taylor A, McKay S, Sloman SB, Morris DM, Mark VW. Tele-rehabilitation of upper-extremity hemiparesis after stroke: Proof-of-concept randomized controlled trial of in-home Constraint-Induced Movement therapy. *Restor Neurol Neurosci.* 2021;*39*(4):303–318. doi: 10.3233/RNN-201100.

34 Ballester BR, Maier M, Duff A, Cameirão M, Bermúdez S, Duarte E, Cuxart A, Rodríguez S, San Segundo Mozo RM, Verschure PFMJ. (2019). A critical time window for recovery extends beyond one-year post-stroke. *J Neural Physiol.* 2019;*122*:350–357. doi:10.1152/jn.00762.2018.

35 Kerr AL, Wolke ML, Bell JA, Jones TA. Post-stroke protection from maladaptive effects of learning with the non-paretic forelimb by bimanual home cage experience in C57BL/6 mice. *Behav Brain Res* 2013;*252*:180–187. https://doi.org/10.1016/j.bbr.2013.05.062

36 Chou R, Peterson K, Helfand M. Comparative efficacy and safety of skeletal muscle relaxants for spasticity and musculoskeletal conditions: a systematic review. *J Pain Symptom Manage.* 2004:*28*(2):140–75. doi: 10.1016/j.jpainsymman.2004.05.002.

37 Chen YT, Zhang C, Liu Y, Magat E, Verduzco-Gutierrez M, Francisco GE, Zhou P, Zhang Y, Li S. The effects of botulinum toxin injections on spasticity and motor performance in chronic stroke with spastic hemiplegia. *Toxins (Basel).* 2020;*12*(8):492. doi: 10.3390/toxins12080492.

6 Stella wants to garden and has Friedreich's ataxia

Neuroscience facilitates our understanding of participation in hobbies

Katherine Dimitropoulou

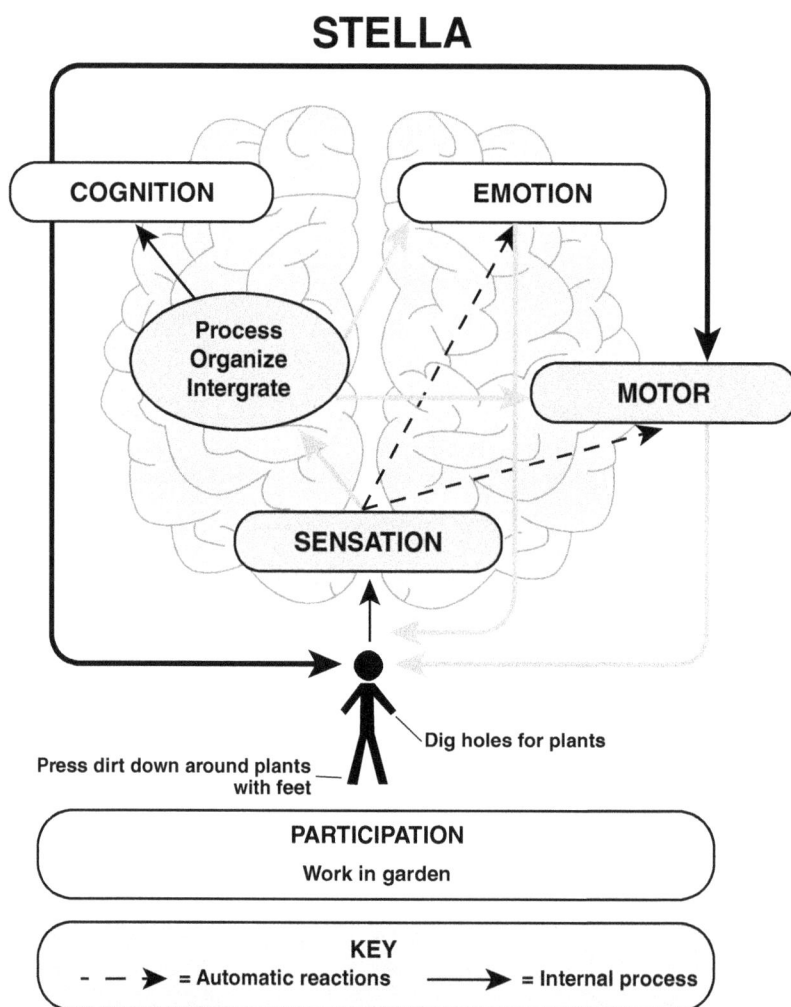

Figure 6.1 Stella brain figure

DOI: 10.4324/9781003524380-8

The purpose of this chapter

The purpose of this chapter is to explore how Stella a 22-year-old, cis-gender female college graduate who wants to grow a flower garden might be affected by Friedreich's ataxia (FA), a condition that impacts the functioning of the cerebellum. Individuals with hereditary cerebellar ataxia experience cerebellar degeneration as they grow and develop, which has consequences for their functional mobility (i.e., walking, climbing stairs, balance, and stability), use of their arms/hands in activities, eye movement control, and speech (difficulty to pronounce words). People with FA can have full lives with their daily routines, relationships, and learning, but may require modifications for function.

The key neuroscience concepts that will be explored in this chapter include the structure and function of the cerebellum. As with all the chapters, these components of the nervous system work with other systems to support overall human function.

Keywords for this chapter are listed in the box below. Be sure you learn what these key features are so you can get the most out of the chapter.

Keywords for this chapter

ataxia	Friedreich's ataxia	spinocerebellum
cerebellar dysarthria	inverse model (backward	superior temporal
cingulate gyrus	planning)	polymodal regions
dysdiadochokinesia	nystagmus	vermis
dysmetria	oral diadochokinesis	vestibulocerebellum
error-based learning	periaqueductal gray	vestibulo-occular reflex
fastigial and interposed	posterior parahippocam-	
nuclei	pal area	
fraxatin	posterior parietal cortex	

Stella, a 22-year-old who loves gardening

Stella is the youngest of two siblings. She lives with her parents in a two-story house in Queens, NYC. She has lived in that house all her life. Stella was diagnosed with FA at the age of 9. FA is a common type of hereditary ataxia. Hereditary cerebellar ataxias encompass a group of rare genetic disorders associated with degeneration of the cerebellum and consequent progressive ataxia (Bird, 2020; Bürk, 2017).

In the last nine months she has transitioned to living independently on the ground floor while her parents reside on the first floor. Her older sister has recently moved to another city. Stella is excited about her independence and is developing strategies to carry out her daily activities with support. Her two-bedroom apartment is modified to accommodate a manual wheelchair with bars in the bedroom and bathroom to help Stella transfer to her bed, and shower chair and toilet. She has a fully customized bathroom and kitchen. She has a home attendant for assistance for 10 hours a day to assist with activities of daily living. She lived in this neighborhood all her life and has friends and relatives that are nearby.

Stella has just finished college (hybrid classes) and is working per diem for a local restaurant managing their social media. She has an adapted keyboard, voice activation system and touch screen to help her work on the computer. She spends approximately 2–3 hours a day working for this company. She wants to gain experience and go to graduate school for her masters in communication studies. Her dream job is to be the public relations person for a large company. She is creative and loves interacting with others.

Her passion is her flower garden and the indoor flowerpots she maintains in her apartment. Stella has indoor flowers in pots in her living room that are raised about 3 feet from the floor. She takes care of them mostly on her own. Stella and her mom maintain a beautiful flower garden in the backyard of her house, with rose bushes, hydrangeas, peonies, and lilies. The backyard is mostly paved (smooth cement walkway) with patches of soil where the plants grow. Stella can navigate from the house to the yard in her wheelchair using a ramp. She can move between plants on the pavement. She loves to participate in all yard work, pruning, cleaning, and watering the plants, as well as mulching (seasonally), adding soil (as needed) and weeding. She prides herself that her flower garden is organic with no fertilizers or other chemicals. On one side of the garden there is a raised flower bed (about 3 feet off the ground) filled with annual flowers. This is her pride and joy as she is the one primarily responsible for it. She spends many hours in her garden taking care of her plants, reading, being with her family and socializing.

Stella moves through her apartment and in and out of her garden with a manual wheelchair that she propels using her wrists, she transfers to an electric scooter (that she can operate) for short distances in her neighborhood. She needs a companion to navigate longer distances and for using a car for transportation. At home she has assistive devices to help her with reaching and grasping objects to carry out her daily activities.

Stella is diabetic, she has vision problems, her speech is slow and lacks clear articulation. She experiences increasing weakness and some loss of sensation in her hands, which makes her worried that she will lose the ability to care for her garden.

Her treatment team focuses on developing a strengthening, balance training program and cardiovascular fitness training to assist with maintaining and increasing functional mobility. The team also works on providing and updating assistive devices to help her maintain her overall lifestyle of independence but primarily her passion: maintaining her flower garden.

Box 6.1   Learning activity

Discuss with your peers:

1. Given this narrative what else do you want to know?
2. What do you need to know more about hereditary cerebellar problems?
3. What is the role of the cerebellum for movement coordination, balance, strength, speech, and cognition?
4. Why is the team thinking of a balance training and fitness program to facilitate Stella's participation in gardening?
5. What are the skills that Stella needs to maintain to be able to take care of her flower garden?
6. How will the team support manipulation ability and other skills that Stella needs to have to do her gardening?

Keywords: hereditary cerebellar problems, hereditary ataxia, young adults with hereditary ataxia, cerebellum, balance, coordination, activities of daily living, instrumental activities of daily living

TIP: Keep a log of your discoveries and discussions and start expanding on them as you explore more in depth the neural processes underlying behavior and function in the subsequent section.

What is Friedreich's ataxia?

FA is a rare inherited disease, that leads to progressive damage in the nervous system. It is caused by a gene mutation, that carries the information for the production of a protein called fraxatin (Bird, 2020; Pilotto & Saxena, 2018). Fraxatin supports the energy producing components of cells (mitochondria). Disruption of this protein production leads to cell death and toxin production that can harm the body (Koeppen, & Mazurkiewicz 2013). In the central nervous system, this process leads to degeneration of the cerebellum (Bürk, 2017).

Box 6.2   Learning activity

1. What are the common signs and symptoms associated with FA?
2. How is the disruption in fraxatin production related to these signs and symptoms?

Keywords: Friedreich's ataxia, symptoms, Fraxatin, cerebellum, degeneration

---

Neuroscience information to guide your thinking about Stella

Box 6.3   Learning activity

Before moving further in this chapter work in small groups to discuss what neural systems support balance, coordination, sensation, and ability to execute complex tasks?

1. How does the cerebellar function relate to these systems?
2. Why does cerebellar function relate to development of diabetes or cardiomyopathy?
3. What systems do you use when engaging in complex tasks that engage functional movement and thinking?

Keywords: cerebellar degeneration, systemic problems, diabetes, cardiomyopathy, functional cognition

---

As indicated previously, FA results in degeneration of the cerebellum. The cerebellum is the largest sensorimotor structure in the brain having extensive connections with the cortex, brainstem, and spinal cord. It is located in the posterior part of the brain close to the spinal cord. The cerebellum affects motor behavior, cognition, speech, vision, and emotional regulation (Bastian & Lisbeger, 2021).

Box 6.4   Learning activity

Find a picture or figure of the cerebellum on the internet that has all of the anatomical regions of the cerebellum (hemispheres and nuclei) and their connections to the cortex, brainstem and spinal cord clearly labelled.

1. What are the names of the structural/anatomical parts of the cerebellum?
2. What parts of the cerebellum make up the cerebellar hemispheres?
3. What are the names of the cerebellar deep nuclei?
4. Which parts of the cerebellum are connected to the cortex?
5. Which parts of the cerebellum are connected to the brain stem?
6. Which parts of the cerebellum are connected to the spinal cord?

Keywords: cerebellum (image-neuroscience atlas), anatomy, nuclei, cortical connection networks, basal ganglia connection, brain stem connection, spinal cord connection

The role of cerebellum in goal directed motor behaviors

The cerebellum is comprised of a series of structures (hemispheres and nuclei) that have specialized functions. For example, the vermis coordinates the trunk, neck movements, the hemispheres coordinate arm/hand(s) and leg(s)/feet muscles. The medial regions (toward the midline of each cerebellar hemisphere assist in accurate execution of movements, whereas the lateral regions (away from the midline of each cerebellar hemisphere) support planning and timing of sequential movements and detection of errors during movement execution (Bastian & Lisbeger, 2021; Cabaraux et al., 2020; Popa & Ebner, 2019).

The most studied connection is that of the cerebellar connection to the sensorimotor cortex and upper motor neuron system. This process affects goal-directed movements and impacts the person's ability to be effective with their movements in the context of functional tasks.

Box 6.5   Learning activity

1. Find a picture of the upper motor neuron tracks (review). Which are they? What is their path?
2. How does the cerebellum connect to the upper motor neuron system?
3. What are the fundamental functions of the cerebellum for control and learning of motor behavior?
4. Think of specific examples in simple and complex daily tasks that the cerebellum may be involved.

Keywords: cerebellum, upper motor neurons, pathways

Cerebellum connections that influence movements

The cerebellum is well known for its connections to several other regions in the brain (cortical and subcortical) forming networks that are important for postural control and to organize and learn functional motor skills. The most studied connection is that of the cerebellar connection to the sensorimotor cortex and upper motor neuron system. This process affects goal-directed movements and impacts the person's ability to be effective with their movements in the context of functional tasks.

The cerebellum connects with cortical and subcortical regions forming reciprocal connections (loops) through which it influences different types of movements. Based on its influence on movement the cerebellum can be divided in three areas: the vestibulocerebellum, the spinocerebellum, and the cerebrocerebellum (Bastian & Lisbeger, 2021; Guell et al., 2018; Guell & Schmahmann, 2020).

Box 6.6   Learning activity

1. Find diagrams of the cerebellar loops.
2. What connections/pathways make up the vestibulocerebellum?
3. What connections/pathways make up the spinocerebellum?
4. What connections/pathways make up the cerebrocerebellum?

Keywords: cerebellum, vestibulocerebellum, spinocerebellum, cerebrocerebellum, degeneration, movement planning, movement execution, balance, precision, activities of daily living, instrumental activities of daily living

---

The vestibulocerebellum is responsible for balance and eye movements (vestibular-ocular reflexive activity—see Chapter 9). It receives information from the inner ear (motion information) and eyes (visual information) and sends signals to a highly specialized area in the brain stem (vestibular nuclei). In this area it influences the motor pathways (vestibulospinal tracks) that control postural muscles and regulate quick adjustments to balance during sitting, standing, and walking. The degenerative process can impact this region of the cerebellum and affects balance but also the person's ability to track a moving object (Bastian & Lisbeger, 2021; Schmahmann et al., 2019).

The spinocerebellum (vermis and medial cerebellar hemispheres, and the fastigial and interposed nuclei) is in close communication with the spinal cord. It receives information related to touch, body position in space, pressure, vision, and auditory stimuli. It connects this information to the cortical regions (e.g. primary motor, premotor cortex) and the brain stem. Through these connections the cerebellum influences the main upper motor neuron pathways (corticospinal and rubrospinal tracks) that control goal-directed movements of the postural muscles and muscles of the extremities and the eyes (Bastian & Lisbeger, 2021; Schmahmann et al., 2019).

The cerebrocerebellum is a region mostly in the outer parts of the cerebellar hemispheres (lateral areas) that communicates with the dentate nuclei. These areas connect to the cortex to mediate spatial navigation, planning, timely execution of voluntary goal-directed movements.

Box 6.7   Learning activity

1. How would a degenerative process affecting each of these systems impact your behavior in simple and complex daily activities that are part of your routine?
2. For example, eating with a fork, putting pants on, brushing your hair, walking in your home. You can use any activity you want and connect it to this discussion.
3. Now think about Stella and gardening, how might damage in each of these systems impact her ability to perform her gardening tasks?

Keywords: cerebellum, vestibulocerebellum, spinocerebellum, cerebrocerebellum, degeneration, movement planning, movement execution, balance, precision, activities of daily living, instrumental activities of daily living

---

Major contributions of the cerebellum in goal directed movements are the processes related to planning and prediction of movement. One of the cerebellar contributions in the process of planning goal directed movements, is known as inverse model (backward planning). In this process, when a desired goal is identified, the system can backward plan the motor commands (movement components) that would be required to achieve this goal. This process supports the ability to carry out sequential tasks efficiently. The second contribution is the process of prediction (feedforward control), which entails the initiation of movement execution based on prior experiences with the specific goal and controlling the muscles that have to contract and the appropriate rate for their contraction or co-contraction for the movement to be successful. This is necessary because sensory information from our movements in space come in with a delay and cannot be readily available to inform ongoing movement. The cerebellum mediates this process by generating plans from prior movement experiences and updating these plans "online" as the sensory information from the movement execution become available. This makes movements look smooth and effective (Bastian & Lisbeger, 2021; Li & Mrsic-Flogel, 2020; Narayanan & Thirumalai, 2019; Parrell et al., 2021).

Box 6.8   Learning activity

1. How would the cerebellar degeneration process affect Stella's movement planning, smoothness, effectiveness?
2. Think of the movements (postures she needs to assume and arm/hand movements needed) Stella needs to carry out when she plants her flowers and waters and prunes her plants.
3. Think of the use of gardening tools as she carries out these tasks.

Keywords: cerebellum, vestibulocerebellum, spinocerebellum, cerebrocerebellum, degeneration, movement planning, movement execution, balance, precision, activities of daily living, instrumental activities of daily living

Individuals with cerebellar lesions present with movements that are jerky, variable and uncoordinated. This process affects arms/hands, legs/feet and their body. It impacts their goal directed actions, their balance, and their reaching/grasping and walking ability. For example, when reaching to touch a target their arm/hand seem to follow a curved rather than a straight line. When they reach the target, they either undershoot or overshoot (this is known as dysmetria). Lack of movement prediction (lack of feedforward control) in the same reaching example, creates slow, jerky movement that appears to be broken in steps, and to be organized at the level of each joint, instead of one smooth reaching motion (Bastian & Lisbeger, 2021; Schmahmann et al., 2019).

The cerebellum is also responsible for steady movements towards a target. Individuals with cerebellar problems often have their hands/fingers oscillate (rhythmic shaking) as they reach a target (intention tremor). This is another example of lack of movement prediction (lack of feedforward control). The person instead of using prediction to organize their movement and use visual feedback to just tune the accuracy of their movement, they use visual feedback for the entire process. The visual feedback needs time to be processed and interpreted before it can inform movement, thus, it provides a time-delayed guidance to limb movement and tremor is the outcome of this process. Lack of cerebellar input to the upper motor neurons (see Chapters 1–3) also impacts the person's ability to carry out fast repeated movements that follow short predictable sequences (this is known as dysdiadochokinesia) (Bastian & Lisbeger, 2021; Schmahmann, 2019).

The cerebellum influences all conjugate eye movements and impacts visual motor control.

Box 6.9   Learning activity

1. What are the cerebellar signs in the visual system?
2. What is the vestibulo-occular reflex?
3. What is nystagmus? Find short videos that demonstrate nystagmus in clients. What do you observe?
4. How does nystagmus affect functional movement? Explore this in tasks like walking, reaching to get a glass of water, carrying a basket across the room.
5. How does cerebellar disfunction affect oculomotor control? Review saccadic eye movements
6. How does cerebellar disfunction affect visual motor control?

Keywords: cerebellum, visual system, vestibulo-occular reflex, nsytagmus, saccades, pursuits, oculomotor system, degeneration

---

The cerebellum is one of the main structures along with the brain stem to regulate the function of the vestibulo-occular reflex. The vestibulo-occular reflex enables eyes to stay fixed on a target as the head is rotating. However, in situations when the eyes need to follow the movement of the head to support visual motor activities such walking and looking around, the vestibulo-occular reflex needs to be suppressed. The cerebellum controls this process and connects it with goal directed actions. Cerebellar degeneration leads to nystagmus, which is the involuntary rhythmic movement of the eyes because of the presence of the vestibulo-occular reflex (no suppression). Specifically, downward rhythmic movements of the eyes (downbeat nystagmus) are clearly observed in clients with cerebellar degeneration (Dickman & Angelaki, 2021; Shemesh & Zee, 2019).

The cerebellum is also important for oculomotor control and has functional implication for visual motor tasks. Specifically, the accuracy and timing of saccadic eye movements are impacted by cerebellar degeneration. Functionally, this process results in increased time, especially when accuracy is important such as when reading (Alexandre et al., 2013; Dickman & Angelaki, 2021; Shemesh & Zee, 2019).

Balance is affected both in sitting or standing without moving and when reaching or walking. The body appears to move constantly, their walking looks awkward with feet apart, no rhythmic steps, appearing to have their body moving first and always trying to catch their balance. The degenerative process eventually makes balance difficult, and individuals need to use wheelchairs for safe mobility. If able to walk, they trip often and can fall easily (Bastian & Lisbeger, 2021).

Cerebellum connections that influence learning of motor skills

The cerebellum contributes to learning movements across body systems such as eye movements, hand/arm, leg movements, sit/stand balance, and actions such as reaching, grasping, and walking. The process of learning involving the cerebellum entails the ability to detect errors (error-based learning) in the predicted movement execution and calibrate the movement to adapt until it accurately matches the task demands and accomplishes the goal. This process can be conscious (i.e., person thinks/plans for it), and/or unconscious (i.e., adaptation occurs without the person thinking about it) (Popa & Ebner, 2019; Narayanan & Thirumalai, 2019). For example, when a person reaches to pick up a small box that appears light in weight, they approach the box with specific force in their hand grip. After they discover that this box is heavy, and the initial plan is not effective to pick up the box, their fingers, hand, arm and posture adapt and increase the grip force accordingly to accomplish the goal. The cerebellum is known to play an important role in detecting the mismatch between the predicted and actual outcome of a movement given the sensory feedback and facilitates quick and effective adaptation (Martin et al., 1996; Diedrichsen et al., 2005; Chen et al., 2006; Spampinato et al., 2017).

Box 6.10 Learning activity

1. Create examples for each other to experience mismatch and the adaptation process. Find examples online.
2. Discuss Stella's case.

   a. What are the consequences of the cerebellar degeneration on her ability to adapt her movements?
   b. How is her ability to care for her flowers affected by it?
   c. Can you think of specific examples?

Keywords: cerebellum, degeneration, learning, adaptation, movement accuracy, movement timing, movement flexibility

---

Cerebellum connections that influence cognition and language

The cerebellum is not only a major sensorimotor hub, but it is also integral to cognitive processes that do not relate to sensorimotor behavior. Specific anatomical cerebellar regions are connected (reciprocally) to association areas of cortex such as the prefrontal cortex, posterior parietal cortex, superior temporal polymodal regions, cingulate gyrus, and posterior parahippocampal area. These connections form distributed networks throughout the brain that support attention, executive functioning, language, verbal working memory, strategy formation, and emotional (limbic) valence, as well as systems related to creativity and imagination (Default mode network) (Schmahmann, 2019; Peterburs & Desmond, 2016; Bernard et al., 2015; Sokolov et al., 2017).

Spoken language problems, such as slow slurred articulation are evident in individuals with cerebellar degeneration known as cerebellar dysarthria (Bodranghien et al., 2016). In clinical tests, when individuals with cerebellar degeneration are asked to repeat as fast as possible a single syllable, they have reduced maximum speaking rate (oral diadochokinesis). The language problems however, extend beyond the articulation of speech. In fact, studies found that issues exist with the production of internal (covert/silent) speech (Bodranghien et al., 2016). Furthermore, impairment on speech perception maybe present (Bodranghien et al., 2016).

Cerebellum connections that influence self-regulation and emotions

---

Box 6.11   Learning activity

1. Discover the functional role of each of the main cortical association regions listed in this section that connect with the cerebellum.
2. Discuss in small groups Stella's case.
3. What are the consequences of the cerebellar degeneration on her cognitive abilities?
4. How might these issues with cognition affect her ability to care for her flowers?
5. Can you think of three specific examples?

Keywords: cerebellum, degeneration, language, cognitive abilities

---

Emerging evidence, currently based on animal studies and some studies in humans with cerebellar lesions, suggest that the cerebellum has projections to and from limbic regions such as the amygdala, hypothalamus, prefrontal cortex and periaqueductal gray (PAG). These structures play a role in self-regulation controlling fight, flight, freezing behaviors as well as emotions (Adamaszek et al., 2017; Carta et al., 2019; Kruithof et al., 2022). The emergent perspective is that cerebellum forms part of neural circuits that are involved in various stages of processing emotions, such as the recognition and evaluation of emotions, and the integration of emotions into behavior. The cerebellum is thought to contribute to associative learning and processing of emotions. This process entails the connection between experiences with objects, sights, sounds, etc., and emotional states. Moreover, the cerebellum modulates processing of emotions for adaptive motor and non-motor behaviors. Specific structures in the cerebellum such as the Vermis areas of the lateral hemispheres, and deep nuclei are considered key regions of emotional processing in the cerebellum. Given the role of the cerebellum for associative learning of emotions, negative emotions appear to have a stronger connection with the cerebellum.

Daily routine: participating in gardening

Stella has had to work with changes in her abilities and her body throughout her adolescence and early adult years. For her, functional motor skills are a puzzle she has to solve every day and in the context of every task. She understands that she has to allocate time and thought to her actions and plan well her day in the garden (as in every other task). She takes difficulties that arise from interacting with the environment in stride and has a positive attitude. Her time with her flower garden, is a rewarding experience of learning about her body each day as well as creating and supporting life.

Stella's tasks in the garden entail getting to the garden from the house, gathering and carrying her tools, working on the garden needs given the season (i.e., planting, pruning, mulching), taking care of her plants (i.e. cleaning, weeding, gathering flowers), cleaning her tools and her hands, and possibly changing her outfit for the next activity.

Within each of these activities there is a set of behaviors (motor, cognitive, emotional) that support her functional abilities and participation in the task. Given Stella's needs it is important to analyze each of these activities. For example, when Stella wants to prune the branches of her rose bush she needs to use tools, visually detect which of the branches she needs to cut, use balance control to lean forward, coordinate arm/hand movements to reach the branch, and apply the right pressure to have the brunch cut. Given the role of the cerebellum in each of these task components we envision that Stella will need to learn how to approach her rose bush so that she maximizes her balance control to lean forward safely from her chair and be able to return to her original posture. She needs to wear gloves because it is likely for her to reach out too far or too close and have her hand caught in the thorny branches. She needs to make sure she has the strength to hold and apply the right pressure to her pruning tool (adaptive devices may be needed here). These considerations become possible when the therapist understands the underlying systems that are involved in the process of executing functional movements for someone with cerebellar degeneration.

Back to the person's life: Stella participating in gardening

Box 6.12   Learning activity

Discuss Stella's case in small groups.

1. What are the sequences of actions she has to do for other gardening tasks (see above)?
2. Analyze two more tasks and create a list of anticipated areas that Stella needs to consider in order to carry out this task?

We have "met" Stella and her goals to take care of her flower garden as independently as possible. We have also analyzed what gardening requires from underlying processes (e.g., motor, cognitive, language, etc.). We have also discussed the neuroscience underpinnings and functional consequences that cerebellar degeneration has for her performance, safety, learning and participation. We are now interested in developing intervention ideas that can support Stella's function and maximize her potential taking under consideration her brain processing skills.

To support Stella's current skills, we need to design the environment and tools she uses to maximize her abilities while accounting for her safety. For example, the family and Stella have already paved the garden and created a ramp to support Stella's ability to get in and out of the garden safely and independently and come close to her plants. We have discovered that she will also need tools to carry out some of the garden care activities such as rakes, and pruning shears, etc.

Box 6.13   Learning activity

Discuss in small groups ways to adapt gardening tools for safe and effective use.

Keywords: cerebellum, degeneration, manipulation skills, instrumental activities of daily living, splints, adaptive tools, safe manipulation

---

Box 6.14   Learning activity

1. Find intervention strategies that target balance/coordination training in individuals with FA.
2. What does the evidence say?
3. Can some of the strategies work for Stella?
4. What intervention strategies you recommended for Stella?
5. How often and how long should she perform them?

Keywords: splints, adaptive tools, movement flexibility, functional mobility, interventions

Note: It is recommended to use PubMed (publicly available) for evidence articles or Google Scholar.

To support motor abilities for Stella we need to assist her in maintaining and increasing balance control and movement coordination. For example, she needs to be able to lean forward while reaching for the flowers, plants, weeds, etc. and apply enough grip pressure to cut, pull, push etc. Although the cerebellar degeneration process is not curable, there is evidence that specific intervention strategies can support Stella in maintaining abilities.

To support her stamina to carry out gardening Stella may need to engage in fitness (cardio) activity. Emerging literature suggests that this type of exercise has also positive impact in the cerebellar processes (see suggestions for further reading).

Box 6.15   Learning activity

Discuss in small groups what type of exercise routine Stella can follow to help her stamina and support cerebellar function.

Keywords: cerebellum, degeneration, exercise, aerobic exercise, strengthening, balance training

Note: It is recommended to use PubMed (publicly available) for evidence articles or Google Scholar.

Box 6.16   Learning activity

Discuss in small groups what types of activities Stella can engage in to allow her to use and practice planning, language skills, and memory skills.

Stella needs to maintain higher level cognitive abilities to support her planning, memory and language skills. Participating in gardening can help her practice these skills. For example, she needs to plan for seasonal activities needed to maintain her garden, she needs to order the right material and equipment, she needs to communicate with others about her needs, safety and success stories of her gardening.

Last but not least, Stella enjoys social interactions and loves to work on her garden with her mom and her friends or spend time in her garden with family and friends. Associating the gardening experience with positive interactions and emotions is significant for her to continue to be motivated. It also supports as we learned from neuroscience network connectivity of cerebellar regions with cognitive and limbic association areas. Maintaining her emotional health supports her cerebellar processes and maintains important neural networks active.

What do we know about ourselves and the population at large from this brain condition and this family story?

Although we do not have cerebellar degeneration understanding the neural processes that the cerebellum supports and their connection to function and participation help us understand how our own bodies engage in motor and cognitive tasks and/or how it reacts to sensory experiences emotionally. For example, we can explain how our body movements adjust after a few tries on a new balance board and we can keep our balance. We can also understand how and why we need to practice a few times and make micro-adjustments to our posture, hand/arm movements, and muscle forces when we shoot a basketball to a hoop before we are able to score.

We also learned that not only movements but cognitive tasks that require strategy building, planning organization and behavioral flexibility are based on learning processes that the cerebellum supports. Although the literature is not clear about what can be effective ways to improve these skills, practice with overt /covert goals of these skills supports cerebellar health.

Learning about the cerebellar neural networks also supports our clinical reasoning skills in other populations (not only hereditary cerebellar ataxias). For example, we have evidence of cerebellar problems increasing with aging. We can then anticipate, assess, and intervene with older adults who present balance coordination issues, and cognitive decline. We have adults with stroke involving cerebellar lesions or affecting the connectivity of the cerebellum to the other networks. We anticipate, assess, and intervene with these individuals to facilitate functional recovery and adaptation to changes in sensorimotor behaviors, but also issues of functional cognition such as executive functioning, working memory, etc., that impact everyday function.

The overall goal is to use our knowledge of neuroscience for clinical reasoning. We can then interpret behaviors effectively and develop hypotheses about underlying processes that guide these behaviors. We can develop assessment and intervention plans that are informed by these hypotheses with expectations for changes in behavior, function and participation that are guided by scientific evidence and not trial and error.

Box 6.17   Learning activity

With your small group, complete the table in the Appendix about the integration of Stella's sensorimotor, cognitive, and emotional needs to successfully complete tasks in a timely manner.

Further reading

If interested for further reading and lived experiences with hereditary cerebellar disorders, consult the following:

Cassidy, E., Naylor, S., & Reynolds, F. (2018). The meanings of physiotherapy and exercise for people living with progressive cerebellar ataxia: an interpretative phenomenological analysis. *Disabil Rehabil*, 40, 894–904.

de Silva, R. N., Vallortigara, J., Greenfield, J. et al. (2019). Diagnosis and management of progressive ataxia in adults. *Pract Neurol*, 19, 196–207.

Friedreich's Ataxia Research Alliance. Meet Sandra, Stella's friend from the FARA network (higher functioning, age on onset of FA 12 years. www.youtube.com/watch?v=CNECMX3AGzc

Ilg, W., et al. (2009). Intensive coordinative training improves motor performance in degenerative cerebellar disease. *Neurology*, 73, 1823–1830.

Ilg, W., et al. (2012). Video game-based coordinative training improves ataxia in children with degenerative ataxia. *Neurology*, 79, 2056–2060.

Keller, J. L., Bastian, A. J. (2014). A home balance exercise program improves walking in people with cerebellar ataxia. *Neurorehabil Neural Repair*, 28, 770–778.

Milne, S. C., et al. (2018). Can rehabilitation improve the health and well-being in Friedreich's ataxia: a randomized controlled trial? *Clin Rehabil*, 32, 630–643.

Seco, C. J., et al. (2014). Improvements in quality of life in individuals with friedreich's ataxia after participation in a 5-year program of physical activity: an observational study pre-post test design, and two years follow-up. *Int J Neurorehabil*, 1, 129.

Synofzik, M., & Ilg, W. (2014). Motor training in degenerative spinocerebellar disease: ataxia-specific improvements by intensive physiotherapy and exergames. *Biomed Res Int*, 2014, 1–11.

Tai, G., et al. (2018). Progress in the treatment of Friedreich ataxia. *Neurol Neurochir Pol*, 52, 129–139.

References

Adamaszek, M., D'Agata, F., Ferrucci, R., Habas, C., Keulen, S., Kirkby, K. C.,... & Verhoeven, J. (2017). Consensus paper: cerebellum and emotion. *The Cerebellum*, 16, 552–576. https://doi.org/10.1007/s12311-016-0815-8

Alexandre, M. F., Rivaud-Péchoux, S., Challe, G., Durr, A., & Gaymard, B. (2013). Functional consequences of oculomotor disorders in hereditary cerebellar ataxias. *The Cerebellum*, 12, 396–405. https://doi.org/10.1007/s12311-012-0433-z

Bastian, A., & Lisberger, S. 2021. The cerebellum. In E. Kandel, J., Koeser, S., Mack, S., Sieglebaum (Eds.), *Principles of Neural Science* (6th ed., pp. 908–931). McGraw Hill.

Bernard, J. A., Leopold, D. R., Calhoun, V. D., & Mittal, V. A. (2015). Regional cerebellar volume and cognitive function from adolescence to late middle age. *Human Brain Mapping*, 36(3), 1102–1120. https://doi.org/10.1002/hbm.22690

Bird, T. (2020). Hereditary ataxia overview. In M. Adam, H. Ardinger, R. Pagan et al., (Eds). GeneReviews® [Internet]. Seattle (WA): University of Washington, Seattle, 1993–2020. www.ncbi.nlm. nih.gov/books/NBK1138/

Bodranghien, F., Bastian, A., Casali, C., Hallett, M., Louis, E. D., Manto, M., & van Dun, K. (2016). Consensus paper: revisiting the symptoms and signs of cerebellar syndrome. *The Cerebellum*, 15, 369–391. https://doi.org/10.1007/s12311-015-0687-3

Bürk, K. (2017) Friedreich ataxia: current status and future prospects. *Cerebellum Ataxias* 2017; 4:4. https://doi.org/10.1186/s40673-017-0062-x

Cabaraux, P., Gandini, J., Kakei, S., Manto, M., Mitoma, H., & Tanaka, H. (2020). Dysmetria and errors in predictions: the role of internal forward model. *International Journal of Molecular Sciences*, 21(18), 6900. https://doi.org/10.3390/ijms21186900

Carta, I., Chen, C. H., Schott, A. L., Dorizan, S., & Khodakhah, K. (2019). Cerebellar modulation of the reward circuitry and social behavior. *Science*, 363(6424) eaav0581. https://doi.org/10.1126/science.aav0581

Chen, H., Hua, S. E., Smith, M. A., Lenz, F. A., & Shadmehr, R. (2006). Effects of human cerebellar thalamus disruption on adaptive control of reaching. *Cerebral Cortex*, 16(10), 1462–1473. https://doi.org/10.1093/cercor/bhj087

Delatycki, M. B., & Bidichandani, S. I. (2019). Friedreich ataxia-pathogenesis and implications for therapies. *Neurobiology of Disease*, 132, 104606. https://doi.org/10.1016/j.nbd.2019.104606

Dickman, J. & Angelaki, D. (2021). Perception. In E. Kandel, J., Koeser, S., Mack, S., Sieglebaum (Eds.), *Principles of Neural Science* (6th ed., pp. 636–648). McGraw Hill.

Diedrichsen, J., Hashambhoy, Y., Rane, T., & Shadmehr, R. (2005). Neural correlates of reach errors. *Journal of Neuroscience*, 25(43), 9919–9931. https://doi.org/10.1523/jneurosci.1874-05.2005

Guell, X., & Schmahmann, J. (2020). Cerebellar functional anatomy: a didactic summary based on human fMRI evidence. *The Cerebellum*, 19, 1–5. https://doi.org/10.1007/s12311-019-01083-9

Guell, X., Schmahmann, J. D., Gabrieli, J. D., & Ghosh, S. S. (2018). Functional gradients of the cerebellum. *elife*, 7, e36652.

Koeppen, A., Mazurkiewicz, J., (2013) Friedreich ataxia: neuropathology revised. *Journal of Neuro-pathology Experimental Neurology*, 72, 78–90. https://doi.org/10.1097/nen.0b013e31827e5762

Kruithof, E. S., Klaus, J., & Schutter, D. J. (2022). The cerebellum in aggression: Extending the cortico-limbic dual-route model of motivation and emotion. *Motivation Science*, 8(2), 150. https://doi.org/10.1037/mot0000251

Li, N., & Mrsic-Flogel, T. D. (2020). Cortico-cerebellar interactions during goal-directed behavior. *Current Opinion in Neurobiology*, 65, 27–37. https://doi.org/10.1016/j.conb.2020.08.010

Manto, M., Bower, J., Conforto, A., Delgado-García, J., da Guarda, S., Gerwig, M., Habas, C., Hagura, N., Ivry, R., Mariën, P., Molinari, M., Naito, E., Nowak, D., Oulad Ben Taib, N., Pelisson, D., Tesche, C., Tilikete, C., Timmann, D. (2012). Consensus paper: roles of the cerebellum in motor control--the diversity of ideas on cerebellar involvement in movement. *Cerebellum*, 11(2), 457–487. [PMC free article: PMC4347949] [PubMed: 22161499]. https://doi.org/10.1007/s12311-011-0331-9

Martin, T. A., Keating, J. G., Goodkin, H. P., Bastian, A. J., & Thach, W. T. (1996). Throwing while looking through prisms: I. Focal olivocerebellar lesions impair adaptation. *Brain*, 119(4), 1183–1198. https://doi.org/10.1093/brain/119.4.1183

Narayanan, S., & Thirumalai, V. (2019). Contributions of the cerebellum for predictive and instructional control of movement. *Current Opinion in Physiology*, 8, 146–151. https://doi.org/10.1016/j.cophys.2019.01.011

Parrell, B., Kim, H., Breska, A., Saxena, A., & Ivry, R. (2021). Differential effects of cerebellar degeneration on feedforward versus feedback control across speech and reaching movements. *Journal of Neuroscience*, 41(42), 8779–8789. https://doi.org/10.1523/jneurosci.0739-21.2021

Peterburs, J., & Desmond, J. E. (2016). The role of the human cerebellum in performance monitoring. *Current Opinion in Neurobiology*, 40, 38–44. https://doi.org/10.1016/j.conb.2016.06.011

Pilotto, F, Saxena, S. (2018). Epidemiology of inherited cerebellar ataxias and challenges in clinical research. *Clinical and Translational Neuroscience*, 2, 2514183X1878525. https://doi.org/10.1177/2514183x18785258

Popa, L., & Ebner, T. (2019). Cerebellum, predictions and errors. *Frontiers in Cellular Neuroscience*, 12, 524. https://doi.org/10.3389/fncel.2018.00524

Salman, M. S. (2018). Epidemiology of cerebellar diseases and therapeutic approaches. *The Cerebellum*, 17(1), 4–11. https://doi.org/10.1007/s12311-017-0885-2

Sarva H, Shanker V. (2014). Treatment options in degenerative cerebellar ataxia: a systematic review. *Movement Disorders Clinical Practice,*1, 291–8. https://doi.org/10.1002/mdc3.12057

Schmahmann, J. D. (2019). The cerebellum and cognition. *Neuroscience Letters*, 688, 62–75. https://doi.org/10.1016/j.neulet.2018.07.005

Schmahmann, J. D., Guell, X., Stoodley, C. J., & Halko, M. A. (2019). The theory and neuroscience of cerebellar cognition. *Annual Review of Neuroscience*, 42, 337–364. https://doi.org/10.1146/annurev-neuro-070918-050258

Shemesh, A., & Zee, D. (2019). Eye movement disorders and the cerebellum. *Journal of Clinical Neurophysiology,* 36(6), 405–414. https://doi.org/10.1097/WNP.0000000000000579.

Sokolov, A. A., Miall, R. C., & Ivry, R. B. (2017). The cerebellum: adaptive prediction for movement and cognition. *Trends in cognitive sciences*, 21(5), 313–332. https://doi.org/10.1016/j.tics.2017.02.005

Spampinato, D. A., Block, H. J., & Celnik, P. A. (2017). Cerebellar–M1 connectivity changes associated with motor learning are somatotopic specific. *Journal of Neuroscience*, 37(9), 2377–2386. https://doi.org/10.1523/jneurosci.2511-16.2017

Therrien, A. S., & Bastian, A. J. (2019). The cerebellum as a movement sensor. *Neuroscience Letters*, 688, 37–40. https://doi.org/10.1016/j.neulet.2018.06.055

7 Torrance wants to be successful in their new job and is autistic

Neuroscience facilitates our understanding of workplace modifications

Olivia Surgent, Lauren Little, Anne V. Kirby, and Anna Wallisch

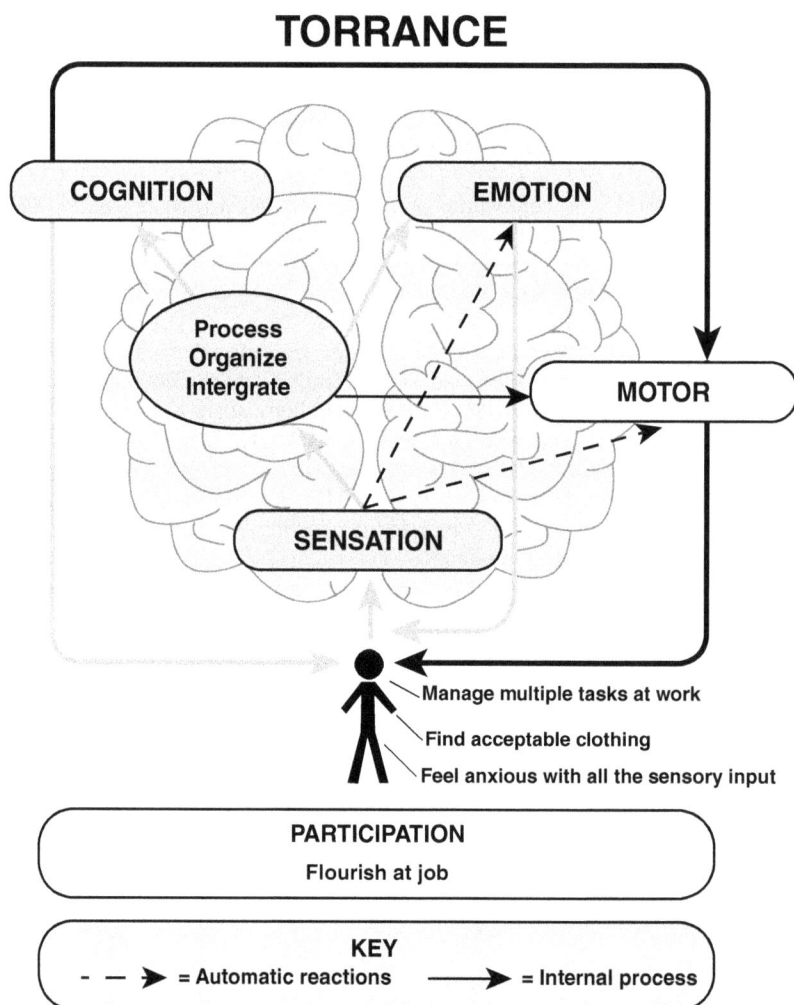

Figure 7.1 Torrance brain figure

DOI: 10.4324/9781003524380-9

Purpose of this chapter

The purpose of this chapter is to explore how Torrance, a 28-year-old autistic adult, can be successful in their new job. We will learn how Torrance's success involves the neuroscience of sensory integration, executive function, and social-emotional processing. We situate these principles in the context of work participation and consider ways to align meaningful employment with nervous system needs. We can learn about the neuroscience principles that may inform work participation from people who experience work tasks and work environments in unique ways. Autistic individuals may have particular interests and strengths that can inform their employment choices; they also can face sensory, executive function, and social-emotional challenges in workplaces not aligned with their needs. Therefore, we can learn from the neuroscience principles that underlie the employment experiences of autistic individuals to understand participation in work more broadly. People on the autism spectrum can have full lives with their daily routines, relationships, leisure, and work, but may require adaptations and accommodations.

The key neuroscience concepts we will explore in this chapter include sensory processing, executive function, and emotional regulation through the lens of an autistic adult. We will examine how these unique neuroscience features affect social-emotional interactions (see also Chapter 11 for more details) and workplace demands. As with all the chapters, these components of the central nervous system work with other systems to support overall human function.

Keywords for this chapter are listed in the box below. Be sure you learn what these key features are so you can get the most out of the chapter.

Keywords for this chapter

amygdala	inhibitory control	set switching
auditory cortex (temporal lobe)	limbic system	somatosensory cortex (parietal lobe)
cortical	olfactory cortex (temporal lobe)	subcortical
emotional regulation	posterior parietal cortex	thalamus
executive functions	prefrontal cortex	visual cortex (occipital lobe)
gustatory cortex (insula/frontal lobe)	sensory gating	
	sensory seeking	

Let's find out about Torrance, their life, and their current employment so we have a context for understanding how their distinct central nervous system influences their life.

Box 7.1   Learning activity

Prior to reading this case:

1. How do you think the characteristics of autistic people will affect Torrance's performance at work?
2. Why is it important for occupational therapy practitioners to understand neurology to help work with autistic people?

Case study: Torrance, an adult who works in an open office company.

Torrance is 28 years old and has just landed their first full-time job in graphic design. After going to community college for two years, and then completing a digital arts bachelor's degree at a state university, Torrance struggled to find a full-time position that met their career goals. Torrance worked freelance for several years, building up their portfolio. Torrance is excited to finally have this job at a start-up company called Cogema.

Torrance identifies as gender nonbinary, meaning that they are not a man or a woman, and asks others to use they/them when referring to Torrance with pronouns. They were diagnosed as autistic at the age of 18 years old and came out as nonbinary when they were 22 years old. In their free time, Torrance likes playing video games, drawing, spending time with their dog, and cooking. They participate in several online communities for autistic people and nonbinary/transgender people. Torrance lives in their childhood home with their mom and younger sibling, since they have not yet been able to afford to move into an apartment. They hope to save up money from this new job and be able to rent an apartment in the next year.

Despite their excitement about the position, Torrance's first few days of work were difficult. After a week of work, Torrance has numerous concerns about being able to stay in this job. Cogema has an "open office"—instead of individual offices or cubicles, workers sit at connected desks in a large open space where they can easily see and hear one another. Torrance's boss told them that this office layout is good for teamwork and creating energy in the office.

The office environment is proving to be overwhelming for Torrance. In the open space, the lights are very bright, and Torrance's colleagues seem to be constantly moving around and talking to one another or on the phone. Their boss told Torrance that the Cogema CEO doesn't like when employees wear headphones because that can segregate employees from the activities of the office. Instead, different employees can take turns playing music over the loudspeaker for everyone to hear. The CEO also wants the office to be a place that's "fun." Employees can shoot Nerf guns to get each other's attention or just to be playful. There is a kitchen next to the office space where employees can eat snacks or cook meals; the noise and smells can be distracting.

Some details about the job are also unclear. Torrance was surprised that even though the job posting said "work from home opportunities," their boss said that employees should only work from home on Fridays. Clothing is another point of confusion. Torrance's boss said they can wear "casual work attire," but they aren't sure what that means. Torrance wore new slacks and a button-down shirt to work on the first day but found it itchy and uncomfortable.

Despite what they were told by their boss on the first day, Torrance has noticed that not everyone in the office follows the guidelines they were given. Many employees have headphones on, some step into conference rooms to make phone calls and for small meetings, and their coworkers seem to wear a wide variety of types of clothes, from sweatshirts to dresses. So, Torrance is unsure about the expectations of the office. They also have noticed that some people seem to be working from home on days other than Fridays.

The demands of the job are also starting to get overwhelming. Because they have only worked freelance before, Torrance usually focused on one project at a time. When Torrance was in college, they usually took a lighter course load to focus on two classes per semester. At Cogema, Torrance has already been assigned three different projects working with three different teams in the company. They are worried about staying on top of multiple projects with different deadlines and different teams. Each group acts like their project should be Torrance's top priority. When Torrance is really overwhelmed, they feel like they start to "shut down," which can mean trouble communicating and doing other important work tasks.

Some things about the job are going well for Torrance so far. Torrance's team uses a chat system to communicate with one another throughout the day, which they like. Torrance communicates well via text. Torrance is excited about the projects they have been assigned to start working on. They also feel welcomed by several employees, including another nonbinary person. Torrance enjoyed eating lunch with some coworkers one day during the week. However, many days Torrance feels like they need a quiet break during lunchtime.

Box 7.2   Learning activity

After reading this case study, discuss the following questions with your peers:

1. What aspects of Torrance's experience stand out to you?
2. What are the employment barriers Torrance is experiencing?

Before you continue reading the chapter, work with your small group to discuss what you already know.

Box 7.3   Learning activity

1. What do you already know about neuroscience that can help understand Torrance's case?
2. What parts of the brain relate to the challenges Torrance is experiencing in the workplace?
3. What neurological processes might help explain Torrance's situation?

Neuroscience information to guide your thinking about Torrance

Autistic people are part of a diverse population with biological and behavioral attributes that vary widely from person to person. Thus, unlike some developmental conditions which can involve a specific set of neurological processes or a certain brain network, autism is not tied to one single brain region or set of brain functions. Instead, autistic people can show a wide variety of developmental and neurological differences, which contribute to a range of different behaviors, experiences, preferences, and needs. In other words, all autistic people vary in their development, neurobiology, and behaviors—just like the variability among non-autistic people.

Sensory processing

Sensory processing refers to how our nervous systems detect sensory information and how we behaviorally respond to stimuli (Dunn, 1997, 2014). Autistic people often have more extreme sensory processing responses as compared to the general population (Baranek et al., 2006; Little et al., 2017; Tomchek & Dunn, 2007). For example, autistic people may experience heightened sensitivity to specific stimuli (e.g., experiencing pain with loud noises; strongly disliking certain textures touching their skin or the smell/taste/texture of certain foods; noticing small changes or errors in surroundings or work products). However, not all responses are heightened. Autistic individuals can also have diminished sensory responses (e.g., not noticing extreme temperature changes; not attending to the sound of their name being called) and/or engage in active sensory seeking behavior (e.g., preference for loud music, intense activity, strong flavors, or movement while working to help concentrate) (American Psychiatric Association, 2013). (For more information on sensory processing, see other chapters in the sensory section of this book and at the end of this chapter.)

While effective sensory processing recruits brainstem, cerebellar, subcortical, and cortical-based systems, the thalamus may especially contribute to differences in the sensory experiences of autistic people. The thalamus functions as a filter that relays only the most critical sensory information from early brainstem-based sensory processing to higher-order processing areas of the cortex. In this way, the thalamus acts as a "gate" that assesses sensory information from the environment and prevents less relevant information from passing through. Imagine what a flood of input you would have to contend with if every single sensory stimulus had to be processed; it would be overwhelming!

Autistic people may have differences in the thalamus-based sensory gating system compared to non-autistic people whereby more information is passed from the environment to cortical sensory processing regions (Marco et al., 2011). This difference in sensory gating is demonstrated through the presence of increased "neural noise," or cortical activation (Dinstein et al., 2012; Dinstein et al., 2015; Haigh et al., 2015; Milne, 2011), and stronger connectivity between thalamic and cortical regions (Green et al., 2016; Iidaka et al., 2019; Woodward et al., 2017) in autistic adults compared to non-autistic adults. This means that autistic people show more neural activity in their thalamic and cortical regions and stronger connections among these regions, representing a more lenient

Table 7.1 Examples of behaviors related to sensory processing patterns

Sensory processing pattern	Definition	Examples of behaviors
Sensory sensitivity	Low threshold for detection of sensory input	Notice details in the environment; like to feel prepared for new environments, are particular about their activities, and may have strong sensory preferences when it comes food or clothing fabric
Sensory avoiding	Low threshold for detection of sensory input with active strategies to reduce input	Notice everything in the environment and may appear vigilant to try to avoid certain sensations; like order, control, and do not like surprises
Sensory seeking	High threshold for sensory input with active strategies to increase input	Prefer intense experiences to focus and learn; like to multi-task and be "on the move"
Sensory registration	High threshold for sensory input	May not notice details and may need extra cues to attend to sensory input

Note: For further reading about Dunn's sensory processing framework, see Dunn (1997, 2001, 2007, 2014).

sensory "gate." It is in this way that autistic people may have excess environmental information pass between the thalamic and cortical regions. As their brains take in more stimuli from the environment, they may experience sensory overload, which can lead to sensory sensitivity and/or avoidance.

Primary sensory processing regions in the cortex also contribute to altered sensory perception in autistic adults. While many regions of the brain process different types of sensory information, the primary sensory cortices have been widely studied and help us understand sensory processing of autistic adults. These regions include:

- **Visual cortex (occipital lobe):** This region of the brain receives, integrates, and processes visual information from the retinas of the eyes.
- **Auditory cortex (temporal lobe):** This region of the brain receives and integrates sound information, allowing us to perform a variety of tasks ranging from detecting a sound in the environment to understanding the complexities of music and speech.
- **Gustatory cortex (insula/frontal lobe):** This region receives input from taste receptors in the tongue, soft palate, and esophagus and is responsible for the perception of taste and its intensity.
- **Olfactory cortex (temporal lobe):** This region receives information from olfactory neurons in the nasal cavity via the olfactory bulb and integrates information regarding smell.
- **Somatosensory cortex (parietal lobe):** This region of the brain is responsible for receiving and processing sensory information from across the body surfaces (e.g., touch, temperature, pain).

Box 7.4   Learning activity

Locate images of the primary cortical sensory areas and identify the locations of the visual cortex and somatosensory cortex.

Keywords: primary sensory, cortex, brain, anatomy

The structural composition and organization of primary cortical sensory areas may be unique in autistic people, with studies suggesting distinct patterns of cortical organization. Among autistic people, these differences in cortical organization may be related to the differences in the thalamus-based sensory gating system (described above). In other words, if the "gate" is allowing excess information to travel past the thalamus, the primary sensory cortices may develop and work differently in autistic people as compared to non-autistic peers. Our primary sensory cortices are important for our brains to create internal representations of the external world, so the differences in these brain regions among autistic adults mean that they may generate such internal representations in a distinct way. In this way autistic people may "see" the world differently, and therefore respond differently.

After initial cortical processing, information is sent to higher-order sensory processing areas which perform multisensory integration. Multisensory integration is a process that uses sensory information from several modalities (e.g., sight, smell, taste, sound, touch), memories of past experiences, along with information about the goals of the task at hand.

The multisensory integration process condenses and manages all of this information so an individual can produce meaningful actions in response to their complete sensory experience. While several brain regions are important for multisensory integration, two particularly important areas are:

- **Posterior parietal cortex:** This region of the brain is involved in spatial attention, translating sensory input into motor responses and motor learning.
- **Insula:** This region of the brain is involved in self-awareness, gustatory (smell), auditory, and vestibular sensorimotor processing, risk-reward behavior, and pain pathways, all of which contribute to the perception of pain and proprioception (awareness of one's body and self).

Ultimately, this processed sensory information is used by the motor cortex (the part of the brain that generates signals to direct body movements) and cerebellum (the part of the brain that regulates fine motor control, precision, and timing) to execute the optimal motor behavior for a situation (e.g., reaching for a glass, walking to another room, dancing with someone). This process is ongoing as each motor action results in taking in new sensory information to adjust our actions and continue towards our goals—and it all happens in an instant! Isn't the brain fascinating?

Together, differences in the organization and neural signaling of the sensory processing network can lead autistic people to respond to sensory cues differently from their non-autistic peers (for reviews see Marco et al., 2011; Schauder & Bennetto 2016). In other words, individuals' motor actions (e.g., covering their ears; not turning when their name is called) in response to sensory stimuli may be related to specific differences in the parts of the brain that underlie sensory processing.

Box 7.5   Learning activity

Discuss with your peers:

1. How would sensory overload influence your ability to perform work activities?
2. What information do we have about Torrance's sensory preferences and/or sensitivities?
3. What brain mechanisms may contribute to Torrance's sensory processing experiences?

Executive function

Brain regions that regulate sensory processing are also strongly connected to those which influence executive function and emotional regulation (Green et al., 2013, 2015, 2019). In other words, our brain's sensory processing networks influence our abilities to carry out goal-directed actions and cope with emotions. The sensory processing networks in our brains may contribute to our abilities related to specific executive functions like attention, decision-making, and emotional control. We can learn from the research on autistic adults to understand the relationships between sensory processing, executive function, and emotional regulation—all of which are related among non-autistic people as well.

Executive functions are the set of brain processes that allow us to select and ultimately perform goal-directed behaviors. (For more information on executive functioning, see Chapter 12 on schizophrenia and integrated chapters at the end of the book). Broadly, executive functioning consists of three components:

- **Inhibition:** the restriction or suppression of automatic responses.
- **Updating:** the constant monitoring and updating of the contents in working memory.
- **Switching:** task or mindset shifting.

Inhibition, updating, and switching processes work together to generate behaviors like planning, decision making, and problem-solving (Friedman & Miyake, 2017). Executive functioning challenges are associated with communication, quality of life, and adaptive functioning (de Vries et al. 2018; Demetriou et al., 2018). For example, when autistic people have executive functioning challenges, they may also have difficulties completing self-care routines or performing new multi-step actions. Further, executive functioning provides contextual, goal-directed information to guide individuals' reactions to environmental features (Fernandez-Prieto et al., 2021). This helps us understand connections between executive functioning and behavioral responses to sensory input.

Box 7.6   Learning activity

Discuss with your peers:

1. What are some aspects of your everyday life that depend on executive functioning?
2. What tasks may be particularly challenging if your executive functioning were impacted?
3. What adaptations could you make to your life to improve your executive functioning (e.g., how could you create supports for better planning or task shifting)?
4. How may your executive function be impacted when you are in different sensory environments? For example, some of you may prefer to study in a quiet library while others may prefer to study in a crowded cafe. Discuss how your ability to attend and task shift is different based on the sensory features of various environments.

Box 7.7   Learning activity

1. Find brain images that illustrate these structures (dorsolateral prefrontal cortex, medial prefrontal cortex, orbitofrontal cortex) so you can see how they fit into the cortex.
2. Find images showing the connections among these regions and how they communicate with each other.

Keywords: frontal lobe, prefrontal cortex, anatomy, executive function

Let's discuss some of the brain regions that are involved in executive functioning processes. The prefrontal cortex, located in the frontal lobe, houses several brain regions that control elements of executive functioning. Research shows differences in executive functioning-related prefrontal cortex processing among neurodivergent populations, including autistic people. There are three key regions in the prefrontal cortex that play central roles in executive functioning: (1) the dorsolateral prefrontal cortex, (2) the medial prefrontal cortex, and (3) the orbitofrontal cortex. Together, these brain regions communicate with one another, as well as with other cortical and subcortical regions to regulate behavior (Fernandez-Prieto et al., 2021).

The dorsolateral prefrontal cortex (dlPFC) is largely responsible for regulating our attention and allowing us to switch from one task to another. In Torrance's case, we see that they find it challenging to switch between projects. This concept, called set switching, is a central function of the dlPFC. Generally, we find that the dlPFC in the autistic population has differences in neurochemical composition (i.e., different *levels* of neurotransmitters present in this part of the brain) (Fung et al., 2021) and activation (i.e., the neural activity of this particular region of the brain) (Zhao et al., 2022). Such differences suggest that the communication between the dlPFC and other brain regions may be distinct in autistic individuals and underlie challenges with certain tasks that require elements of executive control, particularly set switching or switching attention between two tasks.

The medial prefrontal cortex (mPFC) and orbitofrontal cortex (OFC)—commonly referred to together as the ventro-medial prefrontal cortex (vmPFC) due to their highly interconnected nature—are related to emotion and executive function. The vmPFC plays an important role in impulse control, maintenance of working memory, and direction of reward and goal-related behaviors. The vmPFC exercises inhibitory control over emotion-based reflexive responses and behaviors to help us reach our goals and avoid negative consequences. Together, the dlPFC and vmPFC help guide behavior by combining sensory information from environmental stimuli with an individual's understanding of the rewards and emotions associated with those stimuli. For example, the sensations of a familiar study spot (the feel of the chair, the rattle of the fan, the smell of the room) may be associated with previous experiences of deep learning and help you to focus more on your work without getting distracted.

While we have discussed the executive functioning difficulties that autistic people may experience, it is important to note that some autistic individuals have strengths in executive functioning. Such strengths can support some autistic adults to maintain a singular focus in sensory-intensive environments or have heightened attention to detail (Baron-Cohen et al., 2009). This phenomenon is supported by neurobiological evidence that suggests that the superior longitudinal fasciculus, a white matter pathway that connects the dlPFC to the posterior parietal cortex (an area central to multisensory integration), is stronger in some autistic adults compared to non-autistic adults (Fitzgerald et al., 2018). These strong frontal-parietal connections in some autistic adults may underlie the relative strengths in being able to, for example, work in busy environments without distraction and finding errors in data that others miss.

Emotion regulation and social engagement

There are distinct parts of our brains involved in emotion regulation and social engagement. In Torrance's work environment, they are experiencing some challenges related to emotion regulation and social engagement, and we can look to particular brain regions to help us understand such challenges. Chapter 11 describes an autistic child (Kareem) who wants to be in a club; this chapter reviews the emotional regulation networks related to a school-aged child.

The limbic system is a network of five key brain regions that each contribute to regulating our emotions. It has strong ties to our ability, desire, and motivation to interact with others. While several brain regions interact with the central limbic system regions, there are five particular structures that are central to limbic control, which include:

- **Amygdala:** This region of the brain is the core of emotional processing, and a system for processing fearful and threatening stimuli, including detection of threat.
- **Cingulate cortex:** This region of the brain is responsible for the integration of action, emotion, and motivation.
- **Thalamus:** This part of the brain is your body's sensory and motor relay station—all information from your body's senses (except smell) must be processed through your thalamus before being sent to your brain's cerebral cortex for interpretation.
- **Hypothalamus:** This region of the brain is involved in autonomic regulation, and the activity of the pituitary, controlling body temperature, thirst, hunger, and other homeostatic systems.
- **Hippocampus:** This part of the brain is the center of learning and memory.

Among autistic people, the limbic system structures and their mechanisms for communicating with one another are distinct, with unique aspects of limbic system structure (organization and architecture of brain regions) and functional connectivity (neural communication among brain regions) corresponding to more prominent autism features (Mei et al., 2020) (just like sensorimotor executive function above). Further, the architecture of the white matter pathways that connect limbic system regions is associated with emotional regulation in autistic populations (Stephens et al., 2021). Together, this evidence demonstrates how general differences in limbic system organization and function may influence emotional regulation in autistic individuals.

Box 7.8   Learning activity

1. Find a picture of the limbic system that delineates the different areas and their connections with one another, so you have a visual reference as you read the next section.
2. What are the unique functions of each region in the limbic system and how might they work together to regulate emotion?
3. What role may the limbic system play in Torrance's experience in their work environment?

Keywords: limbic system, anatomy, brain, connections

While all aspects of the limbic system are important for emotion regulation and social engagement, the amygdala in particular plays a large role in the regulation of stress and anxiety. Anxiety disorders are highly prevalent among autistic people (White et al., 2009) and may stem from social, sensory, and neuroanatomical roots (South & Rodgers, 2017). Within the autistic population, distinct patterns of amygdala development during childhood and adolescence have been linked to autism features and are thought to greatly contribute to the presence of higher anxiety rates in this population. Specifically, faster amygdala growth during childhood is associated with heightened anxiety in autistic populations (Andrews et al., 2022). While the brain is capable of change throughout life (see Chapters 18, 22) for more information on brain plasticity), childhood is a key time for brain development and sets the stage for how your brain will function as an adult. Therefore, altered patterns of amygdala growth and development during childhood can lead to the presence of more anxiety later in life.

As you've learned above, the amygdala is the brain's core for assessing if environmental or sensory stimuli are threats. If individuals perceive environmental or sensory stimuli as a threat, they may have intense emotional responses that manifest as anxiety. In other words, when individuals have consistent increases in amygdala function, they may perceive threat in situations that others with less active amygdala would not consider threatening. This consistent perception of threat in the environment often contributes to an overall sense of anxiety and even an anxiety disorder. (For more information on anxiety, see Chapter 13.)

The amygdala, however, is not the only brain region associated with anxiety. While the amygdala plays a large role in regulating anxiety, several other brain regions such as the cingulate, prefrontal cortex, and insula (each discussed in earlier parts of this chapter) additionally contribute to stress responses. Brain regions in this anxiety network may have weaker connectivity among autistic adults (Tung et al., 2021), suggesting that they may not communicate with each other as efficiently in autistic populations compared to non-autistic populations. This less efficient neural communication can lead to more challenges in regulating responses in the face of anxiety.

Importantly, this anxiety network does not act in isolation. Instead, these altered network mechanisms both contribute to and are influenced by the alternative neural mechanisms underlying sensory processing and executive. This is supported by research showing that anxiety disorders often co-occur with sensory sensitivities, especially in the autistic population (Kotsiris et al., 2020). From this, we can draw from the link between how consistent differences in amygdala function, sensory processing, and executive functioning contribute to the distinct behavioral profiles of autistic adults. We can then use this information to understand how work environments can mismatch or align with individuals' neurological needs.

Daily life routine: Torrance completing individual and group work in the open office

As you read previously, Torrance works in an open office and has encountered some difficulties with the sensory environment of their workplace. Torrance is also concerned about having to manage multiple projects at once since they are used to working on one project at a time (e.g., when taking college courses). These challenges combine to result in feelings of overwhelm which can make emotion regulation and social functioning more difficult. Let's turn our attention to using principles of neuroscience to outline how parts of Torrance's brain may be reacting to the open office environment and some potential strategies to support their successful work participation.

Back to the person's life … Torrance negotiating the work environment and completing work tasks

In this chapter, we have discussed the evidence about brain functions that underlie sensory processing, executive function, and social-emotional processing. How can we use scientific reasoning to guide our thinking about how to support Torrance in their work? In your future studies, you will learn more about specific intervention strategies.

Box 7.9   Learning activity

1. In class or small groups, discuss some recommendations a clinician could make to support Torrance in their current work environment. Use your neuroscience knowledge and what you know about Torrance to guide your idea generation.
2. Based on your understanding of the interplay between sensory processing and executive functioning, what adaptations to Torrance's work situation may be beneficial?
3. What strategies may be helpful in supporting Torrance's planning and managing work projects?
4. What could help Torrance prevent becoming overwhelmed while at work?

What do we know about ourselves and the population at large from this case example?

By studying Torrance's case, we can understand that all individuals have unique sensory responses that influence how, where, and in what conditions we work most comfortably. Some of us need quiet work environments to focus and call upon our executive function skills. For others, our executive functioning may be enhanced by working in busy environments such as an open office space. Our experiences also may differ depending on the kind of work we are doing and the nature of the stimuli around us. But for each of us, the neural mechanisms that support our sensory processing work alongside executive functioning to support our participation.

We can also learn from Torrance's case about the links between sensory processing, executive function, and social-emotional processing. Our sensory gating systems filter specific sensory information through to higher-order processing, and our executive functions support attending and responding to important information in our environments. However, there can be barriers to executive functioning that make certain actions—such as switching between tasks—more challenging. Highly stimulating sensory environments combined with complex executive functioning demands can contribute to overwhelmed emotional reactions such as anxiety and difficulty functioning.

By understanding the links between sensory processing, executive functioning, and social-emotional responding, we see the importance of adapting work environments to help align with individuals' neurological needs to support their ability to participate in meaningful employment.

Box 7.10   Learning activity

With your small group, complete the table in the Appendix about the integration of Torrance's sensory and cognitive needs to be successful in his new job.

Further reading

The references below provide additional insights into the concepts from this chapter if you are interested.

Dunn, W. (2001). The sensations of everyday life: Empirical, theoretical, and pragmatic considerations. *The American Journal of Occupational Therapy, 55*(6), 608–620. https://doi.org/10.5014/ajot.55.6.608

Dunn, W. (2007). Supporting children to participate successfully in everyday life by using sensory processing knowledge. *Infants & Young Children, 20*(2), 84–101. https://doi.org/10.1097/01.IYC.0000264477.05076.5d

Dunn, W. (2007). *Living Sensationally: Understanding Your Senses.* Jessica Kingsley Publishers.

Dunn, W., Little, L., Dean, E., Robertson, S., & Evans, B. (2016). The state of the science on sensory factors and their impact on daily life for children: A scoping review. *OTJR: Occupation, Participation and Health, 36*(2_suppl), 3S–26S.

Little, L. M., Dean, E. E., Wallisch, A., & Dunn, W. (2018). Sensory Processing. In Schell, B. & Gilen, G (Eds.). *Willard and Spackman's Occupational Therapy* (13th edition). Philadelphia, PA: Lippincott, Williams, & Wilkins.

Shore, S. (2015). *Beyond the Wall: personal experiences with Autism* (2nd Edition) Future Horizons publishing.

Sapperstein, J. (2010). *Atypical: Life with Asperger's in 20 1/3 chapters.* TarcherPerigee, NY.

Zaks, Z. (2006). *Life and Love: Positive Strategies for Autistic Adults.* AAPC Publishing, KC.

References

American Psychiatric Association. (2013). *Diagnostic and statistical manual of mental disorders* (5th ed.). American Psychiatric Association.

Andrews, D. S., Aksman, L., Kerns, C. M., Lee, J. K., Winder-Patel, B. M., Harvey, D. J., Waizbard-Bartov, E., Heath, B., Solomon, M., Rogers, S., Altmann, A., Nordahl, C. W., & Amaral, D. G. (2022). Association of amygdala development with different forms of anxiety in autism spectrum disorder. *Biological Psychiatry, 91*(11), 977–987. https://doi.org/10.1016/j.biopsych.2022.01.016

Baranek, G. T., David, F. J., Poe, M. D., Stone, W. L., & Watson, L. R. (2006). Sensory Experiences Questionnaire: Discriminating sensory features in young children with autism, developmental delays, and typical development. *Journal of Child Psychology and Psychiatry, 47*(6), 591–601. https://doi.org/10.1111/j.1469-7610.2005.01546.x

Baron-Cohen, S., Ashwin, E., Ashwin, C., Tavassoli, T., & Chakrabarti, B. (2009). Talent in autism: Hyper-systemizing, hyper-attention to detail and sensory hypersensitivity. *Philosophical Transactions of the Royal Society of London. Series B, Biological Sciences, 364*(1522), 1377–1383. https://doi.org/10.1098/rstb.2008.0337

de Vries, M., Verdam, M. G., Prins, P. J., Schmand, B. A., & Geurts, H. M. (2018). Exploring possible predictors and moderators of an executive function training for children with an autism spectrum disorder. *Autism, 22*(4), 440–449. https://doi.org/10.1177/1362361316682622

Demetriou, E. A., Lampit, A., Quintana, D. S., Naismith, S. L., Song, Y. J. C., Pye, J. E., Hickie, I., & Guastella, A. J. (2018). Autism spectrum disorders: A meta-analysis of executive function. *Molecular Psychiatry, 23*(5), 1198–1204. https://doi.org/10.1038/mp.2017.75

Dinstein, I., Heeger, D. J., & Behrmann, M. (2015). Neural variability: Friend or foe? *Trends in Cognitive Sciences, 19*(6), 322–328. https://doi.org/10.1016/j.tics.2015.04.005

Dinstein, I., Heeger, D. J., Lorenzi, L., Minshew, N. J., Malach, R., & Behrmann, M. (2012). Unreliable evoked responses in autism. *Neuron, 75*(6), 981–991. https://doi.org/10.1016/j.neuron.2012.07.026

Dunn, W. (1997). The impact of sensory processing abilities on the daily lives of young children and their families: A conceptual model. *Infants & Young Children, 9*(4), 23–35.

Dunn, W. (2014). *Sensory Profile 2.* Bloomington, MN, USA: Psych Corporation.

Dunn, W. (2001). The sensations of everyday life: Empirical, theoretical, and pragmatic considerations. *The American Journal of Occupational Therapy, 55*(6), 608–620. https://doi.org/10.5014/ajot.55.6.608

Dunn, W. (2007). Supporting children to participate successfully in everyday life by using sensory processing knowledge. *Infants & Young Children, 20*(2), 84–101. https://doi.org/10.1097/01.IYC.0000264477.05076.5d

Fernandez-Prieto, M., Moreira, C., Cruz, S., Campos, V., Martínez-Regueiro, R., Taboada, M., Carracedo, A., & Sampaio, A. (2021). Executive functioning: A mediator between sensory processing and behaviour in autism spectrum disorder. *Journal of Autism and Developmental Disorders, 51*(6), 2091–2103. https://doi.org/10.1007/s10803-020-04648-4

Fitzgerald, J., Leemans, A., Kehoe, E., O'Hanlon, E., Gallagher, L., & McGrath, J. (2018). Abnormal fronto-parietal white matter organisation in the superior longitudinal fasciculus branches in autism spectrum disorders. *The European Journal of Neuroscience, 47*(6), 652–661. https://doi.org/10.1111/ejn.13655

Friedman, N. P., Miyake, A. (2017). Unity and diversity of executive functions: Individual differences as a window on cognitive structure. *Cortex, 86,* 186–204. http://dx.doi.org/10.1016/j.cortex.2016.04.023

Fung, L. K., Flores, R. E., Gu, M., Sun, K. L., James, D., Schuck, R. K., Jo, B., Park, J. H., Lee, B. C., Jung, J. H., Kim, S. E., Saggar, M., Sacchet, M. D., Warnock, G., Khalighi, M. M., Spielman, D., Chin, F. T., & Hardan, A. Y. (2021). Thalamic and prefrontal GABA concentrations but not GABAA receptor densities are altered in high-functioning adults with autism spectrum disorder. *Molecular Psychiatry, 26*(5), 1634–1646. https://doi.org/10.1038/s41380-020-0756-y

Green, S. A., Hernandez, L., Bookheimer, S. Y., & Dapretto, M. (2016). Salience network connectivity in autism is related to brain and behavioral markers of sensory overresponsivity. *Journal of the American Academy of Child and Adolescent Psychiatry, 55*(7), 618–626. https://doi.org/10.1016/j.jaac.2016.04.013

Green, S. A., Hernandez, L., Tottenham, N., Krasileva, K., Bookheimer, S. Y., & Dapretto, M. (2015). Neurobiology of sensory overresponsivity in youth with autism spectrum disorders. *JAMA Psychiatry, 72*(8), 778–786. https://doi.org/10.1001/jamapsychiatry.2015.0737

Green, S. A., Hernandez, L., Lawrence, K. E., Liu, J., Tsang, T., Yeargin, J., Cummings, K., Laugeson, E., Dapretto, M., & Bookheimer, S. Y. (2019). Distinct patterns of neural habituation and generalization in children and adolescents with autism with low and high sensory overresponsivity. *The American Journal of Psychiatry, 176*(12), 1010–1020. https://doi.org/10.1176/appi.ajp.2019.18121333

Green, S. A., Rudie, J. D., Colich, N. L., Wood, J. J., Shirinyan, D., Hernandez, L., Tottenham, N., Dapretto, M., & Bookheimer, S. Y. (2013). Overreactive brain responses to sensory stimuli in youth with autism spectrum disorders. *Journal of the American Academy of Child and Adolescent Psychiatry, 52*(11), 1158–1172. https://doi.org/10.1016/j.jaac.2013.08.004

Haigh, S. M., Heeger, D. J., Dinstein, I., Minshew, N., & Behrmann, M. (2015). Cortical variability in the sensory-evoked response in autism. *Journal of Autism and Developmental Disorders, 45*(5), 1176–1190. https://doi.org/10.1007/s10803-014-2276-6

Herrington, J. D., Miller, J. S., Pandey, J., & Schultz, R. T. (2016). Anxiety and social deficits have distinct relationships with amygdala function in autism spectrum disorder. *Social Cognitive and Affective Neuroscience, 11*(6), 907–914. https://doi.org/10.1093/scan/nsw015

Iidaka, T., Kogata, T., Mano, Y., & Komeda, H. (2019). Thalamocortical hyperconnectivity and amygdala-cortical hypoconnectivity in male patients with autism spectrum disorder. *Frontiers in Psychiatry, 10.* https://doi.org/10.3389/fpsyt.2019.00252

Kotsiris, K., Westrick, J., & Little, L. (2020). Sensory processing patterns and internalizing behaviors in the pediatric and young adult general population: A scoping review. *The Open Journal of Occupational Therapy, 8*(1), 1–13. https://doi.org/10.15453/2168-6408.1624

Little, L. M., Dean, E., Tomchek, S. D., & Dunn, W. (2017). Classifying sensory profiles of children in the general population. *Child: Care, Health and Development, 43*(1), 81–88. https://doi.org/10.1111/cch.12391

Marco, E. J., Hinkley, L. B., Hill, S. S., & Nagarajan, S. S. (2011). Sensory processing in autism: A review of neurophysiologic findings. *Pediatric Research, 69*(5 Pt 2), 48–54. https://doi.org/10.1203/PDR.0b013e3182130c54

Mei, T., Llera, A., Floris, D. L., Forde, N. J., Tillmann, J., Durston, S., Moessnang, C., Banaschewski, T., Holt, R. J., Baron-Cohen, S., Rausch, A., Loth, E., Dell'Acqua, F., Charman, T., Murphy, D. G. M., Ecker, C., Beckmann, C. F., Buitelaar, J. K., & EU-AIMS LEAP group (2020). Gray matter covariations and core symptoms of autism: The EU-AIMS longitudinal European autism project. *Molecular Autism, 11*(1). https://doi.org/10.1186/s13229-020-00389-4

Milne, E. (2011). Increased intra-participant variability in children with autistic spectrum disorders: Evidence from single-trial analysis of evoked EEG. *Frontiers in Psychology, 2*(51), 1–12. https://doi.org/10.3389/fpsyg.2011.00051

Schauder, K. B., & Bennetto, L. (2016). Toward an interdisciplinary understanding of sensory dysfunction in autism spectrum disorder: An integration of the neural and symptom literatures. *Frontiers in Neuroscience, 10.* https://doi.org/10.3389/fnins.2016.00268

South, M., & Rodgers, J. (2017). Sensory, emotional and cognitive contributions to anxiety in autism spectrum disorders. *Frontiers in Human Neuroscience, 11.* https://doi.org/10.3389/fnhum.2017.00020

Stephens, K., Silk, T. J., Anderson, V., Hazell, P., Enticott, P. G., & Sciberras, E. (2021). Associations between limbic system white matter structure and socio-emotional functioning in children with ADHD + ASD. *Journal of Autism and Developmental Disorders, 51*(8), 2663–2672. https://doi.org/10.1007/s10803-020-04738-3

Tomchek, S. D., & Dunn, W. (2007). Sensory processing in children with and without autism: Comparative study using the short sensory profile. *The American Journal of Occupational Therapy 61*(2), 190–200. https://doi.org/10.5014/ajot.61.2.190

Tung, R., Reiter, M. A., Linke, A., Kohli, J. S., Kinnear, M. K., Müller, R. A., & Carper, R. A. (2021). Functional connectivity within an anxiety network and associations with anxiety symptom severity in middle-aged adults with and without autism. *Autism Research, 14*(10), 2100–2112. https://doi.org/10.1002/aur.2579

White, S. W., Oswald, D., Ollendick, T., & Scahill, L. (2009). Anxiety in children and adolescents with autism spectrum disorders. *Clinical Psychology Review, 29*(3), 216–229. https://doi.org/10.1016/j.cpr.2009.01.003

Woodward, N. D., Giraldo-Chica, M., Rogers, B., & Cascio, C. J. (2017). Thalamocortical dysconnectivity in autism spectrum disorder: An analysis of the autism brain imaging data exchange. *Biological Psychiatry: Cognitive Neuroscience and Neuroimaging, 2*(1), 76–84. https://doi.org/10.1016/j.bpsc.2016.09.002

Zhao, H.-C., Lv, R., Zhang, G.-Y., He, L.-M., Cai, X.-T., Sun, Q., Yan, C.-Y., Bao, X.-Y., Lv, X.-Y., & Fu, B. (2022). Alterations of prefrontal-posterior information processing patterns in autism spectrum disorders. *Frontiers in Neuroscience, 15.* https://doi.org/10.3389/fnins.2021.768219.

8 Branden wants to run errands and is blind

Neuroscience facilitates our understanding of running errands

Sondra Stegenga

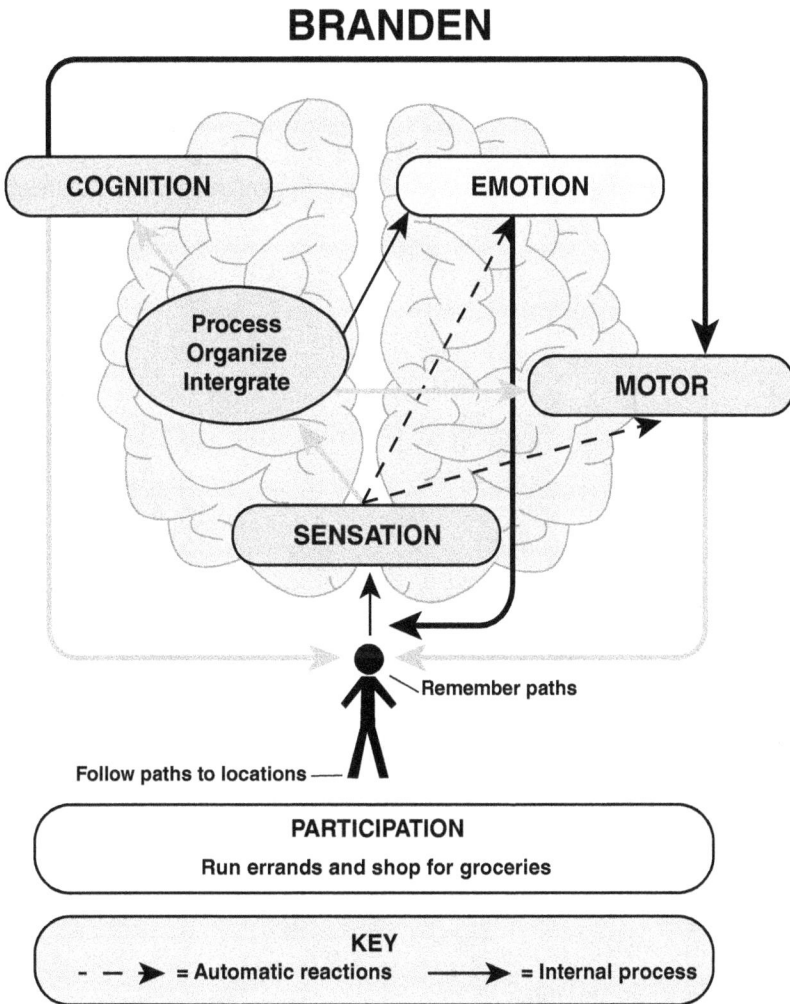

BRANDEN

COGNITION

EMOTION

Process
Organize
Intergrate

MOTOR

SENSATION

Remember paths

Follow paths to locations

PARTICIPATION

Run errands and shop for groceries

KEY

- — ➤ = Automatic reactions   ——➤ = Internal process

Figure 8.1 Branden brain figure

DOI: 10.4324/9781003524380-10

The purpose of this chapter is to discover how Branden, a 21-year-old woman who would like to increase community independence for running errands, might be affected by blindness, a condition that affects her ability to take in visual information from her environment. People with blindness have full lives with their daily routines, relationships, and learning, but may require adaptations or modifications to optimize participation in daily routines.

The key neuroscience concepts we will explore in this chapter include the visual cortices as well as the anatomy of the eye and visual pathways. Particularly, we will discuss the structures and functions of the brain that are linked to the condition of blindness. Recent research indicates there are over 39 million people in the world (Lee & Mesfin, 2022) and over 8 million individuals in the United States (US Census Bureau, 2021) who are blind. Despite these large numbers, many people do not realize there are a variety of neurological causes and conditions underlying blindness and that individuals diagnosed with blindness do not necessarily have total vision loss. In this chapter, students will learn about not only the neurology behind these conditions but the link to functional participation in the meaningful occupation of running errands.

As with all the chapters, these components of the nervous system work with other systems to support overall human function. Keywords for this chapter are listed in the box below. Be sure you learn what these key features are so you can get the most out of the chapter.

Keywords for this chapter

blindness	lateral geniculate	retina
cones	nucleus	retinopathy of prematurity
cornea	macular degeneration	rods
cortical visual	occipital lobe	universal design
impairment	optic nerve	vision association areas
fovia	primary visual cortex	visual field loss
iris	pupil	visual impairments

Box 8.1   Learning activity

Prior to reading the case:

1. How do you think blindness will affect Branden's performance of running errands?
2. Why is it important for an occupational therapy practitioner to understand the neurology of blindness?

Let's find out more about Branden

Branden is a 21-year-old woman who would like to increase her independence with running errands. Specifically, she would like to learn a new neighborhood and new strategies for community mobility. Branden lives in her own apartment with her guide dog, Max.

She enjoys getting together with friends and family, cooking, taking walks in the local park, and going birding with the local aviary club where she is an expert in identifying a range of different bird calls. Branden has a diagnosis of "legal blindness" due to retinopathy of prematurity from being born early at 30 weeks. She currently works from her home as a customer service representative for an online home goods supply store.

Branden loves to cook. She even has her own online blog whereby she provides detailed instructions and videos for recipes she creates. She often receives requests for foods to make from her online followers and, hence, regularly needs to get to the grocery store and other local markets for the specialty ingredients. After living in the same apartment and community for two years she recently had to move to a new apartment in the next town about 10 miles away due to her current building being renovated and rent raised. Although she is excited to be in a town closer to some family and friends, she must learn a new neighborhood and now also navigate public transportation to be able to get to the grocery store since it is no longer in walking distance.

In Branden's new neighborhood, the grocery story is a mile away, requiring use of public transportation to get to the store. She can access paratransit, a bus that provides door to door service for individuals with an established disability. In her community, this service is convenient, but there is a small fee associated with all paratransit rides. Therefore, she prefers to learn the mainline bus route, if possible. She has a bus stop only a quarter block from her apartment building and a stop right at the grocery store, making it a feasible commute if she could become comfortable with the route and accessibility features of the bus system. As the bus comes every 15 minutes during typical business hours during the week, it also would give her flexibility of times to be able to get to the store in case she needs an added ingredient or last-minute item from the store when cooking a new dish for her blog or developing a new recipe.

Branden has connected with workforce services and rehabilitation in her state to sign up for courses to help her learn new skills with public transportation. These classes are specialized and specifically for individuals over 18 years of age and have a diagnosis of legal blindness. The services are paid for through a combination of state and federal money to help in improving independence of individuals who are blind.

Box 8.2   Self-directed learning activity

Discuss with your peers:

1. Having read the narrative, what are some of the things you know about Branden that will be relevant to her running errands? *Hint: Branden's strengths and key interests.*
2. What might be some barriers to running errands in her community?
3. Having read the narrative, what are you curious about?
4. What do you need to know more about?

Thinking functionally about blindness

Communities and cities have historically been built to meet the needs of individuals with a full range of sensory inputs (e.g., 20/20 vision, hearing, touch) and movements (e.g., being able to walk up and down stairs and curbs). This means that navigating most communities is heavily reliant on visual inputs. Therefore, when an individual has sensory loss (e.g., blindness) or other disabilities (e.g., individuals with cerebral palsy or other motor impairments you have learned about earlier in this book) adaptations may be needed to optimally engage in activities in the community.

Individuals with blindness offer a unique perspective on how communities are focused on meeting the needs of the general population and how communities often overlook meeting the needs of a broader range of individuals. For example, if you take a moment to reflect on daily routines, it quickly becomes evident how readily vision is required for many tasks.

Box 8.3   Self-directed learning activity

Take a moment to reflect on going to the grocery store:

1. Write down at least three key tasks of grocery shopping that rely heavily on vision?
2. When navigating sidewalks and street crossings, what aspects rely on vision?
3. What are some accommodations that might already be available in communities to allow use of senses other than vision?

Individuals with neurological or structural conditions that limit access to vision, such as having a cortical visual impairment (CVI) or complete blindness, bring to the forefront the immense need for integration of universal design principles throughout all communities. Universal design is the idea that communities, tasks, and our world at large can be better designed and planned to meet the needs of ALL individuals (e.g., Burgstahler, 2009). Some examples of universal design include having curb cuts and ramps versus only stairs allowing access entry to buildings via wheelchair or by foot or having auditory instructions for when it is safe to walk at crosswalks versus just a visual walk sign.

Box 8.4   Self-directed learning activity

Pause here and take a moment to search out the following information:

1. Find and write down the definition of universal design.
2. What websites and resources did you find on universal design?
3. What are some universal design options that would help Branden get around her community?
4. If more communities and homes used principles of universal design, how would that improve Branden's ability to navigate public transportation and go to the grocery store?

Keywords: universal design, universal design definition, accessibility, inclusive design, barrier free

---

Overall, when considering how our individual neurology makes each of us unique, it becomes important to understand not only how our differences impact one's conditions or diagnoses but even more importantly how that might impact, either as a strength or potential barrier, our function and participation in a range of meaningful daily life activities within our communities. Many times, a sensory difference may only be a barrier due to the way our environments are built and set up for reliance on particular senses, such as vision. If we start to think beyond our current structures, we realize there are many ways of going about an activity, such as running errands, that do not always require vision.

Neuroscience information to guide your thinking about Branden

Now that you have had some time to learn about Branden's routines and preferences and the impacts of the design of our communities on how it might affect individual access to routines and functional access, let's learn some more about blindness. Specifically, in the following we will cover the definitions, important functional characteristics, relevant information on the structures and functions within the brain, and then link this all to what running errands requires from the nervous system, particularly related to individuals with blindness.

Defining "blindness"

Recent research and census information indicate there are 39 million people in the world who are blind (Lee & Mesfin, 2022) and over 8 million of these individuals live in the United States (US) (US Census Bureau, 2020). See Figure 8.1 for an example of a visual field deficit that would qualify as "legal blindness." Blindness is not necessarily total vision loss; in fact, only 15% of individuals diagnosed as being "legally blind" have complete lack of light perception and subsequent total vision loss (Lee & Mesfin, 2022).

It is important to mention that there are not consistent definitions of "blindness." Let's take a moment to search on the internet "visual field cuts" or "central or peripheral vision loss" to see what it might look like to have a significant loss of vision that would qualify as "legal blindness."

Box 8.5   Self-directed learning activity

Stop and discuss the following with a peer:

1. Look up the United States definition of legal blindness.
2. Look up the definition of blindness according to the World Health Organization (WHO). What is their definition of blindness?
3. How does the WHO definition differ from the above definition of "legal blindness" in the United States?
4. What do you think are the benefits and potential barriers of each definition?
5. Before reading this chapter and reading these definitions, how did you define blindness? Did you know there were differing definitions?

Keywords: blindness, legal blindness, United States legally blind, World Health Organization blindness, definition

---

Overall, when you hear the term "blindness," one must always consider what context and definition of "blindness" is being used. Also, it is important to be aware that these definitions may change over time as more research is conducted or as new policies arise. Often definitions for blindness, or other disability categories, are linked to accessing services or funding in particular countries or contexts. For example, meeting the definition of "legal blindness" in the US qualifies individuals for a range of services both in school and beyond (e.g., Workforce Services and Rehabilitation). Due to this funding link, there have been calls from experts in the field of ophthalmology to reconsider the definition of "blindness" to better capture all types of visual deficits that significantly impact life function, particularly with the rise of conditions such as cerebral/cortical visual impairment (i.e., CVI; Kran et al., 2019) that impact function but do not fall under current criteria for "blindness" in most states in the US. This need to better recognize functional impact in definitions of and eligibility criteria related to blindness has been discussed for years, with the International Congress of Ophthalmology already calling for a change in definition back in 2002 emphasizing that criteria for blindness should include function versus just acuity or field deficits (International Council of Ophthalmology, 2002).

Related conditions and causes

Blindness can be caused by a range of conditions and may happen at birth or later in life. It can happen quickly or slowly over time. The most common causes of blindness are age related. In fact, over 82% of people who are blind are over age 50 (Lee & Mesfin, 2022). Although only 4% of individuals experience blindness from causes or conditions at birth, these conditions are important to understand because of the large number of years the individual will be living with blindness. Stop here and let's take a moment to look up more specific details on the different causes of blindness and learn more about the neurological uniqueness of each condition.

Box 8.6   Self-directed learning activity

1. What are the common causes of blindness at birth or in children?

Keywords: Causes blindness, signs and symptoms, age-related blindness, childhood blindness, micronutrient deficiencies

2. What are the common causes of age-related blindness in individuals over age 50?
3. Childhood blindness can be caused by micronutrient deficiencies, such as lack of vitamin A. What happens to the cornea if a child does not have enough Vitamin A? What is the diagnosis for this?

Keywords: Cornea and blindness, vitamin A and blindness, conjunctivitis and blindness, infections and blindness, blindness at birth, retina and blindness

4. Childhood blindness can also be caused by severe eye infection (conjunctivitis) due to exposure to pathogens at birth. What are some infections that might cause blindness if exposed to them during birth?
5. What are some possible issues with the retina in retinopathy of prematurity (ROP)?
6. Cortical visual impairment (CVI) is unlike other visual conditions because often the eye structures are normally developed. What then causes blindness or visual difficulties in an individual with CVI?

Retinopathy of prematurity (ROP) is the condition that Branden has. She does not have any sight in her left eye due to full retinal detachment but does have central vision in her right eye due to only partial damage. Due to advancements in health care supporting more children through premature birth, CVI and ROP have become the primary causes of visual impairments and blindness in young children in high income countries, such as the US (Lueck et al., 2019).

Eye and neural neuroscience anatomy

The first step in "seeing" requires being able to take in information through the eye. The eye is a very delicate structure made up of a cornea, iris, lens, retina, rods, and cones. A complex interaction of all these structures is required to take visual information from the environment and send it via the optic nerve and optic pathways to the brain. The retina is particularly important as it contains millions of light sensitive rods and cones that help to organize and take in all the visual information. If this becomes detached, as with Branden's one eye, an individual will experience total blindness in that eye. A partial detachment or degeneration of part of the retina, can result in visual field loss, such as with Branden's other eye. In other conditions of the retina, such as macular degeneration, the central part of the retina deteriorates with subsequent blurred central visual or complete central field loss or what looks like a central blind spot (Mayo Clinic, n.d.). Macular Degeneration is the most common cause of blindness in adults (Flaxman et al., 2017).

Box 8.7 Learning activity

Before going further, find a detailed picture of (1) the structure of the eye, and (2) the pathways to the brain.

1. Find the lens, cornea, pupil, aqueous humor, and vitreous humor. While not part of the nervous system, their role is to allow light to fall on the retina in which the visual receptors, which are part of the nervous system, are located.
2. Where is the retina located?
3. Identify and compare and contrast the two types of photoreceptors in the retina.
4. Locate the fovia. What is its purpose?
5. Why does a detached retina result in blindness?
6. What is the blind spot. Why is it a blind spot in our field of view? Make sure you can find its location.
7. Define "visual field."
8. What does a central field loss look like compared to a left or right visual field loss? Hint: Keep your picture up of the structure of the eye. You will return to it in another activity.

Keywords: Anatomy of the eye, anatomy of the visual pathways, photoreceptors, retina, lens, cornea, pupil, aqueous humor, vitreous humor, visual receptors, fovia, location of retina, 3D eye model, free eye anatomy quiz

---

Being able to "see" requires a complex interaction between the eyes and the brain. Kran et al. (2019) explain this in terms of not only our structures but the interaction with the inputs of our environment:

> What one "sees" begins with visual processing in the eyes that continues along the anterior visual pathway, lateral geniculate nucleus, retrogeniculate visual pathways, primary visual cortex, and vision association areas. An individual's view of the world is further influenced by other sensory inputs, environment, experience, and attention.
>
> (Kran et al., 2019, p. 25)

After reading this, return to the pictures you downloaded above.

Box 8.8   Learning activity

Return to look at the detailed picture of (1) the structure of the eye, and (2) the pathways to the brain:

1. What are the key structures of the visual pathways? *Hint: What is the difference between the optic nerves, optic tract, and lateral geniculate nucleus of the thalamus?*

Keywords: Optic tract, lateral geniculate nucleus, thalamus, optic nerves, structures of the visual pathways

2. Trace the visual pathways of the brain. What do you notice about the visual pathways relative to the visual fields? *Hint: Does the visual pathway from the right side of the brain control the right or left visual field?*
3. What is the difference between a visual field and the eyes?
4. Why is it important to understand how the visual pathways cross to different areas of the brain? *Hint: keep your picture up of the structure of the eye. You will return to it in another activity.*

Each of the structures are critically important to vision and breakdown can occur in a range of areas. Therefore, knowing the function of each of these areas is important because where a breakdown or disruption occurs due to an injury or dysfunction determines the particular types visual of deficits.

Occipital lobe and association areas

The occipital lobe is one of the smallest brain regions, but it has a very important job. This is where your brain processes the information that was sent from your retina, through the pathways to your brain. The occipital lobe translates the visual information into functional use (Cleveland Clinic, n.d.). Both the primary visual cortex (also known as striate cortex, Broadman's area 17, or V1) and secondary visual cortex (also known as V2) are located in the occipital lobe (Hannan, 2006).

Box 8.9   Learning activity

Return to your detailed picture of the structure of the eye.

1. Where is the occipital lobe located?

Keywords: occipital lobe, color and brain visual systems

2. When you look at an apple, what part of your brain processes the color? What part of your brain would help you to understand whether the apple is lying on its side or standing straight up?
3. What kinds of information are processed in the primary visual cortex and what kinds in the secondary visual cortex?

Keywords: occipital lobe, color and brain visual systems

Some signals are also sent to the lateral geniculate nucleus (LGN) from the primary visual cortex which then transfers the information to parts of the brain outside of the occipital lobe. The parietal visual cortex is one area that receives this information. Here, the brain interprets object motion and spatial relationships. These are very important skills that can impact participation in daily living activities, such as running errands, and all stem from important interactions in the occipital lobe and related pathways. For example, if an individual had difficulty with spatial processing, it may be difficult to accurately grasp items off a shelf at the grocery store. If there was a difficulty with facial recognition, they may not recognize a close friend at the grocery store unless they could hear their voice or have another means to recognize them.

Although the occipital lobe is an important visual processing center of the brain, it is still active in individual with congenital blindness. Studies have shown that the brain adapts in individuals with congenital blindness due to neural plasticity. Interestingly, it becomes a center for assisting with processing sensations such as smell, hearing, and touch (Hannan, 2006; Ortiz-Terán, 2016). This may explain why some individuals with blindness have heightened abilities with other sensations (Ortiz-Terán, 2016).

The role of the occupational therapist

Occupational therapists play an important role in the lives of individuals with visual impairments, including blindness (American Occupational Therapy Association, 2011). For example, occupational therapists may play a role in ensuring older adults are able to age in place. They may also conduct an activity analysis or environmental assessment to identify accommodations or modifications that would be beneficial to the individual's unique needs, such as you practiced in this chapter. Occupational therapists may also collaborate with a variety of related service providers and professionals in the community who specialize in supporting and enhancing the lives of individuals with blindness such as orientation and mobility services, teachers of the visually impaired, ophthalmologists or medical professionals, or transition or workforce services.

We have learned a lot of information so far. Let's take a few minutes to think back about what you learned.

Box 8.10   Learning activity

What have you learned from the information (reflecting back)?

1. What are the defining criteria for the diagnosis of "legal blindness"? *Hint: it is not only total vision loss.*
2. What different health conditions may lead to blindness?
3. Do all individuals with retinopathy of prematurity have a detached retina and subsequent blindness?
4. What do occupational therapists know about serving individuals with blindness or other vision loss?
5. Is it in the occupational therapist's scope of practice to work with individuals who are blind?
6. What other team members might be involved in working with someone like Branden?
7. Who should occupational therapists consider collaborating with when working with individuals who are blind on improving their participation in meaningful daily occupations?

Keywords: occupational therapist, scope of practice, blindness

---

Now that you know more about brain functioning in individuals with blindness, how can we use this scientific reasoning to support Branden in running errands in her community? You will certainly spend a lot more time in other courses exploring details but knowing the neuroscience underpinnings provides a solid foundation to select intervention options that will be supported by brain processing.

Daily life routine: running errands

Running errands is a regular part of the lives of people who are blind, just as it is for most adults. However, this may look very different and require different demands for the person who is blind depending on the location and community that an individual lives in. For example, someone who is blind and lives out in a rural community may have to go many miles to get to a grocery store and hence will require increased planning to be able to have someone drive them to the store and also gather and organize items that can last for several weeks. Differentially, an individual who lives in a large city may have a grocery store only a few blocks away but would require making more frequent trips to the grocery store because they need to walk to the grocery store and also carry home all the groceries. This could be difficult when also working with a guide dog or having a cane in one hand due to their mobility aids for vision. It also could potentially require skills for navigating public transportation or utilizing a local small street market that may only take cash payment and have few accommodations for someone who is blind (e.g., signs with braille or verbal prices versus written/posted signs at the marked). Overall, it is critical to look at every task individually to fully understand the demands and skills required in each unique environment and for every person who has their own individual strengths and needs. With this, we must also consider specific neurologic impacts, such as the effects of blindness and the type of visual condition on the activity. For example, Branden, who has retinopathy of prematurity with complete blindness in one eye and a field deficit in the other, may need different considerations than an individual who has an acuity deficit or CVI when navigating transportation and shopping at the grocery store.

Box 8.11   Learning activity

With your small group, complete the table in the Appendix about the integration of Branden's demands related to running errands and the neuroscience that affects her participation.

Back to the person's life: Branden wants to run her errands

Now that we know more about the brain and integration with the visual system in individuals with blindness and have considered the neuroscience underpinnings (e.g., brain structures and interactions/pathways) and their impact on function, how can we use this information to support Branden in running errands?

Box 8.12   Learning activity

In class or small groups, discuss what accommodations the disability specialists through support services can make to support Branden in being successful when running errands, specifically riding the bus to get to and from the grocery store to obtain groceries.

Use your neuroscience knowledge and what you know about Branden in small groups right now to guide your idea generation.

What do we know about ourselves and the population at large from this brain condition and Branden's story?

First, we all have strengths and areas of greater difficulty depending on the combination of our biological makeup, our life experiences, and our environmental exposures. Hence, we may rely more on certain types of sensory input (e.g., rely more on our vision or hearing) over others depending on our strengths; just like how Branden often leverages her skills and strengths of hearing or touch instead of vision to navigate her community. It is important for us all to be thinking about our strengths so we can optimize performance in daily occupations and meaningful activities routines.

Next, by understanding more about how the brain works and thinking about how our environments are often set up to support individuals with particular sensory inputs, such as vision, it enables us to begin to think about new ways we could universally design our communities to better meet the needs of all individuals instead of only catering to the skills and sensory inputs of the majority population. By providing multiple means and modes of input across different features of our communities, we can decrease barriers for individuals and increase opportunities for participation ultimately creating more opportunities for involvement. For example, if we include auditory "walk" prompts in addition to the visual lighted walk sign, individuals with or without vision or hearing can participate safely in crossing the street. Overall, on the topic of inclusion, it is important to think about our communities and whether they are truly inclusive and welcoming of all the strengths and needs of individuals in our communities. Before we go on, let's take a moment to reflect.

Box 8.13   Learning activity

Reflecting on our experiences:

1. Think of a time when you were in a place or event that you felt "uncomfortable," "not welcome," or "not included"? What was it about the place or event that made you feel this way? *Hint: Was there something you were unfamiliar with? Did navigating the environment or place require skills or knowledge you did not have?*
2. What could have been done to make you feel more comfortable?
3. What other knowledge, skills, or supports would have improved your experience or made you feel more welcome in the space?
4. How could the environment or space have been modified or change to make you, and perhaps many other people, feel more comfortable?
5. What parts of the brain control our feelings of anxiety or fear when we get into situations where we do not feel welcome or included?

Keywords: brain and anxiety, brain and fear

Inclusion often requires three key components to be truly inclusive: access, participation, and supports (Council for Exceptional Children Division for Early Childhood and the National Association of the Education of Young Children, 2009). Merely being in a place is not enough to be considered inclusion. One must be able to authentically participate with people and activities. Too often in schools people consider inclusion to merely be a place, like a general education classroom. However, to achieve true inclusion, an individual must be able to authentically and meaningfully participate in activities. This may require individualized supports or redesigning of the environment to remove barriers and optimize participation. These premises of inclusion are applicable not only to individuals who have an identified disability but for any of us. For example, when we are learning new tasks, such as wanting to join a tennis team or community card playing group, we might initially need some supports to learn about and optimally engage in the new activity. However, to truly feel included and have a sense of belonging, we must be able to access the activity (can I get into the activity or club), participate (do I know and understand the task? Do I have the needed skills?), and have the supports necessary for participation (is there a coach to teach me the rules and skills? Do I have the equipment needed to participate)?

Overall, these topics of universal design, inclusion, and understanding foundations and functional implications of blindness are vast topics and can become an area of specialization in your career as an occupational therapist. Ongoing and continuing education is an ethical obligation of occupational therapists according to the American Occupational Therapy Association Code of Ethics (2020). In fact, section 5 on Professional Competence, Education, Supervision and Training competency 5D states that occupational therapists are to "maintain competence by ongoing participation in professional development relevant to one's practice area" (p. 8). It is also arguably one of the things that makes a career in occupational therapy so much fun—there is always something new and interesting to learn and improve practices. If you are interested in learning more about any of these topics discussed in this chapter, please see the range of resources below including podcasts, online free learning modules, and additional readings! Your faculty can provide other options as well.

Further reading

Blindness

- American Foundation for the Blind: www.afb.org/blindness-and-low-vision/eye-conditions/low-vision-and-legal-blindness-terms-and-descriptions
- General information on Guide Dogs and sanctioned trainers by the International Guide Dog Federation: www.igdf.org.uk
- Guide Dogs for the Blind: www.guidedogs.com/explore-resources/faq
- Perkins School for the Blind: www.perkins.org
- National Federation of the Blind blindness statistics: https://nfb.org/resources/blindness-statistics

Cortical visual impairments

- Online Modules for Learning About CVI from Perkins School for the Blind: www.perkins.org/what-is-cvi/

The brain and occipital lobe

- Detailed information on the Occipital Lobe from the Cleveland Clinic: https://my.clevelandclinic.org/health/body/24498-occipital-lobe

Lived experiences of individuals with blindness and visual impairments

- Morris Frank—History of the Guide Dog (3min 06 seconds). https://vimeo.com/568841913/83dd5446f2?embedded=true&source=vimeo_logo&owner=12308416
- Perkins School for the Blind (n.d.). 10 fascinating facts about the white cane. www.perkins.org/10-fascinating-facts-about-the-white-cane/

Training and workforce services

- Video demonstrating skills learned in Training and Adjustment Classes by the Utah Department of Workforce: www.youtube.com/playlist?list=PLC7xoL4RFgn-wXjCBDblInXYFSoSRxF5z

Universal design

- Universal Design for an Individual with Vision Impairment (Macular Degeneration)—Podcast 06—Mail and Macular Degeneration on the UDL Project https://universaldesign.org/podcast/006-mail-macular-degeneration
- The UD Project: https://universaldesign.org/definition

References

American Occupational Therapy Association (2011). Occupational therapy's role with persons with visual impairment. www.aota.org/-/media/corporate/files/aboutot/professionals/whatisot/pa/facts/low-vision-fact-sheet.pdf

American Occupational Therapy Association (2020). Occupational therapy code of ethics. *American Journal of Occupational Therapy*, *74*(3). https://doi.org/10.5014/ajot.2020.74S3006

Burgstahler, S. (2009). Universal Design: Process, Principles, and Applications. *DO-IT*. www.washington.edu/doit/sites/default/files/atoms/files/Universal_Design_04_12_21.pdf

Cleveland Clinic (n.d.). Occipital Lobe. https://my.clevelandclinic.org/health/body/24498-occipital-lobe

Council for Exceptional Children Division for Early Childhood and the National Association of the Education of Young Children (2009). Early childhood inclusion. www.naeyc.org/sites/default/files/globally-shared/downloads/PDFs/resources/position-statements/ps_inclusion_dec_naeyc_ec.pdf

Flaxman, S. R., Bourne, R. R., Resnikoff, S., Ackland, P., Braithwaite, T., Cicinelli, M. V.,... & Zheng, Y. (2017). Global causes of blindness and distance vision impairment 1990–2020: a systematic review and meta-analysis. *The Lancet Global Health*, *5*(12), e1221–e1234.

Hannan, C. K. (2006). Review of research: neuroscience and the impact of brain plasticity on Braille reading. *Journal of Visual Impairment & Blindness*, *100*(7), 397–413.

International Council on Ophthalmology (2002). Visual Standards: Aspects and Ranges of Vision Loss ICO report. 29th International Congress of Ophthalmology. Sydney, Australia, April 2002.

Kran, B. S., Lawrence, L., Mayer, D. L., & Heidary, G. (2019, October). Cerebral/cortical visual impairment: a need to reassess current definitions of visual impairment and blindness. In *Seminars in pediatric neurology*, 31, pp. 25–29. WB Saunders. https://dx.doi.org/10.1016/j.spen.2019.05.005

Lee & Mesfin (2022). Statpearls—Blindness. National Institutes for Health—National Library of Medicine. www.ncbi.nlm.nih.gov/books/NBK448182/#:~:text=Total%20blindness%20is%20a%20term,have%20some%20level%20of%20vision.

Lueck, A. H., Dutton, G. N., & Chokron, S. (2019, October). Profiling children with cerebral visual impairment using multiple methods of assessment to aid in differential diagnosis. *Seminars in Pediatric Neurology* (31), 5–14. https://doi.org/10.1016/j.spen.2019.05.003

Mayo Clinic (n.d.). Retinal diseases. www.mayoclinic.org/diseases-conditions/retinal-diseases/symptoms-causes/syc-20355825#dialogId2995641

Moodley, A. (2016). Vision and the brain. *Community Eye Health*, *29*(96), 61–63.

Ortiz-Terán, L., Ortiz, T., Perez, D. L., Aragón, J. I., Diez, I., Pascual-Leone, A., & Sepulcre, J. (2016). Brain plasticity in blind subjects centralizes beyond the modal cortices. *Frontiers in Systems Neuroscience*, *10*, 61. https://doi.org/10.3389/fnsys.2016.00061

United States Census Bureau (2020). 2020 American community survey—variable S1810 disability characteristics. https://data.census.gov/table?q=disability&g=0100000US&tid=ACSST1Y2021.S1810

United States Census Bureau (2021). Disability glossary. www.census.gov/topics/health/disability/about/glossary.html#par_textimage_317496440

9 Chloe wants to be successful entering college and has Ménière's disease

Neuroscience facilitates our understanding of attending college

Gaye W. Cronin

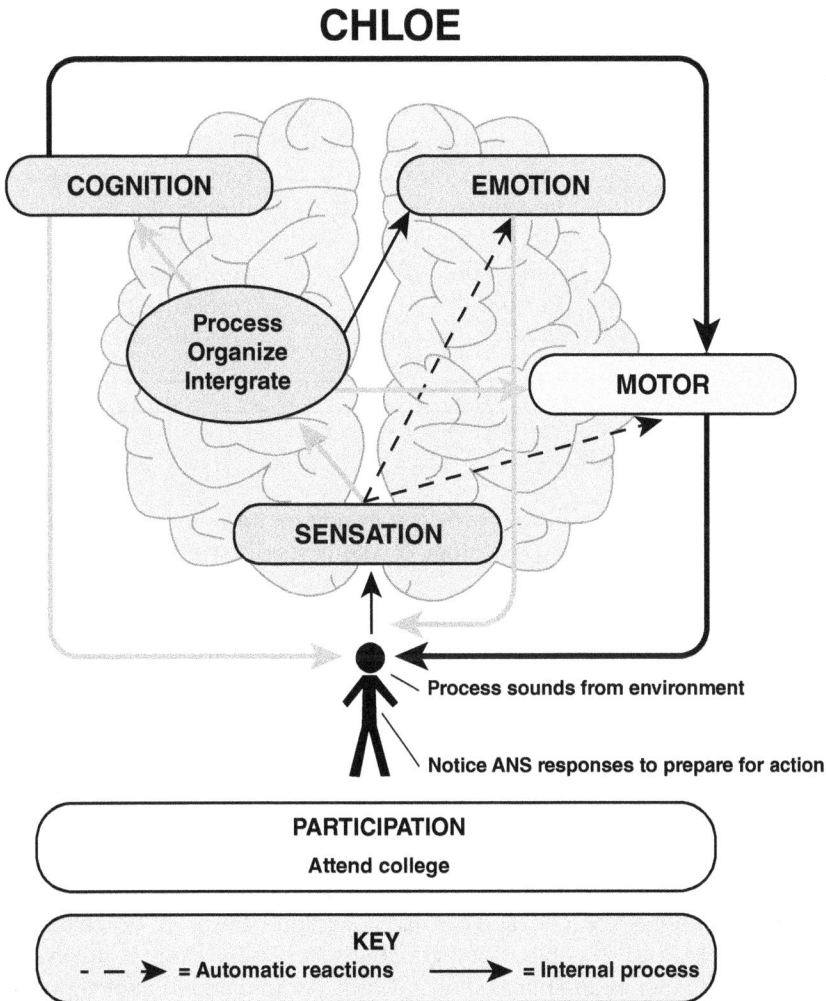

Figure 9.1 Chloe brain figure

DOI: 10.4324/9781003524380-11

Purpose of this chapter

The purpose of this chapter is to explore how Chloe, an 18-year-old getting ready for college, might be affected by Ménière's disease, a condition that changes how the vestibular and auditory systems work. People with Ménière's disease can have full lives with their daily routines, relationships and learning, but may require modifications for function.

The key neuroscience concepts we will explore in this chapter include functions of cranial nerve VIII, the vestibular (balance) and cochlear (hearing) receptors, pertinent neural pathways, the reflexes that are involved and the cortical pathways that support balance and hearing. As with all the chapters these components of the nervous system work with other systems to support overall human function.

Keywords for this chapter are listed in the box below. Be sure you learn what these key features are so that you can get the most out of this chapter.

Keywords for this chapter

cerebellar fixation suppression	hyperacusis	tinnitus
	Ménière's disease	tympanic membrane
cochlea	nystagmus	utricle
cranial nerve VIII	otolith organs	vertigo
cristae ampullae	perilymph	vestibulo-cerebellum
cupula	saccule	vestibulo-spinal reflex
endolymphatic fluid	semicircular canals	vestibulo-ocular reflex

---

Box 9.1   Learning activity

Prior to reading the case, consider: why is it important for an occupational therapy practitioner to understand the physiology of Ménière's disease?

Keywords: Ménière's disease, endolymph, vestibular disorders

Chloe, an 18-year-old cis-gender woman that is college bound

Chloe applied to the University of Georgia and was accepted for Fall admission of 2023. She was diagnosed with left Ménière's disease when she was 16 years old and has managed the disease process with the help of her parents, an otolaryngologist, teachers, an occupational therapist who is a vestibular rehabilitation specialist, and an audiologist. Her maternal aunt also has Ménière's disease, and her mother has a history of vestibular migraine. Chloe's mom is a teacher and her dad is a graphic designer. Chloe has one sister who is 14 years old, and she enjoys being a "big sister." The family is involved in their church and all volunteer at an animal shelter. Chloe participated in contemporary dance in high school that helped her vestibular system by moving with coordination and ankle stability for balance. Chloe is an excellent student and with accommodations completed advanced placement courses and finished high school with a 3.96 grade point average. Her goal is to obtain a college degree in a healthcare field.

What is Ménière's disease?

Ménière's disease (MD) affects a person's ability to stay balanced and to hear all sounds in the environment. MD is associated with Cranial Nerve (CN) VIII (vestibulocochlear) and is classified as an episodic vestibular disorder presenting with four classic manifestations: (1) aural fullness (ear pressure); (2) low-medium frequency sensorineural hearing loss in the Ménière's ear; (3) tinnitus (ear noise) in the Ménière's ear; and (4) episodes of vertigo (some refer to as "attacks") usually associated with nausea and vomiting for greater than 20 minutes in duration (Brookler, 1996). MD is believed to be due to a buildup of the endolymphatic fluid resulting in the irritation of the hair cells (sensory receptors) of the cochlea and vestibular apparatus. To understand MD, the structure and function of the ear must be briefly reviewed.

Box 9.2   Learning activity

1. Find images of the cochlea and vestibular apparatus. Find out how the vestibular/auditory structures look and how they work and be ready to discuss.
2. Find articles on unilateral and bilateral MD and share with your study group. Create a list of key features of MD that might affect daily routines. Use this information to discuss the following questions:
3. How can the context of a college campus affect a student that is experiencing vertigo?
4. How could tinnitus affect learning?

Keywords: bilateral Ménière's disease, oscillopsia, hearing loss, vertigo episodes, vestibular imbalance

---

Neuroscience information to guide your thinking about Chloe

Structure and function of the ear

The ear is a very complicated organ and has three distinct parts: outer (external), middle and inner (internal) and contributes to two extremely important sensory functions: hearing and balance. The outer ear includes the auricle (i.e. the ear you see) and the external auditory canal. Its function is to capture sound waves and convey them to the middle ear. The middle ear consists of the tympanic membrane (ear drum) and the auditory ossicles (ear bones): the incus, malleus and stapes. The oval window houses the stapes footplate and the round window in the middle ear has a thin membrane that separates the tympanic cavity from the scala tympani (fluid filled chamber of the cochlea). The function of the middle ear is to preserve the energy contained in a sound wave as it moves from an air medium to a fluid medium (Hughes, 1985). The inner ear develops structurally for specific functions: hearing, balance, motion perception, head orientation, and reflex movements. To be upright against gravity on a small base of support is a remarkable ability and is directly attributable to the vestibular apparatus. The vestibular apparatus consists of the semicircular canals and the otolith organs: utricle and saccule. Our ability to interpret the pitch and volume of sound is dependent on the cochlea. The vestibular apparatus and the cochlea are housed in the labyrinths of the inner ear and are encased in the temporal bone.

The outer and middle ear are air filled and the inner ear is fluid filled. There are two types of fluid in the inner ear: perilymph, which is high in sodium and low in potassium and endolymph, which is high in potassium and low in sodium. The differences in the ionic concentrations between the fluids, coupled with fluid movement caused by head motion or sound waves are the key to the electrical signaling of the hair cells. This is extremely important in the understanding of occupations of movement, communication, safety, and the importance of hydration and diet to keep the electrolyte balance in the inner ear.

Box 9.3   Learning activity

Think about these questions and be ready to discuss with your group.

1. What is the significance of the chemical composition of the endolymph for managing MD?
2. What is the significance of the outer and middle ear being air filled in regard to environmental inputs?

Keywords: Endolymph, anatomy/physiology of ear, air vs fluid balance of ear

---

Box 9.4   Learning activity

Go to the internet and find images of the outer, middle and inner ear and how they lie in the skull. Be sure the images show the relationship between the vestibular (semicircular canals and otolith organs), and auditory (cochlea) receptors including the nerve fibers and hair cells.

Keywords: anatomy of outer, middle and inner ear, outer and inner ear hair cells

---

Box 9.5   Learning activity

In preparation of reading the next section, find an image, figure, or diagram that clearly labels the organ of Corti, auditory portion of CN VIII and the various parts of the brain (i.e., pons, inferior colliculi, thalamus, Heschl's gyrus, Wernicke's area and the supramarginal gyrus) involved with the processing of sound so you can follow the discussion.

Keywords: cranial nerve VIII, central and peripheral ear portions, organ of Corti, vestibular nuclei

Function of the auditory system

The auditory system contains the sense of hearing. It is composed of the sensory organs in the ears. (cochlea) and the auditory processing center in the brain (i.e. the primary auditory cortex and the auditory association areas) in the central nervous system. The pinna receive sound waves as vibrations then transmits these vibrations via the auditory canal to the tympanic membrane (eardrum) in the middle ear. The middle ear bones amplify the vibration sound pressure. In this context sound is an alteration of pressure propagated in as elastic medium. The stapes bone sends vibrations through the oval window to the cochlea causing movement of the perilymph fluid and vibration (because of the fluid movement) of the hair cells in the inner ear. This causes a transformation of acoustic (sound) energy from an air medium to a fluid medium These vibrations bend the hair cells in the organ of Corti and the hair bundles create an electrical signal which is carried along CN VIII (vestibulocochlear nerve). Specific interpretation of sound frequencies occurs along the length of the cochlea. Other hair cells are housed in the tectorial membrane to assist with cochlear amplification (Levine & Oron, 2015).

The information from CN VIII is then sent to the pons and then to the inferior colliculi in the brainstem for auditory processing. The primary auditory cortex brings sound into awareness or gives perception of sounds: harmonies, timing and pitch, identifies sounds, and the location of sounds. The Heschel's gyrus (find on your images) includes Wernicke's area, which assist with emotions associated with sound and memory of sounds. The supramarginal gyrus aids in language comprehension, links sounds to words, and aids in word choice. It is important to note that sounds are integrated in the brain with other types of information. For example, auditory input is integrated with motor signals (involving the cerebellum, cranial nerve motor nuclei and the spinal cord) producing eye movements that allow you to look toward a sound and when necessary, to move toward or away from a sound. Other structures (e.g. the pons and the thalamus) get involved with sound and learning.

If a functional problem occurs within the cochlea or areas of the brain that interpret sound, the person may develop hearing loss, tinnitus or hyperacusis (Wertz et al., 2024). Tinnitus is the hearing of sounds when no external sound is present. The sound can be described as ringing, roaring, air escaping or "crickets." The sound can be very annoying and can affect concentration and be stressful in attempting to fulfill occupations. Tinnitus can be caused by hearing loss, disease, trauma, infection, neurological disorders, vascular insufficiency, medication side effects, or noise exposure. There is subjective and objective tinnitus. The most frequent is subjective where the person hears the noise inside their head. Conversely, objective tinnitus involves sounds that can be heard by other people and is often caused by involuntary twitching of muscles or vascular conditions. Hyperacusis is a severe sensitivity to some frequencies of sound. Hyperacusis can cause anxiety and phonophobia. (fear of noise). This condition can moderately affect a person's participation in social, educational, or work situations.

Hearing terms

Sound is measured by pressure, displacement, and velocity. Two terms associated with sound are intensity and frequency. The intensity of sounds is usually measured in decibels (dB) or pressure measurement. A dB represents the difference between the two sounds. The frequency of sound is referred to as pure tone and is used to describe auditory sensitivity and measures the number of cycles per unit of time reported in hertz (Hz). Pitch is what a person perceives when the frequency of a tone changes. Loudness is psychological perception of intensity. Noise is a periodic, complex, sound. White noises (broad or narrow band) contain all frequencies of the audible spectrum, randomly distributed. White noise is often used for sound habituation training to treat tinnitus and hyperacusis.

Box 9.6   Learning activity

1. Find some examples (APPs) of white noise and how it can be used to treat tinnitus.
2. Find some resources to support your ideas. Think about noises in your environments that you have adapted to such as trains, airplanes, a clock, car noises, etc.
3. Discuss in your small group how white noise helps you and creates distractions.

Keywords: sound habituation, tinnitus treatment, ear-head noises, white noise

---

Function of the vestibular system

The vestibular apparatus sits deep in the temporal bone. It consists of three semicircular canals (anterior, posterior, horizontal) which encode the direction and speed of angular head motions and the otolith organs that give perception of linear motion and head orientation relative to gravity. When the head moves, the endolymph fluid moves in the semicircular canals and stimulates the hair cells that sit at the base of each canal, and this fires the CN VIII (vestibulocochlear). The message is transmitted via this neural pathway to the brainstem and cerebellum for interpretation and processing of movement and balance. The vestibular system then interacts with the sensory systems of vision and proprioception, allowing for our sense of balance. The vestibular system functions are to maintain balance upright against gravity, monitor position and movements of the head, direct and stabilize the gaze of the eyes, and send signals to the brainstem and cerebellum where it is processed and integrated with visual and spinal responses for motor control of the eyes, body and extremities. It is the first sensory system to develop in humans (Hughes, 1985). As the system continues to mature and develop it can have a direct effect on the development of motor performance skills, performance in occupation including work and play, and performance patterns that develop and mature with time. The vestibular system is fully developed at birth and matures rapidly. The following section will break down the vestibular apparatus into anatomy and function.

Key points to remember about the vestibular system include its maturity even during fetal development, and its important role in motion and gravity experiences. Remember the vestibular portion of CN VIII innervates the utricle, saccule and the semicircular canals.

Box 9.7   Learning activity

Find out more about:

1. The differences in function of the otoliths and SCCs.
2. The distinct functions of the peripheral and central vestibular systems.

Keywords: vestibular receptors, otoliths, ear gravity receptors, ear rocks, semicircular canals, peripheral-central vestibular mechanisms

Semicircular canals

The two sets of three semicircular canals (SCCs) (one set on each side of your head), lie at 90-degree right angles (orthogonal) of each other. Find them on the images you found on the internet (Box 9.4). The names of the canals are the anterior (also referred to as the superior), the posterior (also referred to as the inferior), and the horizontal (also referred to as the lateral). There is an enlarged base of each canal called the cristae ampullae. Hair cells (stereocilia) sit on the crista and protrude into a gelatinous wedge called the cupula which is the sensory end organ. Hair cells are motion detectors, and they move with head movements. The degree of hair cell excitation or inhibition is related to how much the fluid moves in response to head and body movements.

Look at the images you gathered: you will see the anterior and posterior canals come together at the top (in an upright person) and form the common crus. The canals are connected in the center to the utricle and saccule and these spaces are filled with endolymphatic fluid. The anterior and posterior canals sit at 45 degrees off the head sagittal plane, with the horizontal canal approximately 30 degrees pitched upward toward the top of the head in a horizontal plane. Each SCC is responsible for certain head movements and together they keep the brain apprised of head position in space. When the endolymph moves in the SCCs they trigger the hair cells, which then sends a message to the brain. The SCCs work in pairs, with one side being inhibited or facilitated when the other is being facilitated: that is how one knows direction of movement. The ipsilateral anterior SCC is paired with the contralateral posterior SCC. It is equal and opposite in motion. In cases such as MD the endolymphatic fluid is imbalanced causing abnormal movement of the hair cells in the canals creating wrong sensations of motion, such as spins or rotation. The alignment is important for assessment of function of this particular part of the vestibular apparatus. For example, if a patient presents with poor tolerances of horizontal head motions with resultant vertigo, the problem could be arising from dysfunction in the horizontal SCC.

Box 9.8   Learning activity

Discuss this question with your group: why does knowing that the semicircular canals sitting at 90-degree angles become important in head alignment for fluid movement in the canals such as in MD?

Keywords: anatomy of the semicircular canals; alignment of SCC for function and perception

---

Otoliths

The utricle and saccule sit in the center of the SCCs and house the otoliths, which contain calcium carbonate crystals often referred to as "ear rocks or stones" that are reported in size of 5–7 µm (Asadi et al., 2016). The otoliths are stimulated by linear, gravitational, and head tilt motions that cause displacement of the otolithic membranes. Look at the images you found on the internet (Box 9.4) and find the following structures as you read.

The utricle lies in a horizontal plane and the saccule sits in a vertical plane. Both organs contain a wedge of hair cells called the macula. The cilia are inside the otolithic membrane, and the otoliths sit on the otolithic membrane. When the head is level against gravity the otolithic membrane presses on the hair cells for vertical alignment. When the head is tilted the otolithic membrane moves the cilia (hair cells). The otolithic membrane is a gelatinous mass that contains hair cells and is covered with the calcium carbonate crystals referred to as otoliths. The otoliths in the utricle respond to head tilts, ocular shift and ocular tilt and the saccule contains the gravity receptors. The otoliths sense acceleration forward and backward, left or right, up and down. Most utricle signals elicit eye movements while most saccule signals send impulses to skeletal muscles for posture (Asadi et al., 2016).

Box 9.9   Learning activity

1. Locate an image of the inner ear "stones" or otoliths.
2. Discuss with peers the importance of the otoliths and motion detectors in the semicircular canals for classroom and environmental interactions.

Keywords: ear "rocks," calcium carbonate crystals, otoliths, gravity ear receptor, linear ear receptor

---

The central vestibular system

Box 9.10   Learning activity

1. Locate images of the vestibulo-cerebellum (the flocculonodular lobe) and the brainstem nuclei.
2. Locate an anatomy brainstem image of the vestibular nerve combining input from cranial nerves III, IV, and VI.

Keywords: vestibular brainstem nuclei, vestibulo-cerebellum, vestibulo-ocular neural pathways

---

The vestibular nerve has two bundles that make the superior and inferior branches. The superior portion provides neural activity from the anterior and horizontal SCCs and utricle to the brain. The inferior portion provides neural activity from the posterior SCC and saccule. These nerve branches join with the cochlear nerve portion at the medulla of the brainstem and travels to the brainstem nuclei (superior, medial, lateral, inferior), the cerebellum (vestibulo-cerebellum), extraocular nuclei and spinal cord. Find the vestibular brainstem nuclei in your images.

Vestibular signals originating from the vestibular apparatus interact with other sensory signals at the vestibular nuclei. The otoliths also have direct projections to the cerebellum to perceive motion, compare sensory input, calculate spatial relationships, and monitor gravitational relationships. The integration of vestibular and visual input is so important there is a special section of the cerebellum dedicated to the integration called the vestibulocerebellum in the flocculonodular lobe. This section is essential for visual fixation for balance. The afferent information (sensory input) is coordinated with the central mechanisms from the cerebellum and brainstem to provide the efferent (output) reflexes to the muscles controlling the eyes, neck and spinal cord. The brainstem nuclei on each side of the brainstem coordinate information regarding movement and body position via these pathways: the cerebellum, the nuclei of cranial nerves III (oculomotor), IV (trochlea), and VI (abducens), the spinal cord, and the thalamus for head and body control. Image all of these actions taking place in milliseconds to keep your head and body oriented in space and time. Isn't it amazing? Because many of these actions need to occur so quickly, there are efferent (output) reflexes that trigger automatically to keep the head and body oriented: if we had to think about these adjustments, we would fall down before we could make them, such as in MD.

Box 9.11   Learning activity

People with Ménière's disease use cerebellar fixation to attempt to stop the nystagmus associated with a Ménière's attack. How would visual motion of a campus influence this ability?

Keywords: cerebellar visual fixation suppression

Vestibular reflexes

The automatic efferent (output) reflexes are the vestibulo-ocular (VOR), vestibulo-spinal (VSR) and the vestibulocollic (VCR). Vestibular reactions are modulated by central nervous system inhibition and adaptation and cerebellar control. As stated above these reflexes provide automatic, quick responses to keep us oriented in space and time.

The vestibulo-ocular reflex

The purpose of the vestibulo-ocular reflex (VOR) is to maintain stable vision on the retina's fovea (fovea fixation or gaze stabilization) during head and body movements and to provide conjugate eye-head coordination to see clearly so the eyes rotate opposite to the head movements. The VOR does not depend upon the visual system even though when people have VOR dysfunction they report blurred vision because the images are not stable on the retina. The VOR can work in the dark and with eyes closed. For example, a visually impaired patient can still experience VOR dysfunction resulting in instability. This reflexive movement stabilizes the images on the retina during and after head movements. Inputs from the otoliths and SCCs go to the brainstem nuclei and projections go the nuclei of cranial nerves III (oculomotor), IV (trochlear), and VI (abducens). This information forms a three-nerve arc and then travels to the paired extraocular rectus and oblique muscles to coordinate eye movements.

VOR tests of function include rotary nystagmus tests and caloric stimulation that are designed to measure the amplitude and direction of nystagmus (jerky eye movements) produced when the vestibular system is stimulated, eye movement to head movement ratio, and symmetry of eye movements. In normal VOR function, the eye motion, amplitude and velocity should be equal and opposite to the head movement for stabilization of gaze. The VOR response is present at birth and is adultlike by two months (Lane, 2005).

Box 9.12   Learning activity

1. Locate VOR images, videos of nystagmus and function to see this in action.
2. Find a video that shows caloric stimulation testing.

Keywords: caloric testing, nystagmus, videonystagmography (VNG)

Dysfunction of the VOR affects occupations resulting in blurred and distorted vision during reading, riding in a car, watching motion such as a computer screen, walking if they perceive bouncing vision, eye-head coordination and balance affecting eye-foot coordination. The VOR works in tandem with other oculomotor systems of saccades (fast eye movements toward a target) mediated by the cerebellum, smooth pursuits (visual tracking) mediated by multiple systems including the optic tract, reticular formation, cerebellum and parietal lobes, and vergence (aligning visual image on equal parts on the retina making eyes work together). The visual motor system of these functions controls the rectus and oblique muscles, and they are constantly giving neural impulses for steady muscle tension necessary for orientation, movement and stability of the eyes. Chapter 8 explains the visual system further.

Box 9.13   Learning activity

The VOR allows the eyes to rotate equal and opposite to head motion (gain 1:1).
   VOR test: hold your finger at arm's length in front of you at eye level. Keep your eyes on your finger and turn your head side to side for 10 counts as you maintain your focus on your finger. The finger should appear clear and in focus. This indicates the VOR is intact and is referred to as gaze stabilization or fovea fixation.

Keywords: gaze stabilization, VOR

Vestibulo-spinal reflex

The purpose of the vestibulo-spinal reflex (VSR) is to stabilize the head and body by stimulating reflexive, automatic postural adjustments to manage one's relationship to gravity. The VSR works in conjunction with the body's kinesthetic, tactile and proprioceptive sensory systems to orient the body in space. Signals generated by the vestibular inner ear receptors travel through the reticulospinal tracts from brainstem vestibular nuclei then send impulses to the anterior horn cells of the spinal cord. These signals stimulate lower motor neurons that drive skeletal muscles of the extremities and trunk for coordination and movement. Because the purpose of the VSR includes stability and postural adjustments, it contributes to developmental milestones of head control, sitting unsupported, crawling and walking. The balance system is complex and multifaceted to maintain one's body and head against gravity and prevent falls.

   The three key points of skeletal muscle control of the VSR are the neck, thorax and lower extremities, particularly the ankles. An example of a VSR response would be when a person is bumped from behind producing a displacement of the center of gravity. The VSR would signal the lower extremity muscles to co-contract for plantar flexion of the ankles so you can take a step. The VSR must adjust the extremity position to orient the head on the body and to right the head-neck in conjunction with the otoliths.

Box 9.14   Learning activity

Find articles on VSR and its effect on balance, stability and ankle mobility. Share them with your study group.

Keywords: Vesibulo-spinal reflex, postural control, peripheral balance

---

Vestibulocollic reflex

The vestibulocollic reflex (VCR) through co-contraction of the neck muscles (particularly the sternocleidomastoids) stabilizes the head on the neck during ambulation so the head does not jar when a person moves around. Walking stimulates neural receptors of the saccule and signals via the vestibular nerve to the brainstem nucle*i*. Signals are then sent by the VSR and spinal accessory nerve to the neck muscles.

Function of balance and equilibrium

The ability to maintain balance is a complex, orderly, multi-tasked process that occurs between the sensorimotor system, brain, and body. Basically, balance is the ability to maintain the center of body mass within the base of support in any situation and the center of foot pressure also with the center of body mass for ambulation. The brain must receive information from the body's sensory systems of vision, somatosensory/proprioceptive and vestibular systems. When the integrated sensory balance systems are nor working properly this can impede the person's ability to manipulate objects, move safely in their environment, perform self-care, or drive.

Box 9.15   Learning activity

1. Find images, articles and assessments of sensory organization for position in space.
2. Discuss with your group so you can list daily life activities that might be more challenging when sensory organization is affected, and ways to manage.

Keywords: Sensory organization for balance, foam balance activities, position in space sense

---

Sensory organization

The visual system provides a physical reference that orients one's body with the environment (Table 9.1). The eyes view the person in relation to the environment and can calculate motion. The visual system can be fooled, and the brain may miscalculate.

The somatosensory/proprioceptive system gives subconscious information from joint receptors, muscles, proprioceptive, and tactile cues allowing orientation to both the person and to the environment. The input provides the body a sense of relationship to the surfaces for standing, sitting, lying and walking with the main function of allowing the person to remain upright. Proprioception is generated by the vestibulospinal tracts and medial reticulospinal tracts and compared with other senses for balance at the cerebellum. Nerve impulses in the ankle and knees tell the brain about the surface of the ground. Somatosensory inputs are always present.

The vestibular system gives the brain accurate information concerning head movements, orientation of head and body to gravity, postural stability and detects the position of the head in space. The vestibular system is paired and works reciprocally with the opposite side and facilitates coordinated movement with the brain. The brainstem and cerebellum determine the difference in nerve impulses for the two sides to determine the direction, speed and rate of head motions and then signal the VSR and VOR appropriately for environmental interaction.

The sensory organization of vision, proprioception and vestibular is often referred to as a two-sided push-pull system. For example, in static balance, each sensory system contributes equally for steady sensory inputs, conversely in a dynamic motion such as turning, a push-pull (excite-inhibit) response occurs transmitting equal and opposite information from the peripheral systems to the brainstem where motor output to the eyes, neck, and limbs are stimulated to maintain position sense. If there is a conflict in inputs, the cerebellum is called upon to compensate or resolve the conflict. The cerebellum is the main organ for compensation of balance disorders.

The vestibular system is a fast-acting sense used to promote reflexes. Due to the many vestibular stimulations, damage to any part of this complex, multi-connected system will produce vestibular imbalance and abnormal motion perception causing a person to be at

Table 9.1 Sensory organization for position in space

Sensory inputs	Central integration	Output reflexes	Results

Vestibular
Equilibrium reactions
Position in space
Gravity receptors
Angular and linear
  rotation
	Brainstem nuclei
	Integration with other
	  cranial nerve nuclei
	Reticular formation
		Vestibulo-ocular (VOR)
		Ocular motor control
		Gaze stability
		Eye-head coordination
			Balance
			Tolerances of motion
			Stability
			Ocular control

Visual	*Cerebellum*	*Vestibulo-spinal (VSR)*	*Balance*

Acuity
Ocular motor
Vergence
	Comparison with
	  other senses for
	  posture, motor skills,
	  coordination and
	  balance
	Motor plan to spinal
	  cord
		Automatic postural
		  adjustments and
		  reflexes
		Equilibrium reactions
		Head-trunk alignment
		Neck-thorax and ankle
		  stability
			Tolerances of motion
			Stability
			Coordination

Somatosensory	*Cerebrum*	*Vestibulo-collic (VCR)*	*Balance*
Proprioception Kinesthetic Tactile Pressure	Memory and cognition Learning and correction	Co-contraction of neck muscles Head-neck stability	Tolerances of motion Head control Stability Motor memory/position

risk for falls, have decreased postural alignment, perceive that they or their environment is moving inaccurately, have abnormal ocular motor control, including nystagmus and they may experience vertigo. Vertigo is an abnormal perception or illusion of motion.

Box 9.16   Learning activity

Think about all the things you have learned about integration of sensory inputs. Now think about being a college student. How can a college campus and classrooms affect sensory organization inputs?

Keywords: Visual, somatosensory, proprioceptive, vestibular inputs

---

Box 9.17   Learning activity

Case in point: with unilateral MD the input to the vestibulocerebellum is distorted because it is only receiving correct input from one side. The cerebellum is accustomed to receiving equal and opposite inputs from the peripheral vestibular receptors to support balance. When one vestibular system is less active (hypoactive), the contralateral system becomes more active (hyperactive) to attempt to equalize. As the cycle continues, the difference between the 2 sides gets bigger and bigger, as the MD side functions less, and the unaffected side tries to compensate by functioning more. The cerebellum keeps trying to bring the messages into alignment and will now be called upon to suppress the contralateral normal system. This is referred to as the cerebellar clamp or cerebellum suppression. The visual system can also get involved with cerebellar suppression. The cycle of distortion results in nystagmus and vertigo. The cerebellum will signal the visual motor system to fixate their eyes to stop the nystagmus. This is referred to as cerebellar visual fixation suppression.
    How can this process affect daily living and energy?

Keywords: cerebellar suppression

Now back to Chloe

Chloe's parents have been instrumental in watching her low sodium diet, making sure she does her home vestibular exercises, taking her diuretic as needed when the ear pressure or tinnitus increases and providing the necessary modifications for function and occupation. Also, they have made certain her high school nurse has her Zofran (anti-nausea) and meclizine (anti-vertigo) available when she has a Ménière's episode. Now prior to beginning her freshman college year, she and her parents have met with the accommodation's coordinator at the University of Georgia to make sure the following accommodations are in place before Chloe begins school:

1. Closed caption computer programs.
2. School amplification devices for classrooms.
3. Instructor education link on MD for awareness on episodes of vertigo and triggers, including lighting and weather, possibly more time to take exams due to her visual

perceptional problems at times, and the ability to do classes remotely on low atmospheric pressure days or days of feeling an impending episode.

4. On campus mobility accommodations for Chloe when she has an episode (she will not have a car at school).
5. Special diet through school cafeteria for low sodium and limited dairy.
6. Medical alerts in dormitory room for Chloe in the event of an episode.
7. Set up schedule with School Infirmary to check Chloe's electrolytes twice monthly due to her taking a diuretic that possibly decreases potassium causing dehydration.
8. Set up appointments for local Otolaryngologist, Audiologist and Occupational Therapist (specializing in vestibular rehab) and coordinate medical management with school infirmary (see Interventions).
9. Contact the school club dance and physical education to determine if accommodations could be in place for Chloe to participate.

Interventions

Chloe began vestibular rehab therapy (VRT) with occupational therapy (Cronin, 2013) with a therapist who specializes in vestibular rehabilitation when she was diagnosed with MD. The therapy concentrated on safety instructions to do when having an episode, such as sitting or lowering herself to the floor/ground when she experiences the aura that occurs prior to the episode. Chloe experiences a loud "roar" in her left ear approximately 20 minutes before an episode. The therapist has helped Chloe to recognize triggers such as barometric pressure changes, foods high in sodium, repetitive head motions, visual motion including florescent or strobing lights, moving in the dark, stress and fatigue. The therapist has also provided her and her parents on information on supplements of B2 (riboflavin) and magnesium that have been shown to help people suffering from MD and vestibular migraine (Teixido & Carey, 2014). Chloe has specific home vestibular exercises to do between episodes to prevent episodes and to improve vestibular function. Exercises include VOR, VSR balance tasks, gravity movements, dynamic gait tasks, and head-body movements to move the endolymph in her inner ear (Cohen et al., 2017).

Box 9.18   Learning activity

1. Socialization is a big part of college life. What activities/modifications would allow Chloe to have fun as a freshman?
2. Explore vestibular habituation exercises and how they can be incorporated.

Keywords: vestibular habituation exercises, Cawthorne-Cooksey exercises

---

Daily life routine modifications provided by occupational therapy

Chloe's therapist set up the following modifications and will need to continue once at college. Chloe experiences nystagmus "jerking" vision when she has an episode, so the occupational therapist has taught her gaze stability and out of phase eye exercises to do between episodes, so the eyes more readily adjust during an episode and to use cerebellar fixation suppression to do during an episode (focus on something stationary). The therapist advised Chloe's parents to purchase a pair of anti-glare/anti-frequency eyeglasses and a wearing schedule was set up for use with computer and while working under high energy lights. These situations can provoke nystagmus and dizziness. Chloe will also use lamps with green lights in her dormitory room to cancel out florescent lights that can be a trigger for Chloe. Lamps can also provide good illumination for work surfaces.

Chloe cannot lie flat during an episode, so she has a bed wedge she sleeps on during the episodes. She also does side-lying and sit up type exercises between episodes to build tolerances and rolling mat exercises to keep the endolymph moving. She allows extra time for self-care to limit abrupt motions and uses "no tears" shampoo for washing her hair so she does not have to close her eyes in the shower to limit risk for falls. She uses her eyes to compensate for balance and is very visually dependent. Chloe has musician ear plugs to wear when she attends concerts or sporting events to prevent hyperacusis and has purchased a sound machine to use while sleeping for a sound enriched environment and to aid in masking the tinnitus. This encourages the brain to hear the machine instead of the tinnitus to aid in sound habituation. The machine will be in her dorm room at college.

Otolaryngology (ear, nose, and throat doctor) and audiology

Chloe's otolaryngologist does annual audiograms to assess her hearing. Chloe has a low frequency hearing loss. She has a hearing aid for her left ear that has also been programmed to mask and habituate the tinnitus. The hearing can decrease during an episode, if this happens, she may need oral steroids to reduce the swelling and irritation caused by the endolymphatic fluid imbalance. If vertigo episodes do not abate, he may inject her ear directly with dexamethasone (steroid). Chloe's had 4 of these injections.

Conclusion

MD can affect all occupational performances, but with proper medical and therapeutic management, accommodations, adaptations and a motivated person it can be managed. Knowing the neuroscience underpinnings of MD helps us to properly treat and support people with MD to live a satisfying life. With all in place, Chloe should be able to begin college and have a positive and hopefully fun learning experience as she works toward her goal of obtaining a college degree possibly in healthcare.

Box 9.19   Learning activity

With your small group, complete the table in the Appendix about the integration of Chloe's sensory, motor, cognitive and emotional needs to begin college and have a positive and fun learning.

Keywords: Vestibular effects on function and cognition

Further reading

If you are interested in learning more about the auditory and vestibular systems and the live experiences of people with MD-here are some additional sources for you.

Auditory system. https://en.wikipedia.org/wiki/Auditory.system. Accessed January 7, 2023.

Ménière's disease book and education materials published by the National Vestibular Disorders As-
   sociation. www.vestbular.org January 2023.
Ménière's disease. http://en.wilipedia.org/Ménière's disease. Accessed January 7, 2023.
Ménière's Society. www.ménière's.org January 2023.
Vestibular system. http://en.wikipedia.org/wiki/Vestibular_system. Accessed January 7, 2023

References

Asadi, H., Mohamed, S., Lim, C., Nahavandi, S. (2016). A review on otolith models in human perception. *Behav Brain Res.* 309: 67–76.
Brookler, K. (1996). CHE Guidelines for Ménière's disease. *Otolaryngol Head Neck Surg.* 114(6):
   836–837.
Cohen, H., Burkhardt, A, Cronin, G., McGuire, M. (2017). Specialized knowledge and skills in adult
   vestibular rehabilitation for occupational therapy practice. *Am J Occup Ther.* 60 (6): 669–678.
Cronin, G. (2013). Vestibular rehabilitation. In: O'Reilly, R., Morlet, T., Cushing, S. eds. *Manual of
   pediatric balance disorders.* San Diego, CA: Plural Publishing.
Hughes, G. (1985). *Textbook of clinical otology.* New York: Thieme-Stratton.
Lane, K. (2005). *Developing ocular motor and visual perceptual skills.* Thorofare, NJ: Slack.
Levine, R., & Oron, Y. (2015). Tinnitus: The human auditory system. *Handbook Clin Neurol.* 129:
   409–431.
Teixido, M., & Carey, J. (2014). Migraine: More than a headache. www.anausa.org/images/2022/
   articles/Migraine_-_More_than_a_Headache.pdf
Wertz J., Ruttiger L., Bender B., Klose, U., Stark R., Konrad D., Saemisch J., Braun C., Singer W.,
   Dalhoff E., Bader K., Wolpert S., Knipper M., Munk M. (2024). Differential cortical activation
   patterns: pioneering sub-classification of tinnitus with and without hyperacusis by combining
   audiometry, gamma oscillations and hemodynamics. *Front Neuroscience*, 4(17), 1232446.
   doi:10.3389/fnins 2023.

10 Lydia wants to volunteer and has fibromyalgia

Neuroscience facilitates our understanding of volunteering

Rose McAndrew and Sarah Doerrer

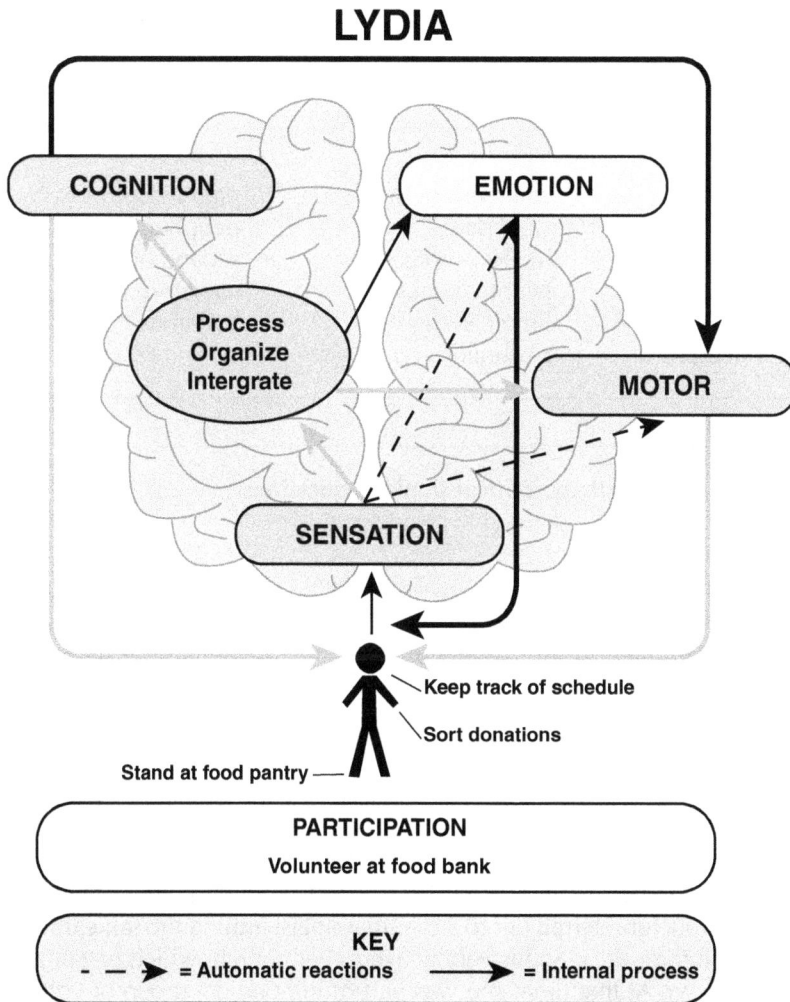

Figure 10.1 Lydia brain figure

DOI: 10.4324/9781003524380-12

Purpose of this chapter

The purpose of this chapter is to discover how Lydia, a 67-year-old woman who wants to continue to volunteer at her local food bank, might be affected by her chronic pain and fibromyalgia. People with chronic pain have full lives with their daily routines, relationships, and learning, but may require modifications for function.

The key neuroscience concepts we will explore in this chapter include exploring the mechanism of nociception and comparing to changes in the brain in chronic pain. We will use fibromyalgia as an example of a chronic pain diagnosis you might encounter when working with people with chronic pain in clinical practice. We will also explore other symptoms that people with fibromyalgia experience and take a deeper dive in the neuroscience behind these symptoms and how they affect a person's ability to participate in volunteering.

As with all the chapters, these components of the nervous system work with other systems to support overall human function. Keywords for this chapter are listed in the box below. Be sure you learn what these key features are so you can get the most out of the chapter.

Keywords for this chapter

allodynia	gate-control theory	pain receptors
amygdala	of pain	peripheral sensitization
central sensitization	hippocampus	second order neurons
cingulate gyrus	hypothalamus	somatosensory cortex
fibromyalgia	limbic system	thalamus
first order neurons	midbrain	

Box 10.1 Learning activity: critical thinking questions

Prior to reading the case:

1. How do you think the symptoms of chronic pain will affect Lydia's volunteer work?
2. Why is it important for an occupational therapy practitioner to understand the neurology of chronic pain?

Let's find out more about Lydia

Lydia retired seven years ago as a home health nurse after muscle pain made it difficult for her to continue to be on her feet all day and to transfer individuals without support. Her primary care doctor referred her to a rheumatologist around the same time who diagnosed her with fibromyalgia. She is very active in her church, which began a food bank about five years ago. At that time, she was part of the original group of volunteers who turned the idea of giving back to their community into action. The foodbank is open three days a week (M-W-F) for individuals to obtain food and is open on Saturday to accept food donations. Additionally, on Tuesdays, volunteers use their own vehicles to make trips to several local grocery stores to obtain perishable items, such as fruit and vegetables, that the stores no longer want to sell but are still viable.

About six months ago, Lydia found that standing for long periods of time increased her fatigue. The day after extended standing periods she also noticed an increase in diffuse pain throughout her body. When she volunteers at the foodbank, Lydia notices that she must stand more on Saturdays than the other weekdays due to needing to sort the donations and placing them on appropriate baker's racks, shelves, or in the small, refrigerated case the food bank uses. She continues to do Tuesday donation pick up as much as she can tolerate, but this activity requires a lot of repetitive movements and moving quickly to load and unload her car's trunk with boxes. She must remain within the established timeline for each stop to ensure the grocery store does not throw away the donations. A couple of weeks ago Lydia forgot the route she needed to take for the pickup. When she returned to the foodbank, she told the staff that there were limited donations that day because she was embarrassed that a simple task she had performed numerous times before had confused her.

On the days that the foodbank is open for people to obtain food, Lydia mostly chats with the families, some of whom are members of her church, or she knows from years of home health nursing. Previously, she knew the inventory well and helped the people find what they might be needing that week, but recently she has had difficulty remembering where certain items are. Nonetheless, she loves this part of her job the most because she can connect with the local community, and she sees how much the food bank is benefiting them.

Lydia is frustrated that she continues to hurt all over her body and is tired all the time. She is scared that she will have to give up volunteering, as just like paid work, volunteering provides her benefits, including social connectedness, contributions to society, and structure and routine to daily life (American Occupational Therapy Association, 2020). If she were unable to participate in this volunteer work, she would experience a loss of a daily routine and social isolation, likely impacting her health and well-being. Thus, she wants to continue volunteering at the food bank, which she now is doing on Monday, Tuesday, and Saturday, for 6–8 hours at a time, depending on the day and the number of volunteers present. She downplays her discomfort to the other volunteers, saying that she doesn't want to "be a burden." No one at her church or at the food pantry knows about her diagnosis of fibromyalgia because she believes there is a stigma attached to this disease. Lydia's pain and fatigue are real and having a disability that no one knows about is stressful. Lydia tried opiates in the past while she was still working as a nurse, but they made her feel sluggish and she did not really get any relief. Lydia is anxious that she will have to give up her volunteer work, something that is important to her socially and spiritually and gives her life productivity. She already had to retire from a job she loved for decades, and she is thinking constantly what her increased symptoms mean for her future.

Box 10.2   Learning activity: peer discussion and active learning

1. Having read the narrative, what are you curious about?
2. What do you need to know more about?
3. As a group, look up the definition and symptoms of fibromyalgia.

Keywords: fibromyalgia, symptoms, neuroscience

Fibromyalgia (FM) is a chronic condition that impacts daily life activities (American College of Rheumatology, 2021). Physicians, usually rheumatologists, rely on careful history and exam to make this diagnosis as there is no specific blood, or other diagnostic, test that can diagnose FM. Unlike other many diseases that rheumatologists treat, FM is not an autoimmune or inflammatory disease, but instead is a disorder of the nervous system.

Box 10.3　Learning activity: critical thinking questions

Prior to exploring the remainder of this chapter consider the following questions:

1. What is the difference between nociception and a pain response?
2. What neurological mechanisms interpret stress or fear, and how does that contribute to interpretation of pain?
3. What is the relationship between pain and cognition? Between pain and fatigue?
4. How do feelings of stress and fear, cognitive changes, and increased fatigue contribute to our ability to participate in productivity roles such as volunteering?

Now that you have had some time to think about these questions and have a preliminary definition of FM, the rest of this chapter will take a deeper dive in the neuroscience of how a person experiences and interprets pain. This chapter will also explore the phenomenon of central sensitization, how stress affects the interpretation of pain, and the specific neuroscientific underpinnings of FM.

Neuroscience to guide your thinking about Lydia

Pain response

Pain is a primary reason many individuals seek out non-routine medical care. It is a necessary survival mechanism to let us know about potential harmful damage to our body. However, pain is a subjective and personal experience that is influenced by not only injury to body structures but also psychological and social factors (International Association for the Study of Pain, 2021). Because of the psychological and social factors effect on the pain experience, we know that the pain network not only involves pain receptors in the body but also pathways in the brain that interpret the meaning of the pain.

Box 10.4　Learning activity: peer discussion

In a small group, discuss your experiences with pain:

1. Have you ever been injured but not notice any pain? What were you doing at that time?
2. Have you ever been in so much pain that you can vividly recall every detail of what happened?
3. Have you ever physically felt uncomfortable when seeing someone else injured or in pain?
4. Have you ever had long-term (chronic) pain that stopped you from doing the things that were meaningful and important to you?
5. How do you think health professionals have historically treated individuals who have pain with no identifiable injury or trauma?

While other chapters of this book discuss symptoms or behaviors that you may not have personally experienced, pain is nearly universal. Pain interpretation is complex, and new discoveries of the neural processes involved occur every day. Pain interpretation involves body structures and neural pathways both within the central nervous system (CNS) and the peripheral nervous system (PNS). Our experience of pain includes an afferent neural pathway via stimulation in the PNS as well as an efferent neural pathway starting in the brain and moving into the spinal cord and the PNS. Both determine how much pain we actually feel—the subjective experience of pain. We will now look at these neural processes before we can take a closer look at how living with FM shapes Lydia's pain experience and contributes to her other symptoms affecting her ability to participate in volunteering.

Afferent pathway

The process of encoding noxious stimuli in the body is known as nociception (processing of harmful stimuli), with designated sensory receptors in the PNS, known as nociceptors, present in muscles, joints, skin, organs, and nerves (Sneddon, 2017). These nociceptors include fast-moving (myelinated) Aδ-fibers, resulting in short-lasting, pin-prick type sensations, and slow-moving (unmyelinated) C-fibers, resulting in the feeling of non-specific, longer-lasting, dull pain (Garland, 2012; Sneddon, 2017; Yam et al., 2018). These signals are transferred from the PNS to the CNS (Garland, 2012).

Box 10.5   Learning activity

1. Find a schematic drawing of the path of a peripheral sensory nerve carrying pain information into the spinal cord. Identify the dorsal horn of the spinal cord, first order neurons, and secondary neurons in this path. Be sure to define these terms.
2. What is the spinal tract that carries pain information to the brain? Diagram its path to the brain. Note whether it stays on the same side of the body or crosses to the other side.

Keywords: peripheral sensory nerve, dorsal horn of spinal cord, schematic drawing

---

First order neurons synapse with second order neurons and ascend to the brain for interpretation. As the signals of noxious (harmful) stimuli ascend to the brain, a phenomenon known as Gate Control is one way to mitigate the signal of strong pain (Melzack & Wall, 1965; Mendell, 2014). An inhibitory neuron at the synapse of the first and second order neurons can "close the gate" to the incoming nociceptive signal if activated.

Box 10.6   Learning activity

Can you connect an experience that you had that illustrates the phenomenon of "closing the gate" in the gate-control theory of pain? *Hint: think of a time when you stubbed your toe or bumped your arm. What are some things that you did when that happened, perhaps subconsciously?*

Pertinent neuro-molecules in the afferent pathway

Throughout this textbook, you will learn about numerous neurotransmitters (chemical messengers between neurons) and their relationship with specific diagnoses and their effect on participation for clients we see in occupational therapy. In relationship to pain transmission, there are several neurotransmitters and neuropeptides (small proteins that modulate information transmission between synapses) pertinent to our understanding of this process. In the afferent pathway, these molecules facilitate the transmission of pain; that is to say, their presence means that pain is perceived.

Although there are many neurotransmitters involved in pain, we will discuss two pertinent to Lydia and FM. Glutamate is a major excitatory neurotransmitter found through the nervous system and is related to pain sensation and transmission (Bán, 2020). Additionally, Substance P is a neuropeptide implicated in nociception (Bán, 2020). It is associated with the emotional connection with pain (Littlejohn, 2020).

Subcortical and cortical areas involved with interpretation of pain: Nociceptive signals reach the thalamus via the second order neuron and then are sent to various other parts of the limbic system and cerebral cortex. These higher-level centers provide the personal experience of pain.

Box 10.7   Learning activity

Describe the basic function of the following structures and in relation to pain:

1. Thalamus.
2. Amygdala.
3. Cingulate gyrus.
4. Hippocampus.
5. Hypothalamus.

In the thalamus pain is filtered taking into account factors psychological and social factors mentioned in the definition provided earlier from IASP. These areas cause us to pay attention (or not) to the incoming sensory information and contribute to how we interpret the pain. Many of us have had experiences where we cut or bruised ourselves and did not realize until hours later. This event occurs because our brains took the incoming nociceptive signals and determined these signals did not require our attention. Maybe we were doing something else fun or even something frightening and the brain simply concluded, "this minor injury is not important to us right now." Perhaps you have experienced the opposite phenomenon. Sometimes our pain is so awful that we avoid that activity (or environment) completely in the future. Experiences with strong emotional content tend to stick, with fearful memories causing a person to avoid this stimulus in the future (Tyng et al., 2017).

To take a deeper dive in to the specific areas of the brain that gives the personal experience of pain, we are going to look closer at the limbic system and the cerebral cortex.

Now let's take a closer look at how the limbic system works regarding pain:

- The **amygdala** connects the process of nociception with emotions and plays a role in forming memories around pain, especially if the event causes fear or aversion. (Urien & Wang, 2019).

- The **cingulate gyrus** (cortex) plays a role in the affective (emotional) process of pain, such as unpleasantness and avoidance and allows us to predict future scenarios that may induce the unpleasantness associated with pain (Xiao & Zhang, 2018).
- The **hippocampus** links current stimulus to previously formed memories regarding pain and is especially implicated in the negative affect and avoidance during chronic pain and chronic stress cycles (Emad et al., 2018; Rolls, 2019).
- The **hypothalamus** links the other brain regions that play a crucial role in chronic pain and its regulation (Pop et al., 2018; Tyng et al., 2017).

Box 10.8   Learning activity: active learning

1. Find pictures showing the location of these structures: (i) primary somatosensory cortex; (ii) orbitofrontal cortex; (iii) insula.
2. Find a picture (or two pictures) that show the limbic system and the cerebral cortex and their relationship to the thalamus and each other, including the pathways between these areas. (in other words, the pain perception network)

The cerebral cortex is also important to consider with the personal experience of pain. As you have been learning throughout this textbook, the cerebral cortex is vast and responsible for many neural processes. We will look at a few pertinent areas relating to this chapter:

- The **primary somatosensory cortex** determines where in the body the nociceptive stimulus occurred (Kim et al., 2015). This process allows us to locate the area of pain.
- The **orbitofrontal cortex** gives value to the stimulus and whether this stimulus is rewarding or punishing (Rolls et al., 2020). Most of the time, we consider pain to be unpleasant and the orbitofrontal cortex helps determine how strongly we perceive the pain.
- The **insula** activates during noxious stimulation, like a pinprick or burn. As such, the insula helps us pay attention to new and novel information among many incoming stimuli (Uddin, 2017). It also assigns subjective feelings and emotion to an experience and is responsible for our ability to physically feel other people's pain, if you recollected the experience at the introduction of this chapter (Xiao & Zhang, 2018). Lastly, the insula is involved with interoception, or our overall internal state, such as hunger or fatigue (Uddin, 2017).

We can now see the close connection of the cerebral cortex which distinguishes, localizes, assigns value, and is responsible for reactions such as empathy for others and the limbic system which connects memory and determines a response. If you look at the pictures you found of the neural connections between these systems, consider them bi-directional: these brain centers influence each other (Urien & Wang, 2019).

Efferent pathway

Lastly, it is important to consider how efferent signals alter the pain experience. The structures of the limbic system and cerebral cortex contribute to the "top-down" modulation of pain, where they assist in determining how many incoming nociceptive signals reach the brain in the first place.

Box 10.9   Learning activity

1. Locate pictures of the periaqueductal gray area, the midbrain, and the medulla.
2. Diagram the descending pain pathway.

This descending neuropathway occurs through activation of an area of the midbrain, known as the periaqueductal gray (PAG), and the medulla (Treede, 2016). These areas receive information from the higher brain structures mentioned above about the location, value, and emotional attachment of pain. You can appreciate how an increase in fear-based emotion, the recollection of old memories of similar pain, or determining that the stimulus is a punishment makes your body ensure all incoming information is interpreted as a necessary for survival.

Pertinent neurotransmitters in the efferent pathway

Like in the afferent pathway, neurotransmitters in the efferent pathway affect how much pain we feel, but conversely, these neurotransmitters act as inhibiters to pain perception, or antinociception (Sawaddiruk et al., 2017). Gamma-aminobutyric acid (GABA) is the main inhibitory neurotransmitter in the CNS (Yam et al., 2018), with the opposite influence of glutamate in the afferent pathway. The presence of the right amount of GABA "slows down" the brain and thus, decreases the amount of pain we feel. Dopamine is an important neurotransmitter related to motor function and pleasure and is discussed in-depth in several chapters in this text. Interestingly, is also involved with antinociception (blocking detection of pain from a harmful stimulus) (Wood et al., 2007) and possibly cognition (Albrecht et al., 2016). Naturally occurring opioids, known as endogenous opioids, including endorphins and enkephalins, also decrease the feeling of pain (Sneddon, 2017). You may have heard of (or experienced) "runner's high," which is the activation of endogenous opioids in our bodies.

Central sensitization

Above you learned the neuroscience underpinning the pain experience. However, sometimes pain continues long after the initial trauma or injury. A phenomenon known as central sensitization is important to understand the neuroscience behind chronic pain.

Box 10.10   Learning activity

1. Look up the definition and mechanism of central sensitization.
2. Look up the definition of peripheral sensitization.
3. Define these terms: hyperalgesia, allodynia, secondary hyperalgesia, and wind-up.

Central sensitization can occur with any injury but is also present in people with chronic diseases, such as Lydia's (Woolf, 2011). Central sensitization includes both pronociception and antinociception. The combination of pronociception (facilitated pain perception) and impaired antinociception results in hyperalgesia (Ichesco et al., 2014; Sawaddiruk et al., 2017; Treede, 2016). Over time this mechanism becomes more pronounced and in individuals with chronic pain, pain can be felt without any stimulus at all.

In a typical pain response, there is a correlation between the amount of input from the peripheral nociceptors and the perception of pain (Lundy-Ekman, 2018). If someone pinches you, you will feel the pinch, and it may hurt for the time it is happening then you would soon forget about it. Now imagine getting kicked in the shin during a soccer match, causing an injury to the soft tissue and a bone contusion. In a normal response to injury, there is a prolonged nociceptive input because of peripheral sensitization (Lundy-Ekman, 2018). For example, a cold pack placed on the area of the kicked shin would feel very painful compared to an area of the leg with no injury. The abnormal input in response to injury in the periphery also produces a large input into the CNS. This large input to the CNS gives us information that we are hurt, and that we should possibly seek medical care or pain medication. Your hypothetical soccer injury may linger months for your pain to subside. However, over time, your post-injury pain diminishes and eventually goes away. You are no longer hypersensitive at the area of injury and are not conscious of pain.

Conversely, in chronic pain when central sensitization has occurred, the perception of pain can arise without any peripheral input (Lundy-Ekman, 2018). This means that you could be watching TV and start to develop aching pain in your lower back. Your body is telling you that you are injured; however, no acute injury has occurred. You reach behind you and touch your lower back and it is painful to the touch. This phenomenon is referred to as allodynia.

Box 10.11   Learning activity

1. In small groups, compare and contrast central sensitization and peripheral sensitization. Be sure to include these concepts: (a) pronociception; (b) antinociception; (c) hyperalgesia; (d) allodynia.
2. Discuss how your life might be disrupted if you were experiencing central sensitization.

To uncover why someone would develop central sensitization, we can draw from what you have been learning in other chapters about neural plasticity. The phenomenon of neural plasticity is responsible for central sensitization. Think back to your hypothetical soccer injury, where you had a soft tissue injury and bone bruise. What if your physician told you that the injury had healed, but you still had pain? Remember, you had already experienced peripheral sensitization as a normal response to injury, which produced a large output to your CNS neurons. At this point you may start experiencing secondary hyperalgesia. Your neurons are in a state of excessive excitability and the threshold needed to elicit a pain signal has been lowered (Latremoliere & Woolf, 2009; Lundy-Ekman, 2018). Additionally, nociceptive-specific neurons convert to non-specific neurons, causing them to respond to both noxious and innocuous stimuli from the PNS (Latremoliere & Woolf, 2009).

Repeated non-painful stimuli in someone experiencing central sensitization, such as individuals with FM, can result in wind-up, where pain is present even after this non-painful stimulus is removed. In the PNS, during wind-up repetitive C-fiber stimulation causes a pain signal that enters the CNS stronger and longer-lasting (Latremoliere & Woolf, 2009; Sawaddiruk et al., 2017).

Neuroscience of fibromyalgia

Now that we've looked at the pertinent structures and processes involved with pain, including a typical pain response and the phenomenon of central sensitization, we will examine the symptoms experienced by clients with FM, like Lydia, and the neurological changes underlying these symptoms. We will explore how her pain as well as other notable symptoms, causes her difficulty in participation in her chosen occupation of volunteering.

Pain

Pain is a major symptom of FM, and as you have just read, there are many mechanisms in the PNS, spinal cord, and brain that contribute to Lydia's personal pain experience. Lydia's afferent pathway changes parallel those noted in central sensitization. In the brain, numerous studies demonstrate decreased gray matter or activity in the thalamus of individuals with FM (Jenson et al., 2012; Sawaddiruk et al., 2017). In the limbic system, the amygdala has increased activity in clients with FM (Sawaddiruk, et al., 2017). People with FM may have structural changes within the hippocampus similar to changes noted when we are under stress (Emad et al., 2018). Lydia is already under stress because she has not disclosed her disability to the other volunteers and is anxious that she must give up this favorite occupation. Additionally, in people with FM, the cingulate cortex is smaller, has decreased activity, and has fewer connections to other parts of the limbic system and brainstem than people without FM (Sawaddiruk et al., 2017; Jenson et al., 2012; Littlejohn & Guymer, 2020).

Box 10.12   Learning activity: critical thinking questions

In small groups discuss the following questions:

1. How does decreased gray matter in the thalamus affect the way Lydia experiences pain? Feel free to refresh your memory on what makes up gray matter.
2. How does increased activity in the amygdala affect the way Lydia experiences pain?
3. When you are under stress, do you tend to have more positive or negative memories? Use your own your personal experience to help you determine what role the hippocampus has in Lydia in linking the daily tasks and activities she does for her volunteer role to her past?
4. What affect does a smaller cingulate cortex with decreased neural activity have on Lydia's ability to accurately assess sensory stimuli while she is volunteering?

Changes are also noted in the cerebral cortex in clients with FM. In the somatosensory cortex, high levels of activity lead to reduced subjective pain ratings (Kim et al., 2015). However, in people with FM, there is decreased activity and decreased connectivity among regions of the somatosensory cortex. The orbitofrontal cortex also has decreased connectivity with the thalamus, limiting its ability to assign appropriate value to incoming noxious stimuli (Jenson et al., 2012), and perhaps overestimating the strength of all incoming signals. Recent research has focused on the role the insula plays in clients with FM and lower pain threshold they experience. The connectivity between the insula and various parts of the brain and metabolism within the insula are increased in clients like Lydia (Ichesco et al., 2014; Littlejohn & Guymer, 2020). Lydia's interoception is also altered due to these changes in the insula (Liu et al., 2022; Sawaddiruk et al., 2017).

Box 10.13   Learning activity

1. What affect does decreased activity in the somatosensory cortex have on Lydia's pain? Choose one activity that Lydia needs to do from the case study. If Lydia's brain overestimates the strength of incoming sensory signals, how would this activity feel to her when she performs it?
2. How does increased activity in the insula affect Lydia's pain? How does it affect interoception?

Lydia also may have an imbalance in the neurotransmitters and neuropeptides noted in the afferent and efferent pathways you read about above. Increased amounts of glutamate and Substance P have been found in clients with FM (Harte et al., 2018; Sluka & Clauw, 2016; Littlejohn & Guymer, 2020; Singh et al., 2019). Additionally, changes in the antinociceptive pathway may also increase Lydia's pain. Studies note decreased amount of GABA in both the brain (Harte et al., 2018) and spinal cord (Singh et al., 2019) in people with FM. Researchers have observed decreased levels of dopamine in various regions of the brain as well (Albrecht et al., 2016). Lastly, the amount of endogenous opioids may also either be decreased in FM clients or they may have decreased ability to bind these natural pain-relievers (Scherpf et al., 2016; Singh et al., 2019).

Box 10.14   Learning activity

1. What affect does an increase in glutamate and Substance P have on Lydia's pain? How does a decreased amount of GABA throughout her CNS affect the amount of pain Lydia experiences?
2. Why do you think that Lydia did not get relief from the opioids her doctor prescribed her in the past?

Fatigue

While chronic pain is the most common symptom of FM, it is not the only symptom that limits participation. Lydia experiences fatigue during and after her shifts at the food bank, especially when she stands. Alterations in thalamus structure and function exist in people with FM (Kim et al., 2021). While standing in and of itself can be physically tiring, in her brain, changes within the thalamus can exacerbate any physical fatigue that she already experiences for long-term standing without breaks. Recall that the thalamus serves as a relay station to other parts of the brain, and changes here affect other parts of the brain as well, including those involved with pain, linking these common symptoms in FM. Altered interoception also leads to overall body fatigue (Liu et al., 2022).

Box 10.15   Learning activity

In a small group, think about a time you felt fatigued (perhaps due to sleeping poorly). How did that affect your ability to perform your daily activities and schoolwork?

Cognition

You have been learning about the importance of functional cognition for participation in occupation, and Lydia's volunteering at her church's food bank is no different. Her volunteer work involves many tasks that requires executive functioning, process skills, and insight within the context of the church community, which would add a social component to this role. Lydia may have difficulty with these factors, which we will explore in-depth.

Repeated research indicates that people with chronic pain have poorer cognition than people without FM.

Box 10.16   Learning activity

1. What kinds of cognitive problems have you experienced when you are in pain or fatigued?
2. What is the common term used by people with FM to describe their cognitive problems?

People with FM have difficulty with executive functioning (Bunk et al., 2019). People with FM often complain of difficulties in mental clarity, attention, multitasking, and memory (Kravitz & Katz, 2015; McCrae et al., 2015). Individuals with FM rate their cognitive problems as having a high impact on their ability to live their daily lives (Kravitz & Katz, 2015). Research focusing on underlying factors needed for process skills like working memory function (Mercado et al., 2021) and reaction time (Martinsen et al., 2014) document decreased function in individuals with FM. In clients like Lydia, there is also decreased activity in the frontal lobe during tasks that require attention (Samartin-Veiga et al., 2019). Additionally, the hippocampus is smaller in volume in clients like Lydia (Mc-Crae et al., 2015). There is emerging evidence for decreased dopamine noted in people with FM affecting cognition (Albrecht et al., 2016).

Box 10.17   Learning activity

In small groups, discuss the following:

1. How does attention, working memory, and long-term memory work together in the specific tasks Lydia needs to do when she volunteers at the food bank?
2. How do the changes noted in people with FM affect the ability to participate in these specific tasks?
3. What is the relationship between dopamine and cognition? How does decreased dopamine in the brain affect Lydia's ability to perform her volunteer work?

Back to the person's life: Lydia wants to continue to volunteer at the foodbank

So now that you know more about the neuroscience and functioning in people with FM, how can we use this scientific reasoning to support Lydia in participating in volunteering? You will certainly spend a lot more time in other courses exploring details but knowing the neuroscience underpinnings provides a solid foundation to select intervention options for Lydia.

Box 10.18   Learning activity

In small groups discuss the following: what interventions you can take to help Lydia manage her symptoms of FM. Use the OTPF-4 to consider different approaches to intervention, such as restore and modify. Use your neuroscience knowledge and what you know about Lydia in small groups right now to guide your idea generation.

What do we know about ourselves and the population at large from this brain condition?

Although this chapter focuses on Lydia's lived experience of participating in volunteering with FM, you might have discovered you had some similar experiences in your own life. Her role as a volunteer, like your role as an occupational therapy student, requires many cognitive processes such as mental clarity, attention, multitasking, and memory. You can recognize how the symptoms that Lydia experiences would affect her ability to participate in volunteering, such as knowing the route to take to collect donations, knowing the updated inventory, and relating to other people. Perhaps you have been in so much pain you have found it difficult to concentrate on your schoolwork due to increased activity in the cerebral cortex and limbic system. Possibly you have been under such extreme stress or experiencing such anxiety that your thalamus exacerbated feelings of fatigue which affected your performance on assignments and tests. Look back at the questions at the beginning of this chapter and reflect now how these examples would affect the things you needed to do as a student if you experienced them every day like Lydia. As occupational therapists, one of our core skills is the ability to connect with our clients. Drawing on personal experiences helps us empathize with what our clients are going through and leads to strong rapport-building.

Box 10.19   Learning activity

With your small group, complete the table in the Appendix about how Lydia can volunteer at her local food bank while managing her chronic pain and fibromyalgia.

Further reading

If you are interested in further exploring the lived experience of chronic pain or fibromyalgia, we recommend the following resources:

- Fibromyalgia Care Society of America (n.d.) Voices of Fibro: www.fibro.org/blog-1
- Melissa vs. Fibromyalgia: www.melissavsfibromyalgia.com
- Fibromyalgia Podcast: https://fibromyalgiapodcast.com/
- Fibromyalgia advocacy in action: https://supportfibromyalgia.org/advocacy-fibromyalgia/
- Abril, A. & Bruce, B. K. (2019). *Mayo Clinic guide to fibromyalgia*. Mayo Foundation for Medical Education and Research.

References

Albrecht, D. S., MacKie, P. J., Kareken. D. A., Hutchins. G. D., Chumin, E. J., Christian, B. T., & Yoder, K. K. (2016). Differential dopamine function in fibromyalgia. *Brain Imaging and Behavior*, *10*(3), 829–839. https://doi.org/ 10.1007/s11682-015-9459-4

American College of Rheumatology. (2021, December). Fibromyalgia. www.rheumatology.org/I-Am-A/Patient-Caregiver/Diseases-Conditions/Fibromyalgia

American Occupational Therapy Association (AOTA). (2020). Occupational therapy practice framework: domain and process (4th ed.) *American Journal of Occupational Therapy*, 74(Supplement_2), 7412410010p1–7412410010p87. doi: https://doi.org/10.5014/ajot.2020.74S2001

Bán, E.G., Brassai, A., & Vizi, E.S. (2020). The role of the endogenous neurotransmitters associated with neuropathic pain and in the opiod crisis: The innate pain-relieving system. *Brain Research Bulletin*, *155*, 129–136. https://doi.org/10.1016/j.brainresbull.2019.12.001

Bunk, S., Preis, L., Zuidema, S., Lautenbacher, S., & Kunz, M. (2019). Executive functions and pain. *Zeitschrift Für Neuropsychologie*, *30* (30), 169–196. https://doi.org/10.1024/1016-264X/a000264

Capone, F., Collorone, S., Cortese, R., Di Lazzaro, V., & Moccia, M., (2020). Fatigue in multiple sclerosis: The role of the thalamus. *Multiple Sclerosis Journal*, *26*(1), 6–16. https://doi.org/1352458519851247

Emad, Y., Ragab, Y., Zeid, A., & Rasker, J. J. (2018). Hippocampus dysfunction may explain symptoms of fibromyalgia syndrome. *Hamdan Medical Journal*, *11*(4), 166–168. https://doi.org/10.4103/HMJ.HMJ_82_18

Garland, E. L. (2012). Pain processing in the human nervous system: A selective review of nociceptive and biobehavioral pathways. *Primary Care*, *39*(3), 561–571. https://doi.org/10.1016/j.pop.2012.06.013

Harte, S.E., Harris, R.E., & Clauw, D.J. (2018). The neurobiology of central sensitization. *Journal of Applied Behavioral Research*, *23*(2), Article 12137. https://doi.org/10.1111/jabr.12137

Ichesco, E., Schmidt-Wilcke, T., Bhavsar, R., Clauw, D. J., Peltier, S. J., Kim, J., Napadow, V., Hampson, J. P., Kairys, A. E., Williams, D. A., & Harris, R. E (2014). Altered resting state connectivity of the insular cortex in individuals with fibromyalgia. *Journal of Pain*, *15*(8), 815–826. https://doi.org/10.1016/j.jpain.2014.04.007.

International Association for the Study of Pain. (2021). Terminology. www.iasp-pain.org/resources/terminology/

Jenson, K. B., Loitoile, R., Kosek, E., Petzke, F., Carville, S., Fransson, P., Marcus, H., Williams, S. C. R., Choy, E., Mainguy, Y., Vitton, O., Gracely, R. H., Gollub, R., Ingvar, M., & Kong, J., (2012). Patients with fibromyalgia display less functional connectivity in the brain's pain inhibitory network. *Molecular Pain*, 8(1), article 32.

Kim, D. J, Lim, M., Kim, J. S., Chung, C. K. (2021). Structural and functional thalamocortical connectivity study in female fibromyalgia. *Scientific Reports*, 11(1), Article 23323. https://doi.org/10.1038/s41598-021-02616-1

Kim, J., Loggia., M.L., Cahalan, C. M., Harris, R. E., Beissner, F., Garcia, R. G., Kim, H., Barbieri, R., Wasan. A. D., Edwards, R. R., & Napadow, V. (2015). The somatosensory link in fibromyalgia: Functional connectivity of the primary somatosensory cortex is altered by sustained pain and is associated with clinical/autonomic dysfunction. *Arthritis & Rheumatology*, 67(5), 1395–1405. https://doi.org/ 10.1002/art.39043

Kravitz, H. M. & Katz, R. S., (2015). Fibrofog and fibromyalgia: A narrative review and implications for clinical practice. *Rheumatology International*, 35(7), 1115–1125. https://doi.org/ 10.1007/s00296-014-3208-7.

Latremoliere A. & Woolf, C. J. (2009). Central sensitization: A generator of pain hypersensitivity by central neural plasticity. *Journal of Pain*, 10(9), 895–926. doi: 10.1016/j.jpain.2009.06.012.

Littlejohn G. & Guymer, E., (2020). Key milestones contributing to the understanding of the mechanisms underlying fibromyalgia. *Biomedicines*, 8(7), 223. https://doi.org/10.3390/biomedicines8070223

Liu, H., Chou, K., Lee, P., Wang, Y., Chen, S., Lai, K., Lin, Ch., Wang, S., & Chen, W. (2022). Right anterior insula is associated with pain generalization in patients with fibromyalgia. *Pain*, 163(4), e572–e579. http://dx.doi.org/10.1097/j.pain.0000000000002409

Lundy-Ekman, L. (2018). *Neuroscience: Fundamentals for rehabilitation* (5th edition). Elsevier.

Martinsen, S., Flodin, P, Berrebi, J., Löfgren, M., Bileviciute-Ljungar, I., Ingvar, M., Fransson, P., & Kosek, E., (2014). Fibromyalgia patients had normal distraction related pain inhibition but cognitive impairment reflected in caudate nucleus and hippocampus during the Stroop Color Word Test. *PLOS ONE*, 9(9), Article e108637. https://doi.org/ 10.1371/journal.pone.0108637

McCrae, C. S., O'Shea, A. M., Boissoneault, J., Vatthauer, K. E., Robinson, M. E., Staud, R., Perlstein, W. M., & Craggs, J. G., (2015). Fibromyalgia patients have reduced hippocampal volume compared with healthy controls. *Journal of Pain Research*, 8, 47–52. https://doi.org/ 10.2147/JPR. S71959

Melzack, R. & Wall. P.D (1965). Pain mechanisms: A new theory. *Science*, 150(3699), 971–979. https://doi.org/10.1126/science.150.3699.971

Mendel, L.M. (2014). Constructing and deconstructing the Gate Theory of Pain. *Pain*, 155(2), 210–216. https://doi.org/ 10.1016/j.pain.2013.12.010

Mercado, F., Ferrera, D., Fernandes-Magalhaes, R., Peláez, I., & Barjola, P., (2021). Altered subprocesses of working memory in patients with fibromyalgia: An event-related potential study using N-Back Task. *Pain Medicine*, 23(3), 475–487. https://doi.org/ 10.1093/pm/pnab190.

Paul, J. K., Iype, T., Dileep, R., Hagiwara, Y., Koh, J. W., & Acharya, U. R., (2019). Characterization of fibromyalgia using sleep EEG signals with non-linear dynamical features. *Computers in Biology and Medicine*, 111, Article 103331. https://doi.org/10.1016/j.compbiomed.2019.103331.

Pop, M. G., Crivii, C. & Opincariu, I. (2018). Anatomy and function of the hypothalamus. In S. J. Baloyannis & J. O. Gordeladze (Eds.), *Hypothalamus in Health and Diseases* (pp. 4–9). Intech Open. https://doi.org/10.5772/intechopen.80728.

Rolls, E. T. (2019). The cingulate cortex and limbic systems for emotion, action, and memory. *Brain Structure and Function*, 224(9), 3001–3018. https://doi.org/10.1007/s00429-019-01945-2

Rolls, E. T., Cheng, W., & Feng, J. (2020). The orbitofrontal cortex: reward, emotion, and depression. *Brain Communications*, 2(2), 1–25. https://doi.org/10.1093/braincomms/fcaa196

Russell, I. J. (2013). Fibromyalgia syndrome and myofascial pain syndrome. In S. McMahon, M. Koltzenburg, I. Tracey, & D. Turk (Eds.), *Wall and Melzack's Textbook of Pain* (6th ed., pp. 658–682). Elsevier/Saunders.

Samartin-Veiga, N., Gonzálex-Villar, A.J., & Carrillo-de-la-Peña, M.T. (2019). Neural correlates of cognitive dysfunction in fibromyalgia patients: Reduced brain electrical activity during the execution of a cognitive control task. *NeuroImage Clinical, 23,* Article 101817. https://doi.org/10.1016/j.nicl.2019.101817

Sawaddiruk, P., Paiboonworachat, S. Chattipakorn, N., & Chattipakorn, S. C. (2017). Alterations of brain activity in fibromyalgia patients. *Journal of Clinical Neuroscience, 38,* 13–122. http://dx.doi.org/10.1016/j.jocn.2016.12.014

Schrepf, A., Harper, D. E., Harte, S. E., Wang, H., Ichesco, E., Hampson, J. P., Zubieta, J. Clauw, D. J., & Harris, R. E. (2016). Endogenous opiodergic dysregulation of pain in fibromyalgia: A PET and fMRI study. *Pain, 157*(10), 2217–2225. https://doi.org/ 10.1097/j.pain.0000000000000633

Singh, L., Kaur, A., Bhatti, M. S., & Bhatti, R., (2019). Possible molecular mediators involved and mechanistic insight into fibromyalgia and associated co-morbidities. *Neurochemical Research, 44*(7), 1517–1532. https://doi.org/10.1007/s11064-019-02805-5

Sluka, K. A., & Clauw, D. J., (2016). Neurobiology of fibromyalgia and chronic widespread pain. *Neuroscience, 338,* 114–129. http://dx.doi.org/10.1016/j.neuroscience.2016.06.006

Smith, M. T., Edwards, R. R., McCann, U. D., & Haythornthwaite, J. A., (2007). The effects of sleep deprivation on pain inhibition and spontaneous pain in women. *Sleep, 30*(4), 494–505: https://doi.org/ 10.1093/sleep/30.4.494.

Sneddon, L. U. (2017). Comparative physiology of nociception and pain. *Physiology, 33*(1), 63–73. https://doi.org/ 10.1152/physiol.00022.2017

Treede, R. (2016). Gain control mechanisms in the nociceptive system. *Pain, 157*(6), 1199–1204. http://dx.doi.org/10.1097/j.pain.0000000000000499

Tyng, C. M., Amin, H. U., Saad, M. N. M., Malik, A. S. (2017). The influences of emotion on learning and memory. *Frontiers in Psychology, 8,* Article 1454. https://doi.org/ 10.3389/fpsyg.2017.01454

Uddin, L.Q., Nomi, J.S., Hebert-Seropian, B., Ghaziri, J., Boucher, O. (2017). Structure and function of the human insula. *Journal of Clinical Neurophysiology, 34*(4), 300–306. https://doi.org/ 10.1097/WNP.0000000000000377

Urien, L. & Wang, J. (2019). Top-down cortical control of acute and chronic pain. *Psychosomatic Medicine, 81*(9), 851–858. https://doi.org/ 10.1097/PSY.0000000000000744

Van Someren, E. J. W. (2021). Brain mechanisms of insomnia: New perspectives on causes and consequences. *Physiology Review, 101,* 995–1046.

von Bernhardi, R., Eugenín-von Bernhardi, L., & Eugenín, J. (2017). What is neural plasticity? In R. von Bernhardi, J. Eugenín, & K. Muller (Eds.), *The Plastic Brain* (pp. 1–18). Springer.

Wood, P. B., Schweinhardt, P., Jaeger, E., Dagher, A., Hakyemex, H., Rabiner, E.A., Bushnell, M.C., & Chizh, B.A. (2007). Fibromyalgia patients show an abnormal dopamine response to pain. *European Journal of Neuroscience, 25*(12), 3576–3582. https://doi.org/ 10.1111/j.1460-9568.2007.05623.x

Woolf, C. J., (2011). Central sensitization: Implications for the diagnosis and treatment of pain. *Pain, 152*(3), S2–S15. https://doi.org/10.1016/j.pain.2010.09.030

Xiao, X. & Zhang, Y. (2018). A new perspective on the anterior cingulate cortex and affective pain. *Neuroscience and Biobehavioral Reviews, 90,* 200–211. https://doi.org/10.1016/j.neubiorev.2018.03.022

Yam, M. F., Loh, Y. C., Tan. C. S., Adam, S. K., Mana, N. A., & Basir, R. (2018). General pathways of pain sensation and the major neurotransmitters involved in pain regulation. *International Journal of Molecular Sciences, 19*(8), 2164. https://doi.org/ 10.3390/ijms19082164

Unit II
Social emotional systems

11 Kareem wants to be in a club and has autism

Neuroscience facilitates our understanding of making friends

Winnie Dunn

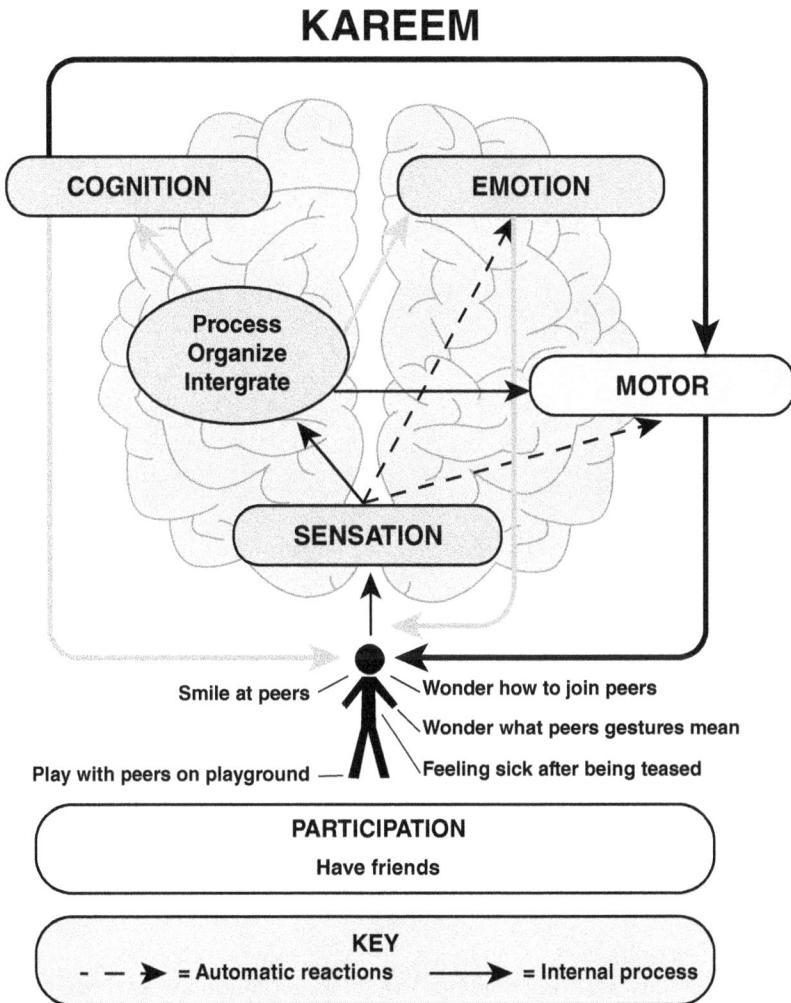

Figure 11.1 Kareem brain figure

DOI: 10.4324/9781003524380-14

Purpose of this chapter

The purpose of this chapter is to discover how Kareem, a third grader who wants to have friends might be affected by autism. Autistic people encounter daily routines, relationships and learning with distinct approaches that help the rest of us understand thinking and engagement more broadly. Autistic people can have full lives with their daily routines, relationships, work and leisure, but may require modifications for function.

The key neuroscience concepts we will explore in this chapter include what the homunculus and synaptic pruning are, how the frontal lobe, hippocampus, amygdala, parietal lobes, basal ganglia and cerebellum operate to support social interactions. As with all the chapters, these components of the nervous system work with other systems to support overall human function.

Keywords for this chapter are listed in the box below. Be sure to learn what these key features are so you can get the most out of the chapter.

Keywords for this chapter

amygdala	homunculus	superior temporal region
basal ganglia	inferior parietal lobe	synaptic pruning
cerebellum	inferior temporal lobe	theory of mind
frontal lobe	parietal lobes	
hippocampus	superior parietal lobe	

Box 11.1   Learning activity

Prior to reading the case:

1. How do you think the characteristics of autism will affect Kareem's social interactions?
2. Why is it important for an occupational therapy practitioner to understand the neurology of autism?

Let's find out about Kareem, his family, and school so we have a context for understanding the impact of his distinct nervous system on his life. As with all the chapters in this text, we learn these relationships from people who have distinct personal experiences in their lives.

Kareem, an 8-year-old who wants to be in a club

Kareem is the oldest of three children in his family. His dad is a teacher, and his mom is a pharmacist. The family likes camping and hiking in their free time. Kareem is particularly interested in plant and animal species, and has started a collection of specimens, pictures and websites that provide more details for him. His parents foster his interest by having part of each family outing include collecting more specimens for Kareem to research when he gets home.

At school, Kareem is in third grade. His brother is in first grade, and his sister is in pre-school in the same school building. Kareem is a successful student academically, and this year he has expressed more interest in playing with other children. In prior years, teachers reported that Kareem seemed content to be alone, exploring the perimeter of the play-ground, sitting alone in the library, and taking little interest in what other children were doing. The teacher and parents are happy that he is more interested in other children, yet early attempts at interaction have been challenging. Kareem doesn't seem to understand other children's social cues or how to join a small group. He barges in, and brings up his own topics, showing little regard for what the children are already doing. Other times group activities in the classroom or at recess seem to overwhelm Kareem; he flees if pos-sible, or sometimes has a meltdown.

Kareem and his family found out he has autism when he was 3 years old. They have had support from teachers, speech therapy, and occupational therapy in preschool, and continues to have these professionals on his school team.

The team wants to focus on Kareem's participation in small group work as a structured strategy for him to learn how to engage with other children successfully. They are also discussing starting an after-school interest group about biology to identify other children/ families that would want to join into nature walks and follow up research.

Box 11.2   Learning activity

Discuss with your peers:

1. Having read the narrative, what are you curious about?
2. What do you need to know more about?

Before you continue reading the chapter, work with your small group to discuss what you already know.

Box 11.3   Learning activity

1. How can scientific reasoning about neuroscience illuminate your insights?
2. What parts of the brain support social awareness and social skill development?

Keywords: autism + neuroscience + social skills

3. How does a person process information while working on a small group project to make meaning out of the situation?
4. What mechanisms in the nervous system explain a sense of being overwhelmed?

Keywords: hyper-responsivity, sensory overload

5. How can the context of a classroom or recess create an overload in the nervous system?

Now that you have had some time to think about all of this, let's consider what small group work requires from the nervous system. You certainly already have some great ideas to build on.

Neuroscience information to guide your thinking about Kareem

Social and biological sciences have contributed a great deal to our current understanding of autism. Since this text is about neuroscience, we will emphasize these aspects here and weave them with our knowledge of associated behaviors and adaptive responses.

Brain development

Some scientists have reported that the cortex expands quickly in first year of life (Askham, 2020) in autistics, including the frontal lobe which supports attention for decision making, the hippocampus, which forms and stores memories (Askham, 2020) and the amygdala which orchestrates emotions (Kandel, 2018). When parts of the brain develop out of sync with each other, this early development can interfere with overall development of other regions that are needed for integrated connections. When there is an imbalance in development, there can also be changes in interpretation of inputs for action. Kandel (2018) discusses three aspects of these changes that matter for autistics. First, there are changes in understanding the emotional aspects of social behavior. Secondly, there are changes to language and communication, and finally there are changes in the way a person understands the relationships between visual perception and movement.

Box 11.4   Learning activity

In small groups, discuss how these changes would affect your behavior.

1. How would your behavior change if you did not recognize the emotional aspect of a social interaction?
2. How would your changed behavior affect others?
3. How would you talk and listen if your brain were processing a small group discussion more slowly?
4. What impact would overfocusing on certain aspects of a conversation have on your interaction?
5. How could misinterpretation of movement of yourself and others affect your social interactions?

Additionally, particularly during development, we expect that the brain will remove brain connections that we don't use (called synaptic pruning) to maintain the efficiency of processing complex information. For autistics, this process seems to be slowed, leaving too many connections, and making it harder to have efficient processing. Imagine trying to hear another person in a quiet place vs a buzzing happy hour; it takes longer to hear, understand, and respond at happy hour.

Social engagement and neuroscience

Social engagement in autism reflects transparent and literal responses. Autistics are honest because they receive information exactly how it appears, rather than through an interpretation filter. They are not concerned with usual social conventions because they are taking behaviors at face value. Autistics can experience stress and anxiety, especially in adolescence and early adulthood as they try to understand the social rules that underlie our choices of behavior. They seem to process the form of the behavior without the meaning it holds for the social group. For example, an adolescent with autism may not recognize the differences in a person approaching for aggression or to have a conversation.

From a neuroscience perspective, social interaction emerges from an integrated network of connections in several areas of the cortex (Gutman, 2017; Kandel 2018). Unlike the primary sensory cortex, which houses sensory maps of the body (called the homunculus), other parts of the sensory cortex integrate input to create appropriate responses.

For Kareem, we are particularly interested in several parts of this network:

- The **superior parietal lobe (area 5)** responds to patterns of motion we make.
- The **inferior parietal lobe** processes movements we observe.
- The **superior temporal region** processes human motion.
- The **inferior temporal lobe** processes faces in coordination with the occipital lobe (visual processing).
- The **amygdala** orchestrates emotional actions, particularly attaching emotional significance to our thoughts and memories.

Box 11.5   Learning activity

1. Find a picture of the parietal and temporal lobes that delineate the different areas, so you have a visual reference as you read the next section.
2. Find a picture of the sensory homunculus in the parietal lobe.

Keywords: homunculus, temporal lobe organization, parietal lobe organization

---

In studies autistic children have the same brain reaction patterns in all the brain areas that process movement. For peers without autism, the superior temporal area responds more strongly when observing human movement. This difference matters because we expect others to understand the meaning of our actions. When people do not recognize the difference in meaning of reaching for a cup (a functional movement with an object) or reaching out to shake hands (a socially driven movement), they may seem out of step with others who easily process the difference in the purpose of these two movements. Differential responding in the superior temporal area for peers gives peers a way to understand the differences.

People with autism also gather different information when looking at faces (inferior temporal lobe); they tend to look around the face, and towards the mouth (seen as avoiding eye contact), while others focus on the eyes to connect and determine what the person might be thinking. This ability to make inferences about what someone else is thinking is sometimes called 'theory of mind'. Autistic individuals interpret the world differently, and neuroscience research has helped us understand how their processing works.

There may also be other centers involved since social engagement since there is such a complex response from integration of brain areas. Functional brain imaging studies demonstrate that this social brain network operates differently for autistic individuals. For example, the basal ganglia processes information related to timing of our responses, which matters for approaching a small group, or for contributing to a conversation (Chapter 23 about Parkinson's disease provides a lot more detail about the functions of the basal ganglia). The cerebellum is involved in coordination, which may also be a factor in active social paradigms such as playground routines or sports activities. A meta-analysis concluded that there are decreased amounts of brain tissue in the cerebellum for autistics (Askham, 2020). Chapter 6 about Cerebellar Ataxia talks about the motoric aspects of the cerebellum. The white matter tracts of the corpus callosum (connection between the left and right brain hemispheres) are lower in autism too, suggesting less efficient connectivity among brain centers.

Sensory processing

Another aspect of social engagement involves how each of us processes the sensory aspects of the people and the contexts. It is common for autistics to be highly sensitive to sounds and touch; each person has their own patterns so we must find out the person's sensory patterns as part of our interviews and assessments. Typically, our brains can filter out extraneous noises; when we hear everything with intensity, we can become depleted, reducing our capacity to manage communication, cognition, and other behaviors. Chapter 7 goes into more details about sensory processing and how it impacts the life of an autistic adult, Torrance.

This sensitivity also makes autistics and others with these sensory patterns very good at noticing small changes in circumstances (even if unable to make meaning out of all that detail). They find patterns more quickly and even see patterns that others might miss.

Remember when we are talking about sensory processing, we are not discussing the sensory organs themselves, but rather the brain's ability to make meaning, interpret, integrate the sensory information so we know what to do next. Sensory processing start in subcortical levels as the brainstem and proceed to and within the cortex, and with the integrating areas of the parietal, temporal, occipital and frontal lobes. As we discussed earlier, when there is less synaptic pruning, there are too many neurons firing to sort out the messages and make sense of a situation.

Daily life routine: Participating in small group work in the classroom

By the time children reach the third grade, there is an increasing focus on cooperative learning groups. The teacher assigns a project and provides a structure for completing the work. With the teacher's guidance available, the students meet in their groups to figure out how they will proceed. Some students might go to the library, or search the internet, while other students prepare visuals or write text to support their project. Students might have some individual tasks to accomplish, but the group provides accountability with frequent check ins. Often, students create the work product (written report, oral presentation, power point summary) and complete the project together

---

Box 11.6   Learning activity

With your small group, complete the table in the Appendix about the integration of Kareem's social participation demands and the neuroscience that affects his participation.

Back to the person/family's life … Kareem participating in small groups at school

So now that you know more about brain functioning in autistics, how can we use this scientific reasoning to support Kareem in his small group work? You will certainly spend a lot more time in other courses exploring details but knowing the neuroscience underpinnings provides a solid foundation to select intervention options that will be supported by brain processing.

Box 11.7   Learning activity

In class or small groups, discuss what accommodations the teacher can make to support Kareem to be successful in small group work. Use your neuroscience knowledge and what you know about Kareem in small groups right now to guide your idea generation.

What do we know about ourselves and the population at large from this brain condition and this family's story?

Even though we learned these things about autistics, it is important to remember that they are human beings just like us. Furthermore, some of us in the general population also use our brains in similar ways even though we don't have autism. Some of us take things more literally, creating some funny moments as we realize (with others' help many times) that we misunderstood some social nuance or larger meaning. We have all misunderstood directions, or even written directions that are well-intentioned but fail to include pertinent details that others need. These moments remind us that our brains can make the same interpretations that autistics make, punctuating the sameness among us rather than our differences.

Many people in the general population are also sensitive to sensory input as well. We make adaptations to suit our needs. Some of us might only buy one brand of socks because others are too tight or get twisted easily. We might time when we go to the grocery store to have a quieter place to shop. These are the same interventions we might suggest to a family that has a member who is autistic because everyone who is sensitive benefits from a more sensory friendly context. Autistics have stronger reactions, so they have shown us how to notice and make adjustments that we all benefit from.

Finally, autistics are better at some tasks because of their brain differences. They notice details and see patterns that the rest of us miss. They are not encumbered by social contexts, and so can focus on their work and their interests more effectively. The references under Further Reading provide additional insights if you are interested.

Further reading

If interested in further reading about the lived experience of autism:

Grinker, R. (2007). *Unstrange Minds: remapping the world of Autism*. Basic Books.
Mottron, L., (03 November 2011) Neuroscience Researcher on Strengths of people with autism for research work. *Nature* 479, 33–35 doi: 10:1038/479033a.
Ne'eman, A. (2010). The future (and the past) of autism advocacy.
Pentzell, N. (2010). Adults with Autism spectrum disorders. in Koenig, K. P., & Kinnealey, M., Eds. Suskind, N, (2014). Life Animated. *New York Times Magazine*. Also a book with the same title.

References

Askham, A. V. (October 15, 2020). Brain structure changes in autism, explained. Spectrum: Autism Research News. Obtained June 3, 2021 from www.spectrumnews.org

Dunn, W. (2011). Sensory Processing: Tools for Supporting Young Children in Everyday Life. Early childhood intervention: Shaping the future for children with special needs and their families, three volumes. S. Maude. Santa Barbara, CA: ABC-CLIO.

Gutman, S. (2017). *Quick Reference Neuroscience for Rehabilitation Professionals*. Third edition. Thorofare, NJ: Slack.

Kandel, E. (2018). *The Disordered Mind: what unusual brains tell us about ourselves*. New York: Farrar, Straus and Giroux.

12 Ian wants to manage his money and has schizophrenia

Neuroscience facilitates our understanding of money management

Antoine Bailliard, Ben Lee, and Valerie Fox

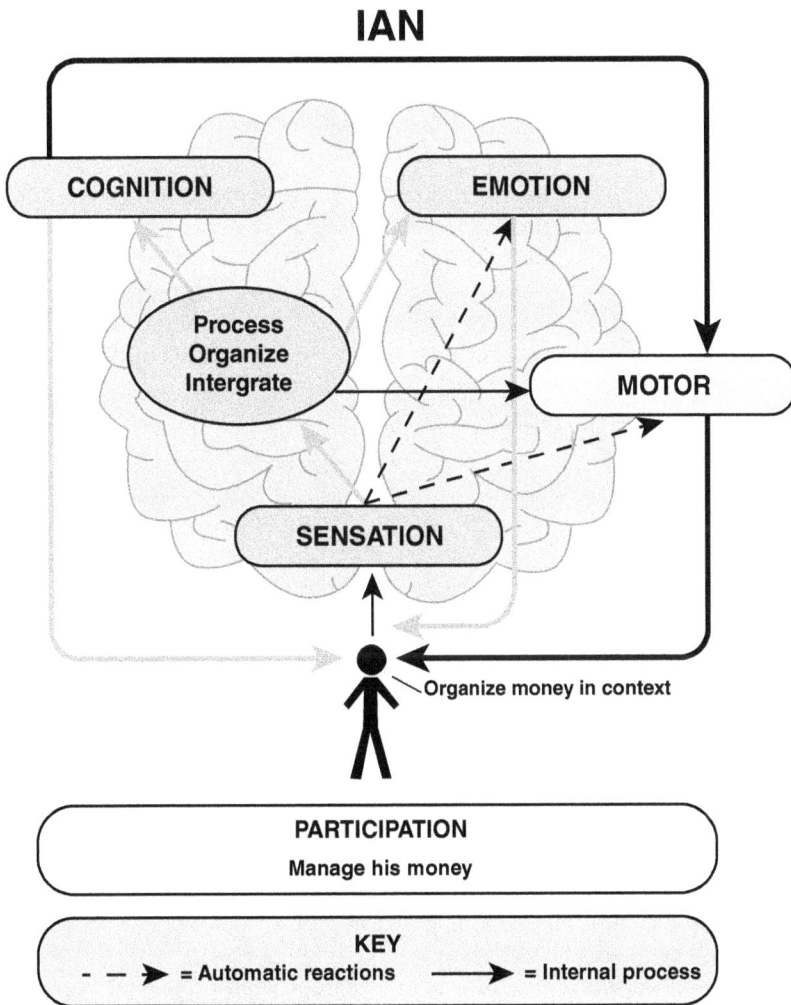

Figure 12.1 Ian brain figure

DOI: 10.4324/9781003524380-15

Purpose of this chapter

The purpose of this chapter is to explore how Ian, a 25-year-old who wants to manage his money, might be affected by schizophrenia, a condition that changes how the brain perceives the world, other people, and one's own sensory, cognitive and emotional experiences. People with schizophrenia can have full lives with their daily routines, relationships, work and leisure, but may require modifications for function.

The key neuroscience concepts we will explore in this chapter include characteristics of schizophrenia including positive and negative symptoms and their neuroscience foundations, how schizophrenia manifests in young adulthood, frontal and prefrontal lobe activity, and how drugs affect the brain to create symptoms and side effects. As with all the chapters, these components of the nervous system work with other systems to support overall human function.

Keywords for this chapter are listed in the box below. Be sure you learn what these key features are so you can get the most out of the chapter.

Keywords for this chapter

anhedonia	interoception	schizophrenia spectrum
auditory sensory gating	mismatch negativity	disorders
avolition	negative symptoms	second generation
delusions	positive psychology	anti-psychotic (SGA)
hallucinations	positive symptoms	medications
first generation	psychotic episode	tardive dyskinesia
anti-psychotic (FGA)	psychosis	
medications	schizophrenia	

Box 12.1   Learning activity

Prior to reading the case:

1. How do you think the symptoms of schizophrenia will affect Ian's performance of money management occupations?
2. Why is it important for an occupational therapy practitioner to understand the neurology of schizophrenia?

Ian, a 25-year-old young man who wants to manage his money

Ian grew up in the city with his parents and two siblings; he was the oldest son in the family. As a child, Ian was outgoing, enjoyed swimming and playing baseball, was active in his church choir, and the editor for his school yearbook. After high school, Ian moved to a nearby state to pursue a college degree in Communications. Ian wanted to be a writer and was involved in publishing a newspaper at his high school. He enjoyed school and was always punctual and engaged in discussions. During the fall semester of his junior year of college, Ian began missing classes and deadlines and failed a few courses. Ian's roommate, a childhood friend, noticed a few changes in Ian's behavior. He was getting little sleep, not showering, increasingly isolated himself, spent a lot of time researching on his computer, and frequently whispered to himself. One night, his roommate woke up to Ian pacing around the room nervously mumbling words about his money and how people had been stealing it from his room when he slept. The next morning, his roommate called Ian's parents to share his concerns about Ian's recent changes in behavior; Ian was hospitalized and subsequently diagnosed with schizophrenia.

After his first episode of psychosis (i.e., experiencing a different reality than others), he left college and moved back home with his parents. Ian was ashamed of his hospitalization and was fearful of reconnecting with his friends after discharge. He felt different and had more trouble focusing on things throughout his day. Simple activities, such as buying a soda at a convenience store, were difficult for him to do because he struggled to focus and would become anxious and more paranoid when experiencing this in public. Ian wanted to return to school, but required additional support to manage his symptoms and stress (which worsened his symptoms). He lived with his parents rent-free and they assisted him with getting to his doctor's appointments for his monthly long-acting injectable medication. His parents also assisted Ian with applying for Supplemental Security Income (SSI) and Medicaid. With SSI, Ian has a monthly income of $914. At first, Ian often ran out of money early in the month due to excessive spending on vaping materials, online computer gaming sites, and loaning others money when he went out. Although his parents encouraged him to develop a budget to manage his SSI, he never followed through due to difficulty focusing and staying organized. As a result, his mother manages his money.

It has been four years since Ian's first psychotic episode. He continues to have auditory hallucinations (especially when he has poor sleep or additional stress); however, he takes his medications as prescribed, engages in healthy eating, avoids alcohol and other substances, and walks daily around his neighborhood. Ian would like to move into his own apartment and feel more independent in his life. He is also lonely and would like to have more friends his age. Recently, he expressed a desire to return to school to complete a degree and find a job in the communications field. He is unsure if he can succeed in school and be a writer because of ongoing difficulties with auditory hallucinations and concentration; nonetheless, he still has a passion for writing and values working. He also realizes he needs more income to achieve his broader life goals, which include purchasing his own home, dating, possibly starting a family, and traveling.

Ian was referred to an occupational therapist to help him address these goals. During the evaluation, Ian identified money management as a priority. Specifically, Ian wants to improve his credit score so he can rent an apartment. He wants to learn how to budget his income, track expenses, and reduce impulsive buying. He also needs to purchase a car and is unsure how to start the process.

Box 12.2   Learning activity

Discussion questions related to Ian:

1. What are Ian's strengths and supports that he can use to reach his goals?
2. What are possible challenges he may face related to reaching his goals?
3. What occupational performance issues should the occupational therapist be considering?

What is schizophrenia?

Schizophrenia is a serious mental illness (SMI) that affects approximately 1% of the global population. People diagnosed with schizophrenia may experience a combination of positive symptoms, such as hallucinations and delusions, and negative symptoms, such as reduced emotional expression, anhedonia (i.e., reduced ability to experience pleasure), and avolition (i.e., decreased ability to initiate and persist in self-directed activities) (van Os & Kapur, 2009). There is a spectrum of diagnoses related to schizophrenia (i.e., schizophrenia spectrum disorders) and diagnostic labels such as schizophrenia and schizo-affective disorder are used to differentiate between people with schizophrenia who have different sets of related symptoms (e.g., mood fluctuations). Currently, there is no effective cure for schizophrenia; the American Psychiatric Association (2020) recommends symptom management through a combination of anti-psychotic medication and psychotherapy as best practice. In addition, there is renewed emphasis on the recovery model and use of positive psychology principles to highlight individual strengths and focus assessments and interventions on quality of life, meaningful positive experiences, and the belief that a person can achieve their goals to live their desired life. Adopting the principles of positive psychology, as an adjunct to medication, have shown to improve outcomes, including improving well-being and symptom reduction (primarily negative symptoms) (Pina et al., 2021).

Box 12.3   Learning activity

1. Look up descriptions of positive and negative symptoms of schizophrenia. Work with your small group to compile an integrated description of positive and negative symptoms.
2. Consider how these positive and negative symptoms would impact your current life and occupations.

Box 12.4   Learning activity

Find an image of the fronto-temporal region of the brain that illustrates cortical thinning. Be prepared to discuss how thinner gray matter might affect the brain's functions.

Keywords: fronto-temporal, cortical thinning, gray matter

Cognitive challenges are also a core feature of schizophrenia and are significant predictors of functional outcomes (Bowie & Harvey, 2006). Typical cognitive symptoms of schizophrenia affect processing speed, working memory, attention, verbal learning and memory, and other executive functions (Bowie & Harvey, 2006). Research suggests that the cognitive symptoms of schizophrenia are related to differences in cortical thickness in the fronto-temporal brain region—people with schizophrenia have a thinner cortex in most fronto-temporal regions (Alkan, Davies, & Evans, 2021) and less gray matter than the general population (Yasuda et al., 2020). The cognitive challenges experienced by people with schizophrenia can be amplified by sociodemographic factors such as gender, education, ethnicity, marital status and employment (Mascio et al., 2021). The combination of cognitive challenges, atypical sensory processing, and positive and negative symptoms of schizophrenia can have a significant impact on participation in meaningful occupations.

Typically, the onset of schizophrenia occurs between the ages of 13 and 25 with a first-episode psychosis; however, there are many instances when people have experienced psychosis at younger and older ages (Fusar-Poli et al., 2017). The content of a person's hallucinations and delusions and their understanding of those experiences can vary across cultures and linguistic backgrounds. For example, qualitative research has shown that people diagnosed with schizophrenia from India and Ghana can have more positive experiences of psychosis (e.g., hearing voices that are supportive) compared to their U.S. counterparts, who typically report antagonistic, hostile comments from their visual and auditory hallucinations (Luhrmann et al., 2015).

Box 12.5   Learning activity

1. Now that you know more about the symptoms of schizophrenia, how do you think they will affect Ian's performance of money management occupations?
2. How might the age of onset of the symptoms of schizophrenia affect the development of money management skills?

Cause of schizophrenia: A set of hypotheses

There are many hypotheses regarding the onset of schizophrenia. One of the oldest hypotheses is the D2 dopamine receptor hypothesis, which proposes that overactivity of specific brain receptors causes positive symptoms (i.e., hallucinations and delusions) (Madras, 2013). Dopamine is a chemical that carries messages across the brain. Based on this hypothesis, scientists developed the first generation anti-psychotic (FGA) medications (e.g., Haldol, Thorazien, Loxapine) in the 1950s to reduce dopamine activity. These drugs were effective in mitigating positive symptoms. However, FGA medications can also cause significant side effects (e.g., muscle stiffness, movement disorders including dystonia, tardive dyskinesia) that affect quality of life. These drugs do not address negative symptoms (McDonagh et al., 2017).

Another hypothesis for the onset of schizophrenia comes from research that demonstrated that other forms of brain activity (e.g., N-methyl-D-aspartate (NMDA) and gamma-aminobutyric acid (GABA) receptors, serotonin) can affect the emergence and severity of schizophrenia symptoms (Coyle, 2006). This hypothesis led to the development of second generation anti-psychotic (SGA) medications in the 1980s (e.g., Risperidal, Clozaril, Seroquel, Zyprexa). SGA medications target both dopamine (target of FGA drugs) and serotonin receptors. As a result, certain SGA medications are more successful in reducing both positive and negative symptoms for people living with schizophrenia. However, SGAs can also cause side effects that negatively affect quality of life such as weight gain and metabolic changes (e.g., diabetes, hyperglycemia, lipid abnormalities). SGAs and FGAs can also cause sexual dysfunction, sleepiness, restlessness, dry mouth, constipation and blurred visions. For many people living with schizophrenia, neither generation of antipsychotics alleviate their symptoms (Miyamoto et al., 2005; Nasrallah & Mulvihill, 2001). Overall, SGAs and FGAs have a limited impact on symptom reduction

(McDonagh et al., 2017; Nasrallah & Mulvihill, 2001) and should always be coupled with non-pharmacological forms of intervention.

The social defeat hypothesis from psychiatry and psychology asserts there is a social cause to the neurological origins of schizophrenia (Hansen et al., 2014; Luhrmann, 2007).

Box 12.6   Learning activity

Select one of the hypotheses about the origin of schizophrenia. Find resources about this hypothesis and be prepared to debate its viability with your peers in class. Your faculty member may have some suggestions re: websites.

This hypothesis argues that stigma and exclusion from society can lead to increased dopamine activity resulting in a higher risk of psychosis (Selten et al., 2013). Indeed, the social context of high-income countries with individualist tendencies (e.g., U.S.) leads to poorer prognoses than in low-income countries with collectivist tendencies (Luhrmann, 2007). A comparison of outcomes for schizophrenia across the world demonstrated that collectivist countries with emerging economies (e.g., India, Nigeria) reported better two- and five-year outcomes than individualist, high-income countries (e.g., U.S.) (Leff et al., 1992). The social defeat hypothesis emphasizes that socio-cultural factors thus have an important role in influencing the daily lives of people living with schizophrenia via neurological mechanisms of increased mesolimbic dopamine activity (i.e., the pleasure and reward circuits).

Sensory processing patterns

Recently, sensory processing has been identified as another neurological difference between people with schizophrenia and typical groups (Bailliard & Whigham, 2017). Neuroimaging has revealed that people with schizophrenia have different auditory sensory gating (i.e., ability to filter out irrelevant auditory stimuli) and different mismatch negativity (i.e., ability to recognize a change in pattern in auditory stimuli) (Javitt & Freedman, 2015; Jahshan et al., 2013). These neurological differences heighten the likelihood of being easily distracted and having difficulty focusing on sounds (i.e., hearing everything all at once without being able to focus on one sound) (Javitt & Sweet, 2015), which can lead to feeling overwhelmed in noisy environments (McGhie & Chapman, 1961). People with schizophrenia also demonstrate differences in visual sensory processing (Yoon et al., 2013), olfaction (i.e., smell) (Bunney et al., 1999; Takashi et al., 2018) and interoception (i.e., sensory processing of internal bodily signals) (Ardizzi et al., 2016; Koreki et al., 2021). Research using the Adult/Adolescent Sensory Profile found that people with schizophrenia have higher scores on low registration and sensation avoiding, and lower scores on sensation seeking than the norm and are, therefore, more likely to miss important sensory information (Brown et al., 2002).

Box 12.7   Learning activity

Now that you know about different hypotheses regarding the cause of schizophrenia, how might an occupational therapy practitioner change their intervention according to each hypothesis?

Impact of schizophrenia on occupational participation

People living with schizophrenia face discrimination and prejudice (i.e., stigma) in society and can be perceived as violent, unstable, and untrustworthy people (Jenkins & Carpenter-Song, 2009; Wood et al., 2014). As a result, social isolation and loneliness are common among people living with schizophrenia and they tend to have fewer friends and narrower social networks compared to the general population (Topor et al., 2016). From a neuroscience point of view, neurological differences in sensory processing of auditory and visual stimuli result in challenges in communicating, including expressing emotions and understanding the emotions of others (Chen & Ekstrom, 2015; Green et al., 2005; Javitt & Sweet, 2015; Kantrowitz et al., 2014). These challenges are significant barriers to engaging in social occupations and maintaining a robust social network of friends and acquaintances who can support a person and make them feel inclusion and belonging (Gur et al., 2006; Mandal et al., 1998; Topor et al., 2016). As a result, people living with schizophrenia typically spend more time being idle (i.e., sleeping or doing nothing) than the general population (Cella et al., 2016), which can further reduce the sensory input needed to foster healthy relationships.

The cognitive challenges and symptomology of schizophrenia (related to differences in gray matter available for processing) can create significant barriers for a person's ability to complete instrumental activities of daily living such as money management, home management, health management, shopping, and meal preparation (Lipskaya et al., 2011). Together, the symptoms of schizophrenia, atypical sensory processing, and cognitive challenges can cause a person to become very disorganized and anxious when attempting to complete a task. Imagine trying to make everyday and important decisions with not enough or convoluted information; it is understandable that people with schizophrenia would feel disorganized and anxious.

In some cases, the symptoms of schizophrenia are so severe that a person has challenges completing basic activities of daily living such as eating or bathing. For many people with schizophrenia, finances are a critical barrier to occupational participation. In the U.S., people who have difficulty finding and maintaining employment are often reliant on Social Security payments and must navigate their way around complex bureaucratic systems to document their illness (Hansen et al., 2014). They are often faced with the complex task of closely monitoring their work hours to avoid losing their Social Security payments for extended periods. Social Security regulates the number of hours a person can work and still qualify for these benefits.

Daily life routine: Managing personal finances

It is easy to take for granted how complex neurological functioning (sensory and cognitive) is deeply involved in a person's ability to perform any occupation, especially one as difficult as managing personal finances. Many of the cognitive challenges experienced by people with schizophrenia make it difficult for them to stay focused on a task and to organize their self and their environment. Challenges with processing speed, working memory, attention, verbal learning and memory, and other executive functions can make money management extremely difficult.

Using money often involves counting, which requires working memory to keep track of numbers and attention to stay focused in an environment with competing stimuli. Counting money in public situations (e.g., buying something from a convenience store) is even more difficult because social pressures (e.g., an impatient clerk or a customer in line behind you) make the activity require more cognitive processing speed. Everyday monetary tasks (e.g., counting change or using an ATM) can be challenging and stressful when a person is having difficulty focusing on the task due to cognitive issues, is distracted by sensory stimuli due to atypical sensory processing, and is preoccupied with positive symptoms such as hallucinations or delusions.

Due to these core dimensions of schizophrenia, a person can also have significant difficulties with monthly budgeting, especially when they receive Social Security benefits that provide limited funds in a lump sum once a month. This requires a person to carefully plan how to distribute their funds across an entire month to support necessary expenditures such as rent, food, and utilities. Often, a person does not have sufficient funds to access leisure or social occupations, which are essential to support a person's recovery. A person in this situation must carefully assess what they need versus want when choosing to spend money. However, when experiencing challenges with processing speed, working memory, attention, verbal learning and memory, and other executive functions, it can be very difficult to plan ahead and calculate a monthly budget. Budgeting also requires a person to assess their habits and routines to see if frequent small purchases add up to consume disproportionate amounts of their monthly Social Security benefits (e.g., buying a coffee shop latte every day).

Other financial occupations that can be challenging for people with schizophrenia include writing and cashing checks and understanding complicated financial processes such as securing loans, paying interest, and paying off debt. Sometimes, people with schizophrenia need support to understand credit and debit cards such as credit scores, credit interest, and how to obtain and use credit or debit cards. Unfortunately, there are many documented instances when people with schizophrenia are cheated out of their money through scams or by loaning money to people. Indeed, sometimes the negative symptoms of schizophrenia lead to difficulty with assertive communication that can lead to hesitancy to saying no when asked for something such as money.

Back to Ian: Budgeting and tracking finances

During the initial evaluation with the occupational therapist, Ian identified a desire to improve his credit score so he could rent an apartment; learn to budget and track expenses; and reduce impulsive buying. Based on clinical observation, informal questioning during the initial evaluation, and results from the Kohlman Evaluation of Living Skills (KELS) standardized assessment, the occupational therapist noted that Ian had a good memory and ability to recall information. He struggled with attention and required additional time for processing and planning. Ian also lacked knowledge about basic budgeting concepts including financial terminology partly because his mother had been managing his finances for a long time. Ian knew how to use a debit card and retrieve money from the ATM but had difficulty anticipating the long-term implications of accumulating debt through credit cards.

The occupational therapist was aware that Ian may have difficulty focusing on verbal instruction, due to potential challenges with processing speed, working memory, attention, verbal learning and memory, and other executive functions and might miss verbal information due to different auditory processing.

Box 12.8   Learning activity

1. What topics might an occupational therapy practitioner discuss with Ian to educate him about money management?
2. How might the practitioner use technology to support Ian with his money management?

The occupational therapist assisted Ian with checking his credit score online. Ian found that his credit score was too low for an apartment because he had never paid rent and had no bills since he lived with his parents. To improve his score, the occupational therapist and Ian collaborated with his mother to open a credit card with a $500 limit. Ian agreed to only use the credit card to buy groceries and initially went to the grocery store with his mother once a week to practice not going over his limit. His mother was present to provide assistance and support if the sensory environment of the grocery store became too overwhelming or if he became too anxious or disorganized to complete the multistep process of buying groceries.

Box 12.9   Learning activity

1. What could an occupational therapy practitioner do to help Ian manage the grocery store sensory environment?
2. What strategies could be used to increase the predictability of grocery shopping for Ian?
3. How could the practitioner prepare Ian for potential challenges he might experience while grocery shopping?

During the next intervention session, Ian and the occupational therapist reviewed a money management app and added budget details on his phone. Ian reported increased awareness of how he spent his money by reviewing the app regularly; however, he continued to struggle with frequently buying. He liked to visit a local videogame store and struggled with frequently buying new games he could play online with others. As one of Ian's only social outlets, online gaming had become increasingly important to him. The occupational therapist affirmed the critical importance of leisure engagement and social participation in promoting mental health and collaborated with Ian to modify his budget to account for leisure expenses. Together, Ian and his occupational therapist discussed and practiced impulse control strategies such as reading a first-person narrative written by Ian to coach himself through impulse control and reviewing his budget prior to visiting the videogame store. They also discussed more affordable ways he could connect meaningfully with others using his interests such as buying used games, purchasing a game streaming service instead, or switching to a more affordable video gaming system.

The occupational therapist worked with Ian through several more sessions to build a routine that included regular monitoring and tracking his finances. Although Ian demonstrated a good understanding of his new money management strategies, he continued to struggle with impulsive buying at times. His credit score was slowly improving, and Ian was more independently managing his finances. He continued to work towards saving for a car and the first and last month's rent for an apartment. Because of the cognitive adaptions and self-management strategies developed with his occupational therapist, Ian felt hopeful about his ability to progress in life and achieve his desired goals.

Box 12.10   Learning activity

There are many possible interventions the occupational therapist could choose to help Ian address his money management.

1. What other intervention ideas might support Ian with budgeting and tracking his finances?
2. How might the targeted occupation be modified?
3. How can the environment be modified?
4. How could adaptations and supports be integrated into Ian's everyday living and daily routines?

What do we know about ourselves and the population at large from this brain condition and this story?

As occupational therapists working with adults with schizophrenia, it is important to understand how atypical neurological functioning (e.g., sensory processing, cognitive) affects their participation in meaningful occupations. To support adults with schizophrenia in achieving their life goals and experiencing wellbeing, occupational therapists can use their expert knowledge to adapt the environment and ways of doing occupation to scaffold their neurological barriers to occupational performance. For example, to address cognitive challenges (e.g., processing speed, working memory, attention, verbal learning and memory, and other executive functions) associated with thinner fronto-temporal cortex and less gray matter, occupational therapists can help implement cognitive supports and structure to scaffold a person's occupational performance. Typical adults routinely implement such cognitive strategies in their daily living; however, positive and negative symptoms of schizophrenia can make it very challenging to do so. Also, the different sensory processing of adults with schizophrenia can further increase the likelihood they miss information and challenge their ability to focus. In addition to helping people develop self-management skills to regulate their sensory arousal, there is a need to adapt the sensory environments of public spaces to make them more inclusive of adults with atypical sensory processing such as people with serious mental illness.

Some of us encounter these same challenges in our everyday lives. Perhaps we also miss important auditory cues in our environments, need more time to process auditory directions, or have difficulty following a fast-paced conversation. This does not mean we have schizophrenia; it does mean that we can use similar adaptive strategies to support our daily routines. Research has shown that sensory processing varies considerably across different people regardless of diagnostic categories. In other words, we all have different sensory capacities and different ways of relating to our worlds sensorially. These natural variations should not be viewed as deficits; instead, they reflect unique ways of being in the world and expressing occupation.

Box 12.11   Learning activity

With your small group, complete the table in the Appendix about the integration of Ian's needs to manage his money.

References

Alkan, E., Davies, G., & Evans, S. L. (2021). Cognitive impairment in schizophrenia: relationships with cortical thickness in fronto-temporal regions, and dissociability from symptom severity. *NPJ Schizophrenia, 7*(1), 20. https://doi.org/10.1038/s41537-021-00149-0

American Psychiatric Association. (2020). *The American Psychiatric Association practice guideline for the treatment of patients with schizophrenia* (3rd ed.). American Psychiatric Association. https://doi.org/10.1176/appi.books.9780890424841

Ardizzi, M., Ambrosecchia, M., Buratta, L., Ferri, F., Peciccia, M., Donnari, S., & Gallese, V. (2016). Interoception and positive symptoms in schizophrenia. *Frontiers in Human Neuroscience, 10,* 379.

Bailliard, A., & Whigham, S.C. (2017). Centennial Topics—Linking neuroscience, function, and intervention: A scoping review of sensory processing and mental illness. *American Journal of Occupational Therapy*: 7105100040.

Bowie, C. R., & Harvey, P. D. (2006). Cognitive deficits and functional outcome in schizophrenia. *Neuropsychiatric Disease and Treatment, 2*(4), 531–536. https://doi.org/10.2147/nedt.2006.2.4.531

Brown, C., Cromwell, R. L., Filion, C., Dunn, W., & Tollefson, N. (2002). Sensory processing in schizophrenia: Missing and avoiding information. *Schizophrenia Research, 55,* 187–195.

Bunney, W. E., Hetrick, W. P., Bunney, B. G., Patterson, J. V., Jin, Y., Potkin, S. G., & Sandman, C. A. (1999). Structured Interview for Assessing Perceptual Anomalies (SIAPA). *Schizophrenia Bulletin, 25,* 577–592.

Cella, M., Edwards, C., & Wykes, T. (2016). A question of time: A study of time use in people with schizophrenia. *Schizophrenia Research, 176*(2–3), 480–484. https://doi.org/10.1016/j.schres.2016.06.033

Chen, Y., & Ekstrom, T. (2015). Visual and associated affective processing of face information in schizophrenia: A selective review. *Current Psychiatry Reviews, 11*(4), 266–272. https://doi.org/10.2174/1573400511666150930000817

Coyle, J. T. (2006). Glutamate and Schizophrenia: Beyond the Dopamine Hypothesis. *Cellular and Molecular Neurobiology, 26*(4–6), 363–382. https://doi.org/10.1007/s10571-006-9062-8

Fusar-Poli, P., McGorry, P. D., & Kane, J. M. (2017). Improving outcomes of first-episode psychosis: An overview. *World Psychiatry: Official Journal of the World Psychiatric Association (WPA), 16*(3), 251–265. https://doi.org/10.1002/wps.20446

Green, M. F., Olivier, B., Crawley, J. N., Penn, D. L., & Silverstein, S. (2005). Social cognition in schizophrenia: Recommendations from the Measurement and Treatment Research to Improve Cognition in Schizophrenia New Approaches Conference. *Schizophrenia Bulletin, 31*(4), 882–887. https://doi.org/10.1093/schbul/sbi049

Gur, R. E., Kohler, C. G., Ragland, J. D., Siegel, S. J., Lesko, K., Bilker, W. B., & Gur, R. C. (2006). Flat affect in schizophrenia: Relation to emotion processing and neurocognitive measures. *Schizophrenia Bulletin, 32*(2), 279–287. https://doi.org/10.1093/schbul/sbj041

Hansen, H., Bourgois, P., & Drucker, E. (2014). Pathologizing poverty: New forms of diagnosis, disability, and structural stigma under welfare reform. *Social Science & Medicine, 103,* 76–83. https://doi.org/10.1016/j.socscimed.2013.06.033

Jahshan, C., Wynn, J. K., & Green, M. F. (2013). Relationship between auditory processing and affective prosody in schizophrenia. *Schizophrenia Research, 143,* 348–353. https://doi.org/10.1016/j.schres.2012.11.025

Javitt, D. C., & Freedman, R. (2015). Sensory processing dysfunction in the personal experience and neuronal machinery of schizophrenia. *American Journal of Psychiatry, 172*, 17–31. https://doi.org/10.1176/appi.ajp.2014.13121691

Javitt, D. C., & Sweet, R. A. (2015). Auditory dysfunction in schizophrenia: Integrating clinical and basic features. National Review of Neuroscience, 16, 535–550.

Jenkins, J. H., & Carpenter-Song, E. A. (2009). Awareness of stigma among persons with schizophrenia: Marking the contexts of lived experience. *The Journal of Nervous and Mental Disease, 197*(7), 520–529. https://doi.org/10.1097/NMD.0b013e3181aad5e9

Kantrowitz, J. T., Hoptman, M. J., Leitman, D. I., Silipo, G., & Javitt, D. C. (2014). The 5% difference: early sensory processing predicts sarcasm perception in schizophrenia and schizo-affective disorder. *Psychological Medicine, 44*(1), 25–36. https://doi.org/10.1017/S0033291713000834

Koreki, A., Funayama, M., Terasawa, Y., Onaya, M., & Mimura, M. (2021). Aberrant interoceptive accuracy in patients with schizophrenia performing a heartbeat counting task. *Schizophrenia Bulletin, 2*(1), sgaa067.

Leff, J., Sartorius, N., Jablensky, A., Korten, A., & Ernberg, G. (1992). The International Pilot Study of Schizophrenia: Five-year follow-up findings. *Psychological Medicine, 22*(1), 131–145. https://doi.org/10.1017/s0033291700032797

Lipskaya, L., Jarus, T., & Kotler, M. (2011). Influence of cognition and symptoms of schizophrenia on IADL performance. *Scandinavian Journal of Occupational Therapy, 18*(3), 180–187. https://doi.org/10.3109/11038128.2010.490879

Luhrmann, T. M. (2007). Social defeat and the culture of chronicity: Or, why schizophrenia does so well over there and so badly here. *Culture, Medicine and Psychiatry, 31*(2), 135–172. https://doi.org/10.1007/s11013-007-9049-z

Luhrmann, T. M., Padmavati, R., Tharoor, H., & Osei, A. (2015). Differences in voice-hearing experiences of people with psychosis in the U.S.A., India and Ghana: Interview-based study. *The British Journal of Psychiatry, 206*(1), 41–44. https://doi.org/10.1192/bjp.bp.113.139048

Madras, B. K. (2013). History of the Discovery of the Antipsychotic Dopamine D2 Receptor: A Basis for the Dopamine Hypothesis of Schizophrenia. *Journal of the History of the Neurosciences, 22*(1), 62–78. https://doi.org/10.1080/0964704X.2012.678199

Mandal, M. K., Pandey, R., & Prasad, A. B. (1998). Facial expressions of emotions and schizophrenia: A review. *Schizophrenia Bulletin, 24*(3), 399–412. https://doi.org/10.1093/oxfordjournals.schbul.a033335

Mascio, A., Stewart, R., Botelle, R., Williams, M., Mirza, L., Patel, R., Pollak, T., Dobson, R., & Roberts, A. (2021). Cognitive impairments in schizophrenia: A study in a large clinical sample using natural language processing. *Frontiers in Digital Health, 3*, 711941. doi: 10.3389/fdgth.2021.711941

McDonagh, M. S., Dana, T., Selph, S., Devine, E. B., Cantor, A., Bougatsos, C., Blazina, I., Grusing, S., Fu, R., Kopelovich, S. L., Monroe-DeVita, M., & Haupt, D. W. (2017). *Treatments for schizophrenia in adults: A systematic review*. Agency for Healthcare Research and Quality (US). https://doi.org/10.23970/AHRQEPCCER198

McGhie, A., & Chapman, J. (1961). Disorders of attention and perception in early schizophrenia. *British Journal of Medical Psychology, 34*, 103–116.

Miyamoto, S., Duncan, G. E., Marx, C. E., & Lieberman, J. A. (2005). Treatments for schizophrenia: A critical review of pharmacology and mechanisms of action of antipsychotic drugs. *Molecular Psychiatry, 10*(1), 79–104. https://doi.org/10.1038/sj.mp.4001556

Nasrallah, H., & Mulvihill, T. (2001). Iatrogenic disorders associated with conventional vs. Atypical antipsychotics. *Annals of Clinical Psychiatry, 13*(4), 215–227. https://doi.org/10.3109/10401230109147385

Pina, I., Braga, C., de Oliveira, T., de Santana, C., Marques, R., & Machado, L. (2021). Positive psychology interventions to improve well-being and symptoms in people on the schizophrenia spectrum: A systematic review and meta-analysis. *Brazilian Journal of Psychology, 43*(4), 430–437.

Selten, J.-P., van der Ven, E., Rutten, B. P. F., & Cantor-Graae, E. (2013). The social defeat hypothesis of schizophrenia: An update. *Schizophrenia Bulletin*, *39*(6), 1180–1186. https://doi.org/10.1093/schbul/sbt134

Takahashi, T., Nakamura, M., Sasabayashi, D., Komori, Y., Higuchi, Y., Nishikawa, Y., Nishiyama, S., Itoh, H., Masaoka, Y., & Suzuki, M. (2018). Olfactory deficits in individuals at risk for psychosis and patients with schizophrenia: Relationship with socio-cognitive functions and symptom severity. *European Archives of Psychiatry and Clinical Neuroscience*, *268*(7), 689–698. https://doi.org/10.1007/s00406-017-0845-3

Topor, A., Ljungqvist, I., & Strandberg, E.-L. (2016). The costs of friendship: Severe mental illness, poverty and social isolation. *Psychosis*, *8*(4), 336–345. https://doi.org/10.1080/17522439.2016.1167947

van Os, J., & Kapur, S. (2009). Schizophrenia. *The Lancet*, *374*(9690), 635–645. https://doi.org/10.1016/S0140-6736(09)60995-8

Wood, L., Birtel, M., Alsawy, S., Pyle, M., & Morrison, A. (2014). Public perceptions of stigma towards people with schizophrenia, depression, and anxiety. *Psychiatry Research*, *220*(1–2), 604–608. https://doi.org/10.1016/j.psychres.2014.07.012

Yasuda, Y., Okada, N., Nemoto, K., Fukunaga, M., Yamamori, H., Ohi, K., Koshiyama, D., Kudo, N., Shiino, T., Morita, S., Morita, K., Azechi, H., Fujimoto, M., Miura, K., Watanabe, Y., Kasai, K., & Hashimoto, R. (2020). Brain morphological and functional features in cognitive subgroups of schizophrenia. *Psychiatry and Clinical Neurosciences*, *74*(3), 191–203. https://doi.org/10.1111/pcn.12963

Yoon, J. H., Sheremata, S. L., Rokem, A., & Silver, M. A. (2013). Windows to the soul: Vision science as a tool for studying biological mechanisms of information processing deficits in schizophrenia. *Frontiers in Psychology*, *4*, 681. https://doi.org/10.3389/fpsyg.2013.00681

13 Alyssa wants to go out with friends and has anxiety

Neuroscience facilitates our understanding of going out with friends

Batya Engel-Yeger

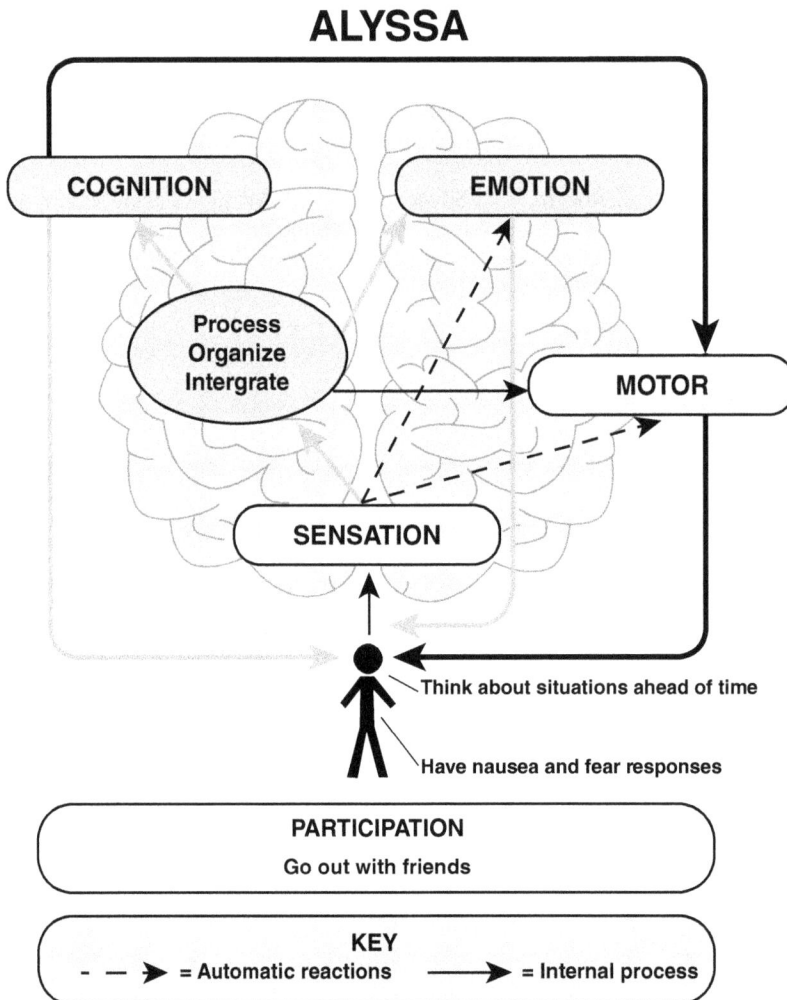

Figure 13.1 Alyssa brain figure

DOI: 10.4324/9781003524380-16

Purpose of this chapter

The purpose of this chapter is to understand how Alyssa, a 20-year-old woman with anxiety and sensory sensitivity, can foster friendships. Alyssa has anxiety and sensory sensitivity. Anxiety is a condition that involves worry about the future; the brain structures and networks responsible for neuro-modulation, with the focus on sensory processing and emotional modulation challenges, can contribute to anxiety. People with anxiety can have full lives with their daily routines, relationships, work and leisure.

The neuroscientific elements will be embedded in examples from daily life experiences. Extreme sensory processing patterns and anxiety are known to be related and result from an un-modulated hyper-aroused nervous system. In people with anxiety, this hyper aroused nervous system may significantly affect various aspects of daily life. This chapter will discuss how Alyssa's hyper aroused nervous system challenges her daily life, with an emphasis on her social participation and relationships. This chapter will help us understand the interrelations between anxiety and sensory processing via the neuroscience lens and how these features affect her friendships. As with all the chapters, these components of the nervous system work with other systems to support overall human function.

Keywords for this chapter are listed in the box below. Be sure you learn what these key features are so you can get the most out of the chapter.

Keywords for this chapter

amygdala	cortisol	multisensory integration
anxiety	executive function	neurotransmitter
arousability	frontal lobe	parasympathetic
ANS	hyper-arousability	prefrontal cortex
central nervous system	hypersensitivity	subcortical
(CNS)	hyposensitivity	sympathetic
cerebral cortex	limbic system	

Box 13.1 Learning activity

Prior to reading the case:

1. How do you think the symptoms of anxiety will affect Alyssa's friendships?
2. Why is it important for an occupational therapy practitioner to understand the neurology of anxiety?

Alyssa, a 20-year-old woman with anxiety and sensory sensitivity, wants to gather with friends and go out to a party

Alyssa is studying medicine at the university. She achieves high grades, but also wants to keep gathering with her friends and even find a new boyfriend. Alyssa has two sisters, both of them are physicians, and so are her parents. Her family wishes that Alyssa will be a physician as well. Alyssa is the youngest sister. Both her sisters are married and have two children. Alyssa decided that she will continue the family heritage and become a physician. She is now in her second year at the university. Her parents and sisters are very happy with this decision; however, her mother is concerned about the fact the Alyssa has not found a boyfriend yet.

Alyssa is studying hard, from early morning till late night. She can meet her friends only during the weekends. Alyssa has five close friends whom she has known since high school. They meet almost every weekend. Her social life is very important to her and she invests all possible efforts to take part in social events such as parties, going to movies, and visits to friends' homes. She is very happy with her friends, but feels it's the right time to have a boyfriend too. Yet, it is quite challenging.

Last year, during her final exams she felt she could not breathe. Her heart raced and her blood pressure was high; her mouth was dry and she got very scared. Alyssa went to see a psychiatrist. The psychiatrist explained that she experienced an anxiety attack. Alyssa realized she has a tendency to be anxious as part of her personality, which is enhanced during stressful life events such as exams, but she didn't know her experience could be defined as a psychiatric disease.

Alyssa also chooses her friends—she has the same social group with five friends for several years. These relaxed quiet people know her sensory sensitivity. Their personality together with their patient and ability to accept her sensory needs, enable them to maintain a good supportive friendship. However, Alyssa wants to elaborate her social circle but this makes her anxious because she is not sure if new people she meets will understand her sensory needs and anxiety tendency. This combination of anxiety and low sensory thresholds is more disturbing during specific periods, such as during exams at the university. In these times, Alyssa becomes more anxious, less patient with people; she responds quickly without allowing others to finish what they have to say, and has a tendency to shout and cry easily. Alyssa is aware of this reactivity and is embarrassed by it. Because her friends know her very well, they accept her and support her in hard times. However, Alyssa wonders what will happen with new people she is going to meet? How will they respond? Will they accept her? Give her a chance? Or maybe run away and decide not to meet her again? And what if this is a man that Alyssa is interested in?

Last week Alyssa met a young man at a party, named John. They started to talk and he asked for her phone number. Alyssa gave him her number and waited for him to call. But some anxious thoughts entered her mind again. What if he wants to meet me? What if we go to a restaurant with lots of people, bright lights, spicy food that will overwhelm me? How will I control my excitement? Will it turn to an anxiety attack?

According to the recommendation of her psychiatrists, Alyssa met an occupational therapist, a psychologist, and together they collaborated on how to create a plan to help her cope with her sensory sensitivity patterns and anxiety in daily life, with a particular focus on how to enhance her social participation and her ability to create a relationship with John. This plan included participating in support groups, and collaborating with professionals in the community that focus on elevating coping strategies (including mindfulness and self-relaxation). Her support group included ten people aged 20–25, who all experienced anxiety. This group made it clear that Alyssa is not alone, that other people experience similar challenges, and that they can support each other to find ways to have satisfying daily life routines and foster social relationships.

Box 13.2   Learning activity

Discuss with your peers:

1. Having read the narrative, what are you curious about?
2. What do you need to know more about?
3. What happens in your body when you are excited/worried?
4. What do you think in this situation?

Now that you have had some time to think about all of this, let's consider what fostering social relationships requires from the nervous system. You certainly already have some great ideas to build on.

Box 13.3   Learning activity

Before you continue reading the chapter, work with your small group to discuss what you already know:

1. How can scientific reasoning about neuroscience illuminate your insights?
2. What brain structures and functions are related to anxiety?
3. What are the mechanisms responsible for anxiety modulation?
4. Why is sensory sensitivity related to anxiety?
5. What are the brain networks that connect between sensory and emotional modulation?
6. What are the brain networks that explain the related behavior?
7. What happens in Alyssa's brain when she meets John?
8. What brain structures and functions support social awareness and social skills?
9. How can the support group assist with the challenges of modulating sensory input and anxiety?

Neuroscience information to guide your thinking about Alyssa

Behavioral and medical sciences provide vast knowledge about anxiety. Here, we discuss brain structures and functions responsible for the interrelations between anxiety, sensory processing and social participation.

First, let's define anxiety. According to the APA dictionary of psychology:

> Anxiety is an emotion characterized by feelings of tension, worried thoughts, and physical changes like increased blood pressure … Anxiety is not the same as fear, but they are often used interchangeably. Anxiety is considered a future-oriented, long-acting response broadly focused on a diffuse threat, whereas fear is an appropriate, present-oriented, and short-lived response to a clearly identifiable and specific threat.
>
> (APA, 2018)

The experience of anxiety creates a perceived need for vigilance; brain pathways begin to work overtime to keep track of all possible sensory input to know all possible aspects of the perceived threat. This over attention to incoming information can make a situation seem more threatening than it actually is, which is why the person's reactions can seem bigger than the situation at hand.

Sensory processing

The ongoing sensory information from our environment and body enters the brain via the sensory systems and tracts. Because there are various sensory modalities, sensory information is first mapped separately in the peripheral parts of each modality (ears, nose, eyes, etc.), entering the brain to the relevant cortexes. For example, visual information from the eyes enters the occipital cortex while the auditory information coming from the ears enters the temporal cortex. As mentioned in Chapter 11 about Kareem:

> when we are talking about sensory processing, we are not discussing the sensory organs themselves, but rather the brain's ability to make meaning, interpret, integrate the sensory information so we know what to do next. Sensory processing start in subcortical levels as the brainstem and proceed to and within the cortex, and with the integrating areas of the parietal, temporal, occipital and frontal lobes.

Sensory information is critical for our survival but also for learning, interacting with the physical and social environments which all leads to meaningful participation in life. The relevant brain structures process the ongoing rich sensory information and create adaptive responses (motor, emotional) as the person interacts with the environment. The adaptive response depends on the ability of the central nervous system (CNS) to properly process sensory information—meaning to treat and to modulate the amount and intensity of the incoming sensory stimuli, i.e., to focus on relevant stimuli and ignore others (Engel-Yeger, 2021). In adequate sensory processing there is a balance between habituation to sensory input (adaptation to an ongoing sensory stimulus) and sensitivity (excitation of the CNS due to a new or changing sensory stimulus) (Miller et al., 2007). Because our environment is dynamic, the CNS has to fluctuate between sensitivity and habitation as is necessary for planning and implementing our activity performance.

While most people have adequate sensory processing, 5–15% of the general population have extreme sensory processing patterns (Galiana-Simal et al., 2020), meaning that there is imbalance between habituation and sensitivity to sensory input in their CNS. When habituation exceeds sensitivity, the person might miss sensory information which is relevant to the activity and be less aware of the environment. This is called "hyposensitivity." When sensitivity exceeds habituation, the person might respond to slight sensory input, whether relevant to the activity or not. This is called "hypersensitivity." Extreme sensory processing patterns are more prevalent in people with psychiatric and neurodevelopmental disorders such as anxiety, schizophrenia, attention deficit hyperactivity disorder and autism spectrum disorder (ASD) (Green et al., 2012) and may significantly impact participation and quality of life (Engel-Yeger et al., 2016).

The processing and modulation of sensory input depends on cellular mechanisms—on receptors and synapse activity; on neurotransmitter balance involved in the function of various brain networks and structures with direct impact on conscious, on arousability, as well as on motor, cognitive and emotional control (Kandel, Schwartz, & Jessell, 2000; Serafini et al., 2017).

For example, people with sensory hypersensitivity are easily overstimulated. In their brain there is over inclusion of stimuli, whether relevant to the environmental demands or not (Davies & Tucker, 2010). This may cause hyper-arousability, anxious and defensive behavior, and withdrawal from specific stimuli and environments (Engel-Yeger & Dunn, 2011).

People with extreme sensory processing patterns may overcome related functional obstacle if they are *aware* of their own sensory profile and apply the right *coping* mechanisms to deal with their sensory patterns. For that, the networks that connect between sensory brain areas, cognitive and emotional areas have to communicate properly. When talking about Alyssa—she is sensory sensitive. Her sensory sensitivity may enhance her anxiety, but her anxiety may cause her to be more alert and sensitive to sensory stimuli. This is because her CNS is hyper-aroused. We may understand it better when we think about us going in a dark alley in an unknown area, to reach a new friend's home. In this situation, our senses are sharp, and our CNS should be on high alert because we must attend to the unfamiliar environment to make the right cognitive decisions (e.g., keep going in the right direction, avoid unpredictable obstacles such as a step, or dangerous animals, etc.). We may be a bit stressed, feel our heart race and might even sweat. We understand cognitively that in order to go safely through the alley and reach our destination, we have to notice stimuli from our environment, and if we hear a sound of a snake, or see an object on the road, we will act accordingly (e.g., quickly move out of the way). Otherwise, we may fall or get bitten.

Alyssa also has low threshold to sensory input. According to Dunn's sensory processing model (Dunn, 2014), she is the "sensitivity" type. That means that sensory input is overwhelming; she perceives sensory input coming from the environment as intensive and sometimes even painful. For example, some clothing textures, as wool, feel itchy; bright neon lights in the room make her eyes painful; loud music in a party hurts her ears. People talking load in a restaurant make her want to run away because of the overwhelming auditory stimuli. Therefore, Alyssa stays away from environments and situations with sensory input that may overwhelm her. These extreme sensory experiences can feed Alyssa's anxiety. Actually, we can refer to this relation as a circle where sensory sensitivity enhances anxiety, and in turn, anxiety enhances sensory sensitivity. In order to control this vicious cycle, and optimally function, Alyssa tries to control her physical and human environment. Therefore, she organizes her room in a convenient way for her sensory systems—the walls as painted in gentle beige, the light is warm, the windows have an option to be covered when the bright sun enters the room.

Box 13.4   Learning activity

1. Read about Dunn's Sensory Processing Framework (DSPF) from one of the references at the end of this chapter (Dunn, 2014; Dunn et al., 2016; Tomchek et al., 2015).
2. Think about what sensory patterns you exhibit in your life. What circumstances bring out these features? What adjustments have you made to accommodate your sensory processing patterns?
3. Talk with your peers about similarities and differences among your sensory experiences.

Keywords: sensory processing, Dunn's Framework, sensory patterns

The next section will discuss brain areas and networks that connect between sensory processing, anxiety and cognition and enable the adaptive behavior people need to function everyday. We will learn how sensory stimuli in a hypersensitive person with anxiety, and the related hyper-arousability, impact the body systems and engage cognitive abilities, including high cognitive functions, named—executive function (EF), so people can cope with the situations they face in their lives.

Brain areas and networks related to sensory processing and anxiety

The amygdala is the brain area that is activated in a stressful situation; the amygdala is more activated in anxiety. The amygdala is responsible for the increased anxious, vigilance-related behavior and for learning and memory related to fear. Dealing with stressful situations demand quick and strong autonomic (autonomic nervous system responses [ANS], such as breathing, heart rate; consists of sympathetic and parasympathetic responses), endocrine (hormonal actions), and motor/behavioral responses. For that, cortical and subcortical areas of the brain must be synchronized. The amygdala has connection with cortical and subcortical brain areas.

The amygdala elicits the autonomic, endocrine, and motor/behavioral responses in several ways. The hypothalamus, pituitary gland, and the adrenal gland are activated in a stressful situation to enable the body to deal with the stress. Activation of this system (called the hypothalamus-pituitary-adrenal [HPA] axis) results in the secretion of cortisol, a hormone naturally released from your adrenal glands, which plays an important role in the stress response. By interacting between glands, hormones, and parts of the brainstem, the HPA axis regulates the use of energy and the digestive system, immune system, mood, emotions and sexuality in the body during stress (Joseph & Whirledge, 2017). The amygdala activates areas in the brainstem that are responsible for visceral functions such as changes in heart rate, blood pressure, body temperature, sweating, in order to enable the body to engage in "fight or flight" reactions (sympathetic reactions of the ANS) when needed.

It should be noted that brain networks communicate via the "brain fuel"—the neurotransmitters. The neurotransmitter-specific fiber systems that target the amygdala and other brain areas, include the locus ceruleus which provides norepinephrine for the brain (McDonald, 2014; Mashour & Pryor, 2015).

Box 13.5   Learning activity

Find a picture of the HPA axis and map the body organs that it affects in order to deal with a stressful event.

Keywords: hypothalamus, pituitary, amygdala, HPA axis

The amygdala activates frontal areas that are responsible for memories, and the prefrontal cortex which directs executive functions such as self-control, attention, and memories to modulate fear and find just the right strategy to cope with the stressor

(Etkin & Wager, 2007). Indeed, dealing with a stressful event requires finding a cognitive solution. Questions such as these run through the prefrontal cortex:

- What happened?
- Do I remember a similar event from the past? What did I do then? Was it effective?
- Should I use similar strategies as before? New ones?
- What should I do first to overcome the stressful event successfully? What next?

We understand that during a stressful event we must be attentive to our environment and not miss any stimulus that may harm us. Therefore, sensory information is integrated in our brain with cognitive and emotional centers to perceive the situation at hand. Sensory information is compared to previous memories to decide what will be the appropriate behavioral responses (Zhou et al., 2021).

Sensory processing and the prefrontal cortex—sensory-cognitive networks

EF enable people to adopt and maintain appropriate problem-solving processes to reach a future goal. EF include working memory, emotion control, initiation, planning, organization, time management, shifting attention, flexibility, all of which are critical for emotion regulation, self-restraint, for surviving and for performing each and every meaningful activity (Barkley, 2012).

The prefrontal cortex covers the front part of the frontal lobe. This brain area is responsible for guiding behavior and social interactions, using the executive functions listed above; the prefrontal cortex connects with structures associated with sensory processing, memory and emotion.

Box 13.6 Learning activity

Find an illustration of the connections among the prefrontal cortex, sensory cortices and the sensory receptors. Explain the connections in your own words using an everyday problem-solving situation you face. Share your ideas with peers (Dresp-Langley, 2023, provides one such image).

Studies explored how the brain processes sensory information to enable people to correctly interpret and flexibly respond to stimuli in the environment. Some of these studies highlighted that the process depends on the context of the situation. For example, in the context of walking in a dark alley in an unfamiliar area, the CNS is hyper-aroused due to the stressful context. In a different context, as when walking safely near our known and familiar home, the CNS is relaxed. The studies mapped neuronal mechanisms responsible for this flexibility and highly context-dependent behavioral responses to sensory events. Neuroscientific evidence revealed that sensory information processing in specific sensory regions (as vision, hearing, somato-sensation) interacts with global mechanisms of multisensory integration, under the control of the prefrontal cortex. That means that the prefrontal cortex, which receives and integrates inputs from diverse sensory modalities, is involved in the modulation of this sensory input, to match the context of the activity—if we walk thought a dark alley, then the sensitivity will be much higher than when we walk near our home. When we meet new friends, we will be highly sensitive as compared to a social meeting with old friends that we already know and can predict their reactions. Thus, the EF creates the behavioral output based on the sensory information and the judgment of the flexibility required for adapting to the context (Dresp-Langley, 2023).

Another brain area that impacts sensory—emotional-cognitive processing is the thalamus. The Thalamus processes information from all senses (except smell). The thalamus filters and organizes sensory information, and then relays information among different subcortical areas and the cerebral cortex, including the prefrontal cortex to enhance attentional control to the most salient sensory information. This is most important in stressful situations.

When people have sensory hypersensitivity and anxiety, there is inefficient inhibition of these thalamus/cortex connections. Habituation to familiar sensory inputs is ineffective, so people continue to get too much sensory input from the environment and all this input may be perceived as overwhelming. This experience may affect the person's EF by interfering with attention, clouding decision making, reducing self-control, and providing faulty information for planning which results in maladaptive behavior and inept social functioning (Green et al., 2018; Halassa & Acsády, 2016). Therefore, the networks between the sensory information via the thalamus and the amygdala to the prefrontal cortex all contributes to a fear response.

Box 13.7   Learning activity

In small groups, discuss:

1. How will a person with anxiety and sensory sensitivity may behave when facing an overwhelming sensory input as intense perfume of a friend he/she just met?
2. How would it affect the person's behavior during this social interaction? What can we see in the person's body and physiological signs?
3. How would this behavioral response affect the friend? How would this behavior change if the friend is aware to the anxiety and sensory sensitivity?
4. What will be the consequences of the anxious—sensory sensitive person?

Social engagement and neuroscience

In a hyper aroused brain, as in people with sensory hypersensitivity and anxiety, the challenges in self-control may affect social relationships and participation. Although they understand the social codes and are deeply motivated to connect with people, the subcortical areas dominate the prefrontal cortex, and the fight or flight behavior (sympathetic responses in the ANS) overrides the adaptive modulated behavior. Therefore, when Alyssa is with friends, her behavior and social interaction may be affected by her hyper-aroused brain as when facing uncomfortable sensory inputs coming from the environment (such as a sudden noise; load music at the party; a smelly person near her;

bright and fast changing lights, as in a party). When Alyssa is overwhelmed because of sensory input she perceives as extreme (in this case from the party environment), she might behave in a fight or flight manner, meaning that the activity of her visceral parts of the body will be enhanced, as expressed in elevated heart rate, blood pressure, and sweaty hands. She may intuitively show fear or a disgusted expression on her face, run away to the toilets or outside the hall, and not be able to pay attention to her friends, to communicate properly with them, to laugh and enjoy the situation and create new relationships with John. Her anxiety may be elevated due to the excitement of meeting John and her worries about her behavior. She may get panicked or behave in a way that other people will consider as odd. To take charge of her responses during social participation, Alyssa can use her EF to understand what happens in her body, how to achieve self-control, what action to initiate, and what cognitive strategies to use to have a more successful and satisfying social life.

As noted by Dunn in Chapter 11 about Kareem:

> from a neuroscience perspective, social interaction emerges from an integrated network of connections in several areas of the cortex (Gutman, 2017; Kandel, 2018). Unlike the primary sensory cortex, which houses sensory maps of the body (called the homunculus), other parts of the sensory cortex integrate input to create appropriate responses.

Let's summarize what brain structures we mentioned till now. For Alyssa, we are particularly interested in several parts of this network:

- The parietal lobe—processes sensory information and contains the somatosensory cortex.
- The thalamus—a subcortical relay for sensory information from periphery to cortex.
- The limbic system (amygdala, hippocampus, septum)—emotional affective control.
- The amygdala orchestrates emotional actions, particularly attaching emotional significance to our thoughts and memories
- The autonomic nervous system (ANS)—(1) its sympathetic part (reacts to a stressed situation—real or imagined, by preparing the body for action) and (2) its parasympathetic part (relaxation).
- Locus ceruleus (the "blue spot")—the principal site for brain synthesis of norepinephrine/noradrenaline (one of the brain and body mobilizer for action). The locus ceruleus is a part of the reticular activating system, and is located in the pons of the brainstem and is involved with physiological responses to stress. Secretion of norepinephrine will increase cognitive function through the prefrontal cortex, increase motivation, activate the HPA axis, and increases the sympathetic discharge/inhibits parasympathetic tone (through the brainstem).
- Reticular formation—visceral connections impact heartbeat, respiration, vasomotor activity
- Prefrontal cortex and the executive functions—the use of high cognitive abilities to control behavior and decide what action should be made to deal with the stressor.
- The orbito-frontal cortex plays a key role in impulse control, monitoring ongoing behavior and socially appropriate behaviors.

Box 13.8   Learning activity

1. Find a picture of each of the brain parts described above.
2. Describe parts of the body that are affected by the autonomic nervous system—what happens to them when the sympathetic part is activated and what happens when the parasympathetic part is activated?
3. List the executive functions.
4. Look at the picture and draw the stages involved in the neuro-sequence of what happens to the persons when seeing a snake (sensory processing and anxiety).

Keywords: names of brain areas, sensory processing and anxiety patterns

---

Life routine: social participation—gathering with friends—Alyssa is going out to a party

During their twenties, young people are extremely interested in participating in social activities, create new social networks, including romantic relationships. For that they may gather with friends daily and even participate in parties as a routine (not necessarily a daily routine but probably a weekly routine). This stage is significant for their wellbeing and for building their future. A successful social interaction highly depends on the person's ability to communicate. Communication begins with the ability to properly perceive input—auditory (as: what do my friends say), visual (keep eye contact, read body language), tactile (react in accordance to the situation, for example when given a hug) etc. Communication also depends on the ability to process all inputs, in accordance to the context and activity demands (e.g., a friendly conversation in the campus vs. Alyssa is invited to the party), monitor emotional responses (e.g., happiness and excitement because of the invitation to the party), and to execute the proper motor acts (e.g., smile and other facial expressions to what is said by her friend; accepting the hug and give back a hug), and the proper communication behavior (e.g., know when to listen, when to answer). The EF orchestrates all of these responses as part of overall behavioral regulation (e.g., inhibition of some responses, initiation of interactions, attention to others, judgement about the meaning of another's behavior, knowing what should be said, what should not). This coordination between the people involved in the social interaction, is critical for the success of relationships and for creating a desire to further communicate and keep in touch.

What happens in the brain of a person with sensory processing challenges and elevated anxiety during social participation?

Alyssa is at the party. Her old friend tells her that John has just arrived; John gets close to Alyssa and starts talking with her. After a few minutes, he asks her to dance with him. The lights on the dance floor are bright, changing quickly, the music is very loud. This intense sensory input elevates Alyssa's emotional stress. Thoughts such as: how will I handle this intense sensory input, what if I cannot adapt to it, how will John react if I run away to the toilet, what will he think about me? Will he still be interested in me?' run through Alyssa's head.

Box 13.9   Learning activity

With your small group, complete the table in the Appendix about the integration of Alyssa's social participation demands and the neuroscience that affects her participation. Refer to possible interactions between her sensory-emotional-cognitive demands and networks.

Back to the person: Alyssa is gathering with friends and they go to a party

After understanding what goes on inside the brain of people with anxiety and sensory processing challenges, think how we can use scientific reasoning to support Alyssa to successfully participate in social activities as during the party. Think of possible intervention direction based on your neuroscientific knowledge to support Alyssa's brain processing and behavior.

Box 13.10   Learning activity

In class or small groups, discuss what strategies should Alyssa apply to successfully participate in the party, gather with her friend and create a good start in her relationships with John? What brain networks can support her behavioral output?

As occupational therapists, we should understand brain activity responsible for sensory processing challenges and anxiety, how sensory processing challenges and anxiety affect the person's ability to perform activities and participate in daily life. Intervention is significantly improved when we understand underlying body mechanisms that explain behavior and participation. By combining our neuroscientific knowledge with the person's story from their own voice, we may optimally tailor the intervention that will best fit the person's specific characteristics, needs, interests and challenges. In that way, we may elevate engagement in therapy and together create opportunities for meaningful participation with a significant positive impact on people's wellbeing in the real context of their lives.

What do we know about ourselves and the population at large from this brain condition and from Alyssa's story?

We should remember that each of us experience anxious situations during our lives. While some of us adapt and cope properly with stressful stimuli and events, other have greater challenges in regulating their response to stressful situations and experience them as anxious for a long time. In our demanding world, anxiety is a worldwide phenomenon. About one-third of the population worldwide suffers from anxiety disorders (Bandelow & Michaelis, 2022). Among individuals with sensory processing challenges, anxiety trend is significantly higher (Cervin, 2023). The COVID-19 pandemic is a good example of how a stressful event elevates people's anxiety, affects our daily lives and behavior, our social participation, our emotional wellbeing (Cénat et al., 2021). Studies note that anxiety is more prevalent in women (Metin et al., 2022). While some people cope with their anxiety and modulate it in an adaptive way (using for example proper cognitive strategies, use the help of others, or create adaptations in their environment to overcome the overwhelming situation), others may experience greater challenges in regulating the way anxiety occurs in their brain and body.

Further reading

If interested in further reading about the lived experience of people with anxiety and sensory sensitivity, consult the following:

Galiana-Simal, A., et al. (2020). Sensory processing disorder: Key points of a frequent alteration in neurodevelopmental disorders. *Cogent Medicine, 7*(1), 1736829. Retrieved February 1, 2023.

Lane, A. E. (2020). Practitioner Review: Effective management of functional difficulties associated with sensory symptoms in children and adolescents. *Journal of Child Psychology and Psychiatry, 61*(9), 943–958.

Martin, E. I., Ressler, K. J., Binder, E., & Nemeroff, C. B. (2009). The neurobiology of anxiety disorders: brain imaging, genetics, and psychoneuroendocrinology. *Psychiatric Clinics, 32*(3), 549–575.

Peng, W., Jia, Z., Huang, X., Lui, S., Kuang, W., Sweeney, J. A., & Gong, Q. (2019). Brain structural abnormalities in emotional regulation and sensory processing regions associated with anxious depression. *Progress in Neuro-Psychopharmacology and Biological Psychiatry, 94*, 109676.

Stoller, C. C., Greuel, J. H., Cimini, L. S., Fowler, M. S., & Koomar, J. A. (2012). Effects of sensory-enhanced yoga on symptoms of combat stress in deployed military personnel. *The American Journal of Occupational Therapy, 66*(1), 59–68.

References

APA (2018). Anxiety. Rerieved from https://dictionary.apa.org/anxiety

Bandelow, B., & Michaelis, S. (2022). Epidemiology of anxiety disorders in the 21st century. *Dialogues in clinical neuroscience, 17*(3), 327–335. https://doi.org/10.31887/DCNS.2015.17.3/bbandelow

Barkley, R. A. (2012). *Executive functions: What they are, how they work, and why they evolved.* Guilford Press.

Cénat, J. M., et al. (2021). Prevalence of symptoms of depression, anxiety, insomnia, posttraumatic stress disorder, and psychological distress among populations affected by the COVID-19 pandemic: A systematic review and meta-analysis. *Psychiatry research, 295*, 113599. https://doi.org/10.1016/j.psychres.2020.113599.

Cervin, M. (2022). Sensory Processing Difficulties in Children and Adolescents with Obsessive-Compulsive and Anxiety Disorders. *Research on Child and Adolescent Psychopathology*, 1–10.

Davies, P. L., & Tucker, R. (2010). Evidence review to investigate the support for subtypes of children with difficulty processing and integrating sensory information. *The American Journal of Occupational Therapy, 64*(3), 391–402.

Dresp-Langley, B. (2023). The Grossberg Code: Universal Neural Network Signatures of Perceptual Experience. *Information, 14*(2), 82. www.mdpi.com/2078-2489/14/2/82.

Dunn, W. (2014). *Sensory profile 2: Strengths-based approach to assessment and planning.* Pearson: San Antonio.

Dunn, W., et al. (2016). Prevalence of sensory characteristics in the general population: A person-centered approach. *American Journal of Occupational Therapy, 70*(4) (Suppl. 1).

Engel-Yeger, B. (2021). The involvement of altered sensory modulation in neurological conditions and its relevance to neuro-rehabilitation: a narrative literature review. *Disability and Rehabilitation, 43*(17), 2511–2520.

Engel-Yeger, B., & Dunn, W. (2011). The relationship between sensory processing difficulties and anxiety level of healthy adults. *British Journal of Occupational Therapy*, *74*(5), 210–216.

Engel-Yeger, B., Gonda, X., Muzio, C., Rinosi, G., Pompili, M., Amore, M., & Serafini, G. (2016). Sensory processing patterns, coping strategies, and quality of life among patients with unipolar and bipolar disorders. *Brazilian Journal of Psychiatry*, *38*, 207–215. https://doi.org/10.1590/1516-4446-2015-1785.

Etkin, A., & Wager, T. D. (2007). Functional neuroimaging of anxiety: a meta-analysis of emotional processing in PTSD, social anxiety disorder, and specific phobia. *American Journal of Psychiatry*, *164*(10), 1476–1488.

Galiana-Simal, A., et al. (2020). Sensory processing disorder: Key points of a frequent alteration in neurodevelopmental disorders. *Cogent Medicine*, *7*(1), 1736829. Retrieved February 1, 2023.

Green, S. A., Ben-Sasson, A., Soto, T. W., & Carter, A. S. (2012). Anxiety and sensory over-responsivity in toddlers with autism spectrum disorders: Bidirectional effects across time. *Journal of Autism and Developmental Disorders*, *42*, 1112–1119.

Green, S. A., Hernandez, L. M., Bowman, H. C., Bookheimer, S. Y., & Dapretto, M. (2018). Sensory over-responsivity and social cognition in ASD: Effects of aversive sensory stimuli and attentional modulation on neural responses to social cues. *Developmental Cognitive Neuroscience*, *29*, 127–139.

Gutman, S. (2017). *Quick Reference Neuroscience for Rehabilitation Professionals*. Third edition. Thorofare, NJ: Slack.

Halassa, M. M., & Acsády, L. (2016). Thalamic inhibition: diverse sources, diverse scales. *Trends in Neurosciences*, *39*(10), 680–693.

Joseph, D. N., & Whirledge, S. (2017). Stress and the HPA axis: balancing homeostasis and fertility. *International Journal of Molecular Sciences*, *18*(10), 2224. https://doi.org/10.3390/ijms18102224. PMID: 29064426; PMCID: PMC5666903.

Kandel, E. R. (2018). *The disordered mind: What unusual brains tell us about ourselves*. Hachette UK.

Kandel, E. R., Schwartz, J. H., Jessell, T. M., Siegelbaum, S., Hudspeth, A. J., & Mack, S. (Eds.). (2000). *Principles of neural science* (Vol. 4, pp. 1227–1246). New York: McGraw-Hill.

Mashour, G. A., & Pryor, K. O. (2015). Consciousness, memory, and anesthesia. In R. D. Miller (Ed.), *Miller's anesthesia*, 8th ed. Philadelphia, PA: Churchill Livingstone, pp. 287–289.

McDonald, A. J. (2014). Amygdala. In M. J. Aminoff & R. B. Daroff (Eds.), *Encyclopedia of the neurological sciences* (second edition), Academic Press, pp. 153–156, https://doi.org/10.1016/B978-0-12-385157-4.01113-1.

Metin, A., Erbiçer, E. S., Şen, S., & Çetinkaya, A. (2022). Gender and COVID-19 related fear and anxiety: A meta-analysis. *Journal of Affective Disorders*. doi: 10.1016/j.jad.2022.05.036.

Miller, L. J., Anzalone, M. E., Lane, S. J., Cermak, S. A., & Osten, E. T. (2007). Concept evolution in sensory integration: A proposed nosology for diagnosis. *The American Journal of Occupational Therapy*, *61*(2), 135.

Serafini, G., Gonda, X., Canepa, G., Pompili, M., Rihmer, Z., Amore, M., & Engel-Yeger, B. (2017). Extreme sensory processing patterns show a complex association with depression, and impulsivity, alexithymia, and hopelessness. *Journal of Affective Disorders*, *210*, 249–257.

Tomchek, S. D., et al. (2015). Sensory pattern contributions to developmental performance in children with autism spectrum disorder. *Am J Occup Ther*, *69*(5). https://doi.org/10.5014/ajot.2015.018044

Zhou, Y., Rosen, M. C., Swaminathan, S. K., Masse, N. Y., Zhu, O., & Freedman, D. J. (2021). Distributed functions of prefrontal and parietal cortices during sequential categorical decisions. *Elife*, *10*, e58782. https://doi.org/10.7554/eLife.58782.

14 Abraham wants to fish and has depression

Neuroscience facilitates our understanding of learning a new activity

Alexandra L. Terrill

ABRAHAM

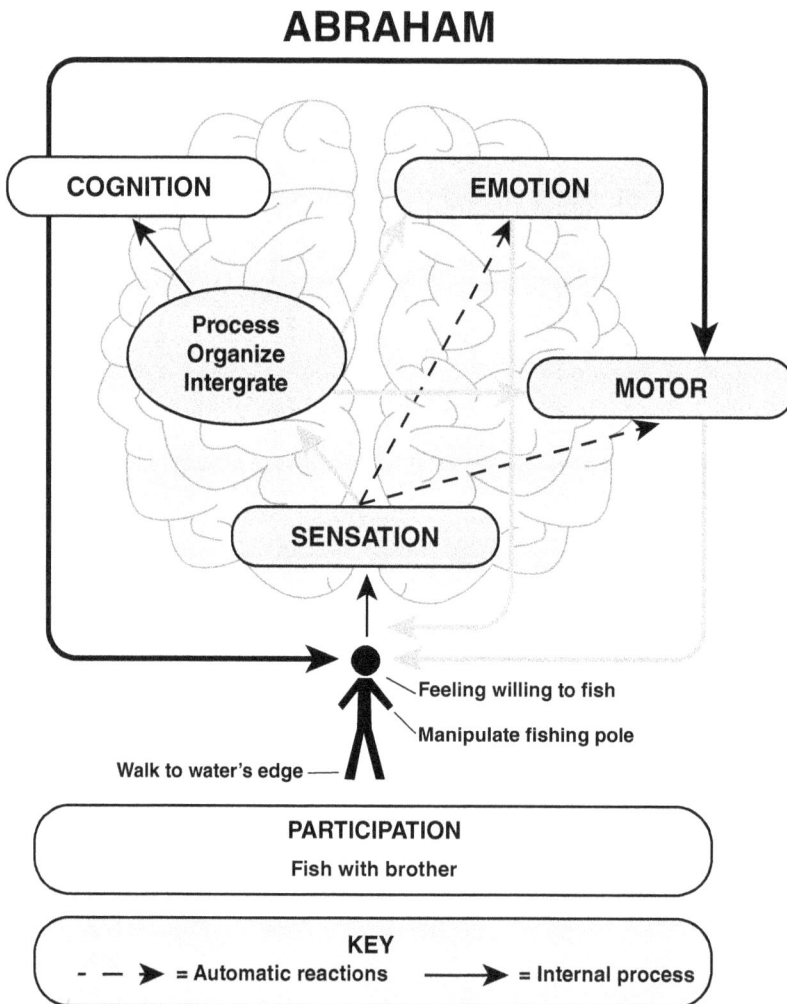

Figure 14.1 Abraham brain figure

DOI: 10.4324/9781003524380-17

Purpose of this chapter

The purpose of this chapter is to discover how Abraham, a 57-year-old man who wants to learn a new activity, might be affected by depression, a condition with neuroscience underpinnings that impact the learning of a new activity. Depression can have a serious impact on our ability to function. As we will learn, depression is the result of a complex interaction of psychological, biological, and social factors that can impact how someone thinks, behaves, and feels. People with depression have full lives with daily routines, participating in meaningful activities, relationships, and learning, but may require modifications for function.

In this chapter, we will specifically explore the connection between depression and the brain, and how learning can be affected when a person is depressed. The key neuroscience concepts we will explore in this chapter include stress's impact on the nervous system and likely role in depression, neurotransmitters in depression, depression's impacts on neural networks involved in learning, learned helplessness, and the monoamine deficiency theory. As with all the chapters, these components of the nervous system work with other systems to support overall human function.

Keywords for this chapter are listed in the box below. Be sure you learn what these key features are so you can get the most out of the chapter.

Keywords for this chapter

amygdala	dopamine	limbic cortex
anhedonia	dorsal striatum	monoamine deficiency
basal ganglia	dorsolateral prefrontal	theory
catecholamines	cortex	neurotransmitter
cingulate cortex	gray matter	norepinephrine
cortisol	hippocampus	serotonin
default network	hypothalamus–pituitary–	striatum
depression	adrenal (HPA) axis	

Let's find out more about Abraham, a man who wants to learn to fish

Abraham, age 57, had a stroke 18 months ago. He has made significant improvements in his recovery, but Abraham continues to have trouble speaking and has some paralysis on his right side, which alters his gait and limits the use of his right hand. Although he is independent in his activities of daily living (ADLs), they now take him longer to complete and he gets easily frustrated because of this. He is being seen by his occupational therapist today to further address his upper extremity impairments. His wife of 19 years is with him.

Prior to his stroke, Abraham was employed as a manager of a marketing firm and was the primary provider for his family. However, he is not currently employed; his former fast-paced job was too high-demand and Abraham has not felt ready to look for other options. Abraham reports that he has been getting fatigued easily, generally lacks energy, and he has trouble concentrating. He says he is having some memory problems: "As soon as I leave a room, I can't remember what I left for to begin with or what I was supposed to be doing." He is considering early retirement due to disability. His wife has had to get a second job to support them. The occupational therapist asks Abraham what his hobbies are. He says he is not sure anymore, that he feels like he can't do anything. His wife interjects, "That's not true! You have made so much progress, but it's like you are just not trying." She then turns back to the occupational therapist and adds, "He just sits on the couch and watches TV for hours on end." When she says this, Abraham shrugs and fixes his gaze on the floor. "I guess my hobby is watching TV."

Abraham discloses that he frequently struggles with feelings of worthlessness because he is "letting his family down," and that he feels like a burden especially on his wife. He says, "Sometimes, I just wish I wouldn't wake up in the morning." The occupational therapist asks Abraham whether he thinks he is depressed. Abraham shrugs and explains that he probably doesn't feel much different than most people who have had a stroke.

Box 14.1   Learning activity

1. Discuss: having read this narrative, what do you know about Abraham?
2. Is Abraham depressed? Look up symptoms for depression and compare these with what Abraham and his wife are reporting.

Keywords: depression, depression symptoms

Now, let's go back to Abraham and find out more

The occupational therapist indicates that Abraham's referring provider noted some concerns about depression. She explains that although depression after a stroke is common, it is not a normal part of the recovery process. There may be some organic causes for Abraham's depression. Many of the issues he is dealing with are related to changes in occupational performance he has experienced as a result of the stroke, which could also contribute to feeling depressed. The occupational therapist assures him that there are things he can do to help him feel better, and that occupational therapy can help him with this. While his wife eagerly nods along, Abraham is a bit skeptical, stating, "I just can't get much joy out of anything. Why would this be any different?" However, he agrees to give it a try.

The occupational therapist asks Abraham what kinds of things he used to enjoy doing before the stroke. Abraham said he loved to camp and hike; there was nothing better to escape his high-pressure job than spending his free time in the outdoors. He often went with his older brother and belonged to an active local hiking club. Since his stroke, Abraham has not spent a lot of time outdoors, especially in the wilderness, because his walking is slow and unsteady. He feels that he cannot do the things he used to do and is not motivated to try. He has not returned any phone calls from his former co-workers and hiking friends because he is very self-conscious about his ability to speak and hold a conversation the way he used to do. His wife says, "He's become very withdrawn, not doing the things he loves to do, and I don't think that's helping his mood."

Neither Abraham nor his wife think that going back to hiking is a great idea for safety reasons. The occupational therapist encourages him to come up with a new outdoors leisure activity. His wife suggests he learn how to fish, because his older brother has been trying to get him to fish with him for years. Abraham is not too sure at first; although fishing wouldn't require a lot of walking, it still requires two hands, and he has trouble with coordination and strength in his right hand. The occupational therapist reassures Abraham that this is something he can learn. Reluctantly, but with a smile on his face, Abraham agrees to give this a try.

Box 14.2   Learning activity

1. Use your activity analysis skills to analyze the demands of learning to fish.
2. Determine the difference in demands between angler fishing and fly fishing.
3. How might depression affect his ability to learn and regularly do this activity?

Box 14.3   Learning activity

1. Look up the symptoms of depression. Write them down and define them.
2. Which symptoms are somatic and which are nonsomatic? What does somatic and nonsomatic mean?

Keywords: depression symptoms, somatic symptoms, nonsomatic symptoms

3. How might these affect a person's ability to participate in day-to-day activities?

What is depression?

Before we go any further, let's learn a bit more about depression. Depression is a highly prevalent and serious mood disorder, contributing to a significant proportion of disease burden and disability worldwide. Depression is more common among individuals who have chronic medical conditions, such as cardiovascular and neurological disorders, including stroke. Depression consists of a number of symptoms that are somatic or nonsomatic.

According to the American Psychiatric Association's Diagnostic and Statistical Manual of Mental Disorders, 5th edition (DSM-5) (APA, 2013), a depression diagnosis requires the presence of at least five out of a possible nine symptoms of depression for at least two weeks and must cause the individual clinically significant distress or impairment in social, occupational, or other important areas of functioning. At least one of these symptoms must be (1) a depressed mood, or (2) anhedonia, which is a loss of interest or pleasure in doing things the person used to enjoy.

Let's go back to Abraham, who is now trying to learn how to fish

After the session with the occupational therapist, Abraham was looking forward to learning how to fish. Based on the therapist's suggestion, he had looked up some "how-to" videos online to learn more about tying lures, but he had some difficulties focusing and the video moved too fast for him to follow along. When his wife asked why he had not called his brother to go fishing, he admitted that he was worried that this would be yet "another task at which he would fail." When his brother showed up at their door the following Saturday morning, angling gear packed in his car, Abraham agreed to give it a try.

Abraham's brother drove them to a nearby lake where they had space to set up and fish off the shore. Abraham struggled to put the lure on the line, his unaffected hand being his non-dominant hand, and his frustration was apparent. When his brother offered to help, Abraham threw the pole down and muttered, "I knew I wouldn't be able to do this!" Abraham's brother finished attaching the lure and handed the pole back to Abraham. Casting the line was yet another challenge, requiring multiple attempts, one resulting in the hook and line getting hopelessly tangled in nearby bushes. Abraham said, "I'll never get this—I want to go home." But Abraham's brother patiently cut the line, re-tied the lure, and handed back the pole, stating, "Let's try just one more time. Remember, it takes time and practice to learn this." This time, the cast was successful. Unfortunately, no fish were biting. After a few more attempts at casting and reeling, Abraham said he was feeling fatigued, and they packed up the gear.

When they arrived at home, Abraham's wife opened the front door and asked how it went. "I didn't catch anything," said Abraham, but his brother was quick to add, "But he learned how to cast a line like a champ!" Abraham felt that anyone could have done that with as much help as he needed from his brother to manage it.

Box 14.4   Learning activity

Think about Abraham's first attempt at learning how to fish and some of the problems he was having with the task. Based on what we have learned thus far, do you think his difficulties are related to symptoms of depression or stroke?

Neuroscience information to guide your thinking about Abraham

Though we typically associate emotions with matters of the heart, the brain is the true seat of your emotions. There have been many advances in our understanding of the biology of depression, but we still have a lot to learn. Some of these major advances include finding links between specific parts of the brain and depression, discovering how neurotransmitters make communication between brain cells possible, and learning how biological factors interact with psychological and social factors to affect risk and symptoms of depression. Although this last point is important, this chapter will mainly focus on areas of the brain and neurotransmitters.

Box 14.5   Learning activity

Before you continue reading the chapter, discuss in small groups:

1. Depression is the result of a complex interaction of psychological, biological, and social factors that can impact how someone thinks, behaves, and feels, and how they will cope with and adjust to something like a stroke. What are some of the ways depression is affecting Abraham's day-to-day function?
2. What do you know about the brain and depression? In thinking about the brain and its structures, which structures do you think are involved in mood regulation and depression?

First, let's look at how certain areas of the brain might be associated with depression, and how this affects day-to-day functioning. The key regions that have gained consensus for an involvement in depression include the limbic cortex (amygdala, hippocampus), the cingulate cortex, dorsal striatum and the frontal lobe (dorsolateral prefrontal cortex and medial prefrontal cortex).

Box 14.6   Learning activity

1. Before reading on, look up each of the brain regions below known to be involved in depression. Note their specific primary function(s) and how they are connected: (i) limbic cortex (amygdala, hippocampus); (ii) cingulate cortex; (iii) striatum; (iv) frontal lobe (dorsolateral prefrontal cortex and medial prefrontal cortex).
2. How do you think these play into some of the symptoms of depression we discussed above? How do you think this affects the way a person functions?

Keywords: Limbic cortex, amygdala, hippocampus, cingulate cortex, striatum, frontal lobe, dorsolateral prefrontal cortex, medial prefrontal cortex

---

As you just discovered, the limbic cortex has a number of important functions. It is also thought to play a critical role in the body's stress response, as it is highly connected to the endocrine and autonomic nervous system (think fight-or-flight response). The hippocampus is primarily associated with being the memory center of the brain, but also plays a role in learning and emotions (Tyng et al., 2017). It is also one of the areas neurogenesis—or the formation of new nerve cells—occurs. The amygdala's main function is in emotional responses, including happiness, fear, and anger. It interacts with the hippocampus in that it attaches emotional content to memories.

Box 14.7   Learning activity

Look up the "default network." Think about the structures involved and what its function is. How might this network be involved in depression?

Keywords: default network, default mode network

The cingulate cortex is made up of the cingulate gyrus and the cortical gray matter lining the superior and inferior borders of the cingulate sulcus. It could be considered a connecting hub of emotions, sensations, and action as it shares extensive neural pathways with other regions of the brain. Some of these pathways are those involved in motivational processing, which is apparent through the connections with the reward centers of the brain (orbitofrontal cortex, basal ganglia, and insula). The cingulate cortex also projects pathways to the lateral prefrontal cortex, which is involved in executive control, working memory, and learning. Because the cingulate cortex also shares neural circuits with the hippocampus and amygdala, it likely also plays a role in consolidating long-term memories and processing emotionally relevant stimuli, respectively (Rolls, 2019).

The striatum is a cluster of interconnected nuclei that form a part of the basal ganglia. It is involved in decision making functions, such as motor control, emotion, habit formation, and reward. As such, it supports goal motivated behavior.

The prefrontal cortex can be divided into dorsolateral and ventromedial sectors based on anatomical connectivity and functional specialization (Koenigs & Grafman, 2009). The dorsolateral prefrontal cortex, which includes portions of the middle and superior frontal gyri on the lateral surface of the frontal lobes, receives input from specific sensory cortices, and has dense interconnections with premotor areas, the frontal eye fields, and the lateral parietal cortex. Conversely, targets of ventromedial prefrontal cortex projections include the hypothalamus and periaqueductal gray, which mediate the autonomic activity associated with emotion, and the ventral striatum, which signals reward and motivational value. In addition, the ventromedial prefrontal cortex has dense reciprocal connections with the amygdala, which is involved in threat detection and fear conditioning. The connectivity patterns of these two regions of the prefrontal cortex are distinct, as is their functionality (Koenigs & Grafman, 2009). Indeed, "cognitive" or "executive" functions are attributed to the dorsolateral prefrontal cortex, whereas the ventromedial prefrontal cortex is primarily associated with "emotional" or "affective" functions.

Box 14.8   Learning activity

Now that you've learned more about the brain structures involved with mood regulation, think about what happens when a person is depressed. What do you think happens to the brain structures, and how might this affect a person's functioning?

Loss of gray matter

Gray matter is a type of tissue in your brain that plays a crucial role in allowing a person to function normally day to day. It makes up the outermost layer of the brain and gets its gray tone from a high concentration of neuronal cell bodies. Gray matter is essential to our ability to think and reason, control voluntary movement, memory, and emotions, as well as process information, sensation, perception, learning, speech, and cognition.

Box 14.9   Learning activity

Look up an image of a healthy brain and one of a "depressed" brain. Compare the two, paying special attention to the gray matter volume. What differences do you notice?

Keywords: depression brain imaging, healthy brain imaging

Research has shown that in persons with depression, several areas of the brain shrink. More specifically, these areas lose gray matter volume (Grieve et al., 2013). Based on converging evidence from cognitive, structural neuroimaging, functional neuroimaging, and postmortem studies, changes in the prefrontal cortex have been observed frequently in association with depression (Bremner et al., 2002; Drevets et al., 2008; Steele et al., 2007).

This is especially true for the dorsolateral subregion of the prefrontal cortex, which plays a pivotal role in self-monitoring and decision making and provides executive control on other prefrontal cortex regions, such as the medial prefrontal cortex, as well as monitoring of the limbic system.

Why does this happen? One explanation for why depression is associated with structural changes in the brain is the hormone cortisol.

Box 14.10   Learning activity

Look up cortisol. What is its primary role? How might it be related to depression?

Keyword: cortisol

When faced with a threat or stressor, the amygdala determines the appropriate response, and—if necessary—sends a signal to the hypothalamus, which activates the sympathetic nervous system, sending out a cascade of hormonal and physiological responses. A surge of catecholamines is released by the adrenal glands, causing increased heart and respiratory rate (think "fight-or-flight"). As the body continues to perceive the stressor, the hypothalamus activates the hypothalamus–pituitary–adrenal (HPA) axis, which regulates both production and secretion of cortisol. As the threat passes, cortisol then helps the body return to its natural state.

Chronic stress, cortisol levels, and mental health issues like depression have a well-established link (Russell & Lightman, 2019). Our brain is well-equipped to handle acute stressors. However, when faced with a constant or chronic stressor that cannot be solved by simply "fighting or fleeing," cortisol remains elevated. You may have heard or read about the detrimental effects of having elevated cortisol levels, including increasing risk of cardiovascular disease. People who are depressed have an overactive HPA axis and release larger amounts of cortisol than people who are not. Sustained high cortisol levels may play the biggest role in changing the physical composition and chemical activities of the brain. This includes loss of gray matter.

Box 14.11   Learning activity

Before you read on, look up a picture of the brain and locate the areas thought to be affected by depression. Think about these structures of the brain and their main functions.

1. What do you think happens when these areas of the brain shrink? What might a decrease in gray matter mean in terms of symptoms a person with depression experiences?
2. How might this affect their ability to function?

Keywords: brain image, brain regions, gray matter, limbic cortex, amygdala, hippocampus, cingulate cortex, striatum, frontal lobe, dorsolateral prefrontal cortex, medial prefrontal cortex

---

Hippocampus and connected regions

Limbic regions have been frequently implicated in the pathophysiology of depression. Neuroimaging studies have demonstrated functional and morphological changes in limbic structures, and particularly the hippocampus in depressed adults (Campbell et al., 2004; Cotter et al, 2001). The hippocampus (as you previously discovered) is important for learning and memory. As part of the limbic cortex, it also connects to other parts of your brain that control emotion and is responsive to stress hormones. That makes it vulnerable to depression. Research has shown that the hippocampus is smaller in some people with depression. For example, a now well-known series of fMRI studies demonstrated that, on average, the hippocampus was 9–13% smaller in women with a history of depression as compared with women who were never depressed (Sheline et al., 1996, 1999). The more episodes of depression a woman had, the smaller the hippocampus. Those with a history of depression also scored lower on tests of verbal memory, a process linked to hippocampal function.

Stress—or more specifically, the stress hormone cortisol—is likely to be a key factor here as it can suppress the production of new neurons (nerve cells) in the hippocampus. People with depression experience long-term exposure to elevated cortisol levels, and decreased production of new brain cells as well as shrinking of existing brain cells in the hippocampus occurs (Dziurkowska & Wesolowski, 2021). This can lead to memory problems in persons with depression.

It is important to note that depression is not the not the result of selective regional dysfunction in the brain. Rather, it involves dysfunction of neural networks that normally modulates mood and emotions (Drevets et al., 2008). For example, disruption in functional connectivity between the prefrontal cortex and amygdala as well as prefrontal cortex and hippocampus have been documented (Kong et al., 2013), suggesting disruption of reciprocal connection between these structures.

Drug actions in the brain

Now that we've learned about areas of the brain that might be affected, let's take a closer look at the role of neurotransmitters in regulating mood. Neurotransmitters are the chemical messengers in the brain that carry signals from one neuron (nerve cell) to the next target cell. As you learned in previous chapters, when a neuron becomes activated, it passes an electrical signal from the cell body down the axon to its terminal, where neurotransmitters are stored and released into the synapse (the space between that neuron and the dendrite of a neighboring neuron). As the concentration of a neurotransmitter rises in the synapse, neurotransmitter molecules begin to bind with receptors in the membranes of the two neurons.

Box 14.12   Learning activity

Look up a video showing how neurotransmitters function in chemical synapses of the brain to send signals from one neuron to the next.

Keywords: chemical synapse video, neurotransmission video

Neurotransmitters are crucial to the biological processes underlying perception, thoughts, and emotions. The exact number of unique neurotransmitters is not known, but more than 100 have been identified in the complex human neural system. Regulation of how many of these neurotransmitters are being sent between neurons at any given time is believed to be involved in mood as they are involved in various neurological functions such as attention, appetite, sleep, and cognitive function.

Box 14.13   Learning activity

One of the major theories of depression is the monoamine deficiency theory (Delgado, 2000).

1. Look up the description of this theory
2. What are the primary functions of the 3 neurotransmitters in this theory of depression?

Now, go back to your list of symptoms associated with depression.

3. How do each of these neurotransmitters map onto these symptoms? Think about the primary function of each of these neurotransmitters—if you have low levels of this neurotransmitter, how might this translate to symptoms and how well you function?

Keywords: monoamine deficiency theory, depression neurotransmitters

---

To be clear, although chemicals are involved in the process, depression doesn't spring from simply having too much or too little of certain brain chemicals. Rather, many chemicals are involved, working both inside and outside nerve cells. There are millions of chemical reactions that make up the dynamic system that is responsible for your mood, perceptions, and how you experience life. But there are some medications that may help manage depression's effects on the brain by helping to realign its neurotransmitter levels. Let's take a look at some of the most commonly prescribed treatments and the associated neurotransmitter function.

Serotonin is the most extensively studied neurotransmitter in depression. A link between lowered serotonin and depression was first suggested in the 1960s, and widely publicized from the 1990s with the advent of the Selective Serotonin Reuptake Inhibitor (SSRI) antidepressants. SSRIs are often used as first-line pharmacotherapy for depression. As the name suggests, SSRIs exert action by inhibiting the reuptake (reabsorption) of serotonin, thereby alleviating symptoms of depression by increasing serotonin activity in the brain. Although the role of serotonin in depression is now widely accepted by the public, science brings it into question. Indeed, a recent systematic umbrella review (Moncrieff et al., 2022) found no convincing evidence that depression is associated with, or caused by, lower serotonin concentrations or activity. Most studies included in the review found no evidence of reduced serotonin activity in people with depression compared to people without, and there were also no studies that were able to induce depression by artificially lowering serotonin levels. What this means is that based on this review, there is no hard evidence that depression is simply the result of a deficit in serotonin.

Similar to serotonin, depression is associated with lower levels of norepinephrine (Moret & Briley, 2011). Tricyclic antidepressants (named for their three-ringed structure) and the serotonin-norepinephrine reuptake inhibitors (SNRIs) that replaced them and are antidepressants that affect both serotonin and norepinephrine levels in the brain.

As we learned earlier, the two hallmark symptoms of depression are depressed mood and anhedonia. Anhedonia is particularly difficult to treat. One reason may be that it involves a different mechanism and as such is less responsive to the more commonly pre-scribed antidepressant medications. In addition to the historically well-known serotonin and norepinephrine-containing circuits, studies using neuroimaging, pharmacological, and electrophysiological methods in humans and animal models of depression have also provided support for the presence of dopamine system dysfunction (Belujon & Grace, 2017; Yadid & Friedman, 2008). The brain releases dopamine while engaging in pleasur-able activities. Anhedonia is not only defined as being unable to experience pleasure but encompasses the complex reward-related deficits observed in depression, such as disrup-tion of the anticipation, motivation, and decision-making processes involved in obtain-ing a reward (Treadway & Zald, 2011). As such, it is not surprising that anhedonia has been linked to dysfunctions in the reward system, and in particular the dopamine system (Der-Avakian & Markou, 2012). Indeed, this downregulation of the dopamine system is perhaps the best explanation of another well-validated model of depression, the learned helplessness model (Seligman & Beagley, 1975).

Box 14.14   Learning activity

1. Look up a video explaining the learned helplessness model. How do you think it relates to the dopamine system?
2. What might learned helplessness look like in a person with depression? Can you think of instances in which we saw this in Abraham?

Keywords: learned helplessness model video

As you just learned, the learned helplessness model posits that when an individual continuously faces a negative, uncontrollable situation, they may stop trying to change their circumstances, even when they have the ability to do so. The model stems from a series of now-classic psychology experiments by Seligman and Maier (1967), in which dogs who learned they could not escape an electric shock stopped trying in subsequent experiments, even when it became possible to avoid the shock by jumping over a bar-rier. This experiment and its findings have been replicated numerous times in different contexts; interestingly, approximately half of animals exposed to uncontrollable stress develop learned helplessness whereas the other half seems to have undergone an adapta-tion to protect them from the detrimental effects of inescapable stress (i.e., seems resil-ient). Indeed, animals who develop learned helplessness show weight loss, altered sleep patterns, changes in HPA axis activity, and a density decrease in hippocampus and the medial prefrontal cortex (Nestler & Hyman, 2010). This, of course, aligns well with what is observed in people who have depression.

Because it involves a different mechanism, a single anti-depressant is usually not very effective against anhedonia. Therefore, augmentation strategies, involving the addition of a second drug to an existing antidepressant therapy, are often used to optimize treatment, such as the addition of an atypical antipsychotic to an SSRI treatment.

Daily life routine: learning a new activity

Learning a new activity can be challenging and rewarding. Regardless of what you are learning, you need to create and strengthen neural pathways in your brain. It involves a number of regions—and interactions between regions—in the brain, including the hippocampus and prefrontal cortex.

Box 14.15   Learning activity

1. Before reading on, find a video that explains how the brain learns. What regions are involved?
2. What do you think happens when these regions are not functioning optimally, like when a person has depression?

Keywords: neuroscience of learning video, how the brain learns video

---

As you learned earlier, depression involves a lot of the same regions of the brain as are involved in learning. It might make it more difficult to focus, to retain, and even to have the motivation to begin learning a new activity.

Box 14.16   Learning activity

With your small group, complete the table in the Appendix about the integration of Abraham's learning a new activity and the neuroscience that affects his participation.

Back to the person's life: Abraham wants to learn how to fish

So now that you know more about brain functioning in persons with depression, how can we use this scientific reasoning to support Abraham in learning how to fish? You will certainly spend a lot more time in other courses exploring details but knowing the neuroscience underpinnings provides a solid foundation to select intervention options that will be supported by brain processing.

Box 14.17   Learning activity

In class or small groups, discuss what interventions you can use to help Abraham manage his depression.

What do we know about ourselves and the population at large from this brain condition and this family story?

From Abraham's specific experience with depression, you may have noticed that it significantly impacted his everyday life. You can tell how depression can affect Abraham's ability to learn a new activity, knowing the symptoms he is experiencing (like difficulties concentrating, lack of energy, and anhedonia) are likely making it more difficult for him to do so. Even if you have never been depressed yourself, you may have had days when how you were feeling emotionally was making it difficult for you to concentrate and engage in learning in the classroom. You may have felt so tired, it was difficult to memorize terms or remember them for a test.

It is important to note yet again that although the focus of this chapter was more on the biological aspects of depression, psychological and social factors should always be considered to create a more holistic picture of the person. For example, the amount of stress someone has in their life and how they manage it could be significant (think back to the role of stress and cortisol in depression). Connecting with others—perhaps through shared activities—can be important. Like with Abraham and learning how to fish so he can spend time with his brother. Think about how you handle stress and manage negative emotions.

Further reading

If interested in further reading about depression:

Jesulola, E., Micalos, P., & Baguley, I. J. (2018). Understanding the pathophysiology of depression: From monoamines to the neurogenesis hypothesis model—are we there yet? *Behavioural Brain Research, 341*, 79–90. doi:https://doi.org/10.1016/j.bbr.2017.12.025
Korb, A. (2016). The Upward Spiral: Using Neuroscience to Reverse the Course of Depression, One Small Change at a Time. ReadHowYouWant
For further reading about stroke and emotional changes, including depression:
Meyerson, D.E., & Zuckerman, D. (2019). *Identity theft: Rediscovering ourselves after stroke*. Andrews McMeel Publishing
Towfighi, A., Ovbiagele, B., El Husseini, N., Hackett, M. L., Jorge, R. E., Kissela, B. M., Mitchell, P.H., Skolarus, L. E., Whooley, M. A., & Williams, L.S. (2017). Poststroke depression: A scientific statement for healthcare professionals from the American Heart Association/American Stroke Association. *Stroke, 48*, e30–e43. https://doi.org/10.1161/STR.0000000000000113

References

APA. (2013). *Diagnostic and statistical manual of mental disorders*, 5th edition (DSM-5). Washington, DC: American Psychological Association.
Belujon, P., & Grace, A. A. (2017). Dopamine system dysregulation in major depressive disorders. *International Journal of Neuropsychopharmacology, 20*(12), 1036–1046. doi:10.1093/ijnp/pyx056
Bremner, J. D. (2002). Structural changes in the brain in depression and relationship to symptom recurrence. *CNS Spectr. 7*(2), 129–130, 135–139. doi:10.1017/s1092852900017442.
Campbell, S., Marriott, M., Nahmias, C., & MacQueen, G. M. (2004). Lower hippocampal volume in patients suffering from depression: a meta-analysis. *Am J Psychiatry, 161*(4), 598–607. doi:10.1176/appi.ajp.161.4.598
Cotter, D., Mackay, D., Landau, S., Kerwin, R., & Everall, I. (2001). Reduced glial cell density and neuronal size in the anterior cingulate cortex in major depressive disorder. *Arch Gen Psychiatry, 58*(6), 545–553. doi:10.1001/archpsyc.58.6.545

Delgado, P. L. (2000). Depression: the case for a monoamine deficiency. *J Clin Psychiatry, 61 Suppl 6*, 7–11.

Der-Avakian, & A., Markou, A. (2012). The neurobiology of anhedonia and other reward-related deficits. *Trends Neurosci., 35*(1), 68–77. doi: 10.1016/j.tins.2011.11.005.

Drevets, W. C., Price, J. L., & Furey, M. L. (2008). Brain structural and functional abnormalities in mood disorders: implications for neurocircuitry models of depression. *Brain Structure and Function, 213*(1), 93–118. doi:10.1007/s00429-008-0189-x

Dziurkowska, E., & Wesolowski, M. (2021). Cortisol as a biomarker of mental disorder severity. *Journal of Clinical Medicine, 10*(21), 5204. doi: 10.3390/jcm10215204.

Grieve, S. M., Korgaonkar, M. S., Koslow, S. H., Gordon, E., & Williams, L. M. (2013). Widespread reductions in gray matter volume in depression. *Neuroimage Clin, 3*, 332–339. doi:10.1016/j.nicl.2013.08.016

Koenigs, M., & Grafman, J. (2009). The functional neuroanatomy of depression: distinct roles for ventromedial and dorsolateral prefrontal cortex. *Behav Brain Res, 201*(2), 239–243. doi:10.1016/j.bbr.2009.03.004

Kong, L., et al. (2013). Functional connectivity between the amygdala and prefrontal cortex in medication-naive individuals with major depressive disorder. *J Psychiatry Neurosci, 38*(6), 417–422. doi:10.1503/jpn.120117

Moncrieff, J., Cooper, R. E., Stockmann, T., Amendola, S., Hengartner, M. P., & Horowitz, M. A. (2022). The serotonin theory of depression: a systematic umbrella review of the evidence. *Molecular Psychiatry*. doi:10.1038/s41380-022-01661-0

Moret, C., & Briley, M. (2011). The importance of norepinephrine in depression. *Neuropsychiatr Dis Treat, 7*(Suppl 1), 9–13. doi:10.2147/ndt.S19619

Nestler, E. J., & Hyman, S. E. (2010). Animal models of neuropsychiatric disorders. *Nat Neurosci, 13*(10), 1161–1169. doi:10.1038/nn.2647

Rolls, E. T. (2019). The cingulate cortex and limbic systems for emotion, action, and memory. *Brain Struct Funct, 224*(9), 3001–3018. doi:10.1007/s00429-019-01945-2

Russell, G., & Lightman, S. (2019). The human stress response. *Nature Reviews Endocrinology, 15*(9), 525–534. doi:10.1038/s41574-019-0228-0

Seligman, M. E., & Beagley, G. (1975). Learned helplessness in the rat. *Journal of Comparative and Physiological Psychology, 88*, 534–541. doi:10.1037/h0076430

Seligman, M. E., & Maier, S. F. (1967). Failure to escape traumatic shock. *Journal of Experimental Psychology, 74*(1), 1–9. doi:10.1037/h0024514

Sheline, Y. I., Sanghavi, M., Mintun, M. A., & Gado, M. H. (1999). Depression duration but not age predicts hippocampal volume loss in medically healthy women with recurrent major depression. *J Neurosci, 19*(12), 5034–5043. doi:10.1523/jneurosci.19-12-05034.1999

Sheline, Y. I., Wang, P. W., Gado, M. H., Csernansky, J. G., & Vannier, M. W. (1996). Hippocampal atrophy in recurrent major depression. *Proc Natl Acad Sci U S A, 93*(9), 3908–3913. doi:10.1073/pnas.93.9.3908

Steele, J. D., Currie, J., Lawrie, S. M., & Reid, I. (2007). Prefrontal cortical functional abnormality in major depressive disorder: a stereotactic meta-analysis. *J Affect Disord, 101*(1–3), 1–11. doi:10.1016/j.jad.2006.11.009

Treadway, M. T., & Zald, D. H. (2011). Reconsidering anhedonia in depression: lessons from translational neuroscience. *Neurosci Biobehav Rev, 35*(3), 537–555. doi:10.1016/j.neubiorev.2010.06.006

Tyng, C. M., Amin, H. U., Saad, M. N. M., & Malik, A. S. (2017). The Influences of Emotion on Learning and Memory. *Frontiers in Psychology, 8*. doi:10.3389/fpsyg.2017.01454

Yadid, G., & Friedman, A. (2008). Dynamics of the dopaminergic system as a key component to the understanding of depression. *Prog Brain Res, 172*, 265–286. doi:10.1016/s0079–6123(08)00913-8

15 Sonya wants to care for her children and has bipolar disorder

Neuroscience facilitates our understanding of caring for children

Katelyn Mwangi

SONYA

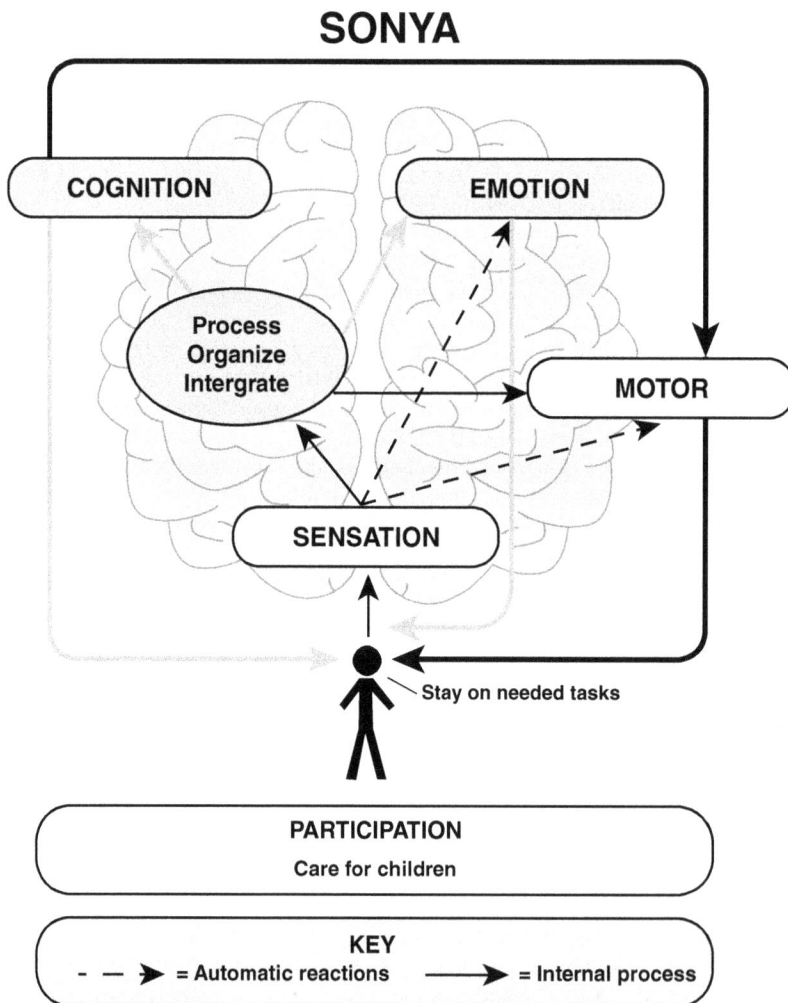

Figure 15.1 Sonya brain figure

DOI: 10.4324/9781003524380-18

Purpose of this chapter

The purpose of this chapter is to understand the implications of neuroscience on the occupation of caregiving for children. Specifically, we will look at Sonya who has a diagnosis of bipolar disorder type II, and how this impacts participation in her valued role as a mother. People with Bipolar disorder can have full lives with their daily routines, relationships, work and leisure, but may require modifications for function.

This chapter highlights the following structures in the central nervous system: prefrontal cortex, neurotransmission, and drug actions on the brain. As with all the chapters, these components of the nervous system work with other systems to support overall human function.

Keywords for this chapter are listed in the box below. Be sure you learn what these key features are so you can get the most out of the chapter.

Keywords for this chapter

amygdala	dorsolateral PFC	neurotransmission
bipolar I disorder	hyperactivity	prefrontal cortex
bipolar II disorder	hypomania	serotonin
cyclothymic disorder	inhibition	ventromedial PFC
depression	lithium	
dopamine	mania	

Box 15.1   Learning activity

Prior to reading the case:

1. How do you think the symptoms of bipolar disorder will affect Sonya's parenting?
2. Why is it important for an occupational therapy practitioner to understand the neurology of bipolar disorder?

Sonya, a mother who wants a plan for caring for her children

Sonya is a 27-year-old female (she/her) who works as a manager at a retail store. Sonya is a mother to two children, Lina (11) and Mikey (8), and recently found out she is expecting a third child with her partner. While the news of the pregnancy is exciting, Sonya is overwhelmed with her growing responsibilities and concerns with how to manage her bipolar disorder during pregnancy.

When Sonya was 25 years old, she began to feel increasingly fatigued throughout the day. While previously upbeat and able to manage her responsibilities, she experienced a lack of interest in many activities, including spending time with Lina and Mikey. Instead of frequent outings to the park, or volunteering at their school, Sonya began spending her free time at home in her room. Sonya's social isolation intensified her feelings of sadness and guilt, particularly related to not being a good enough mother. Throughout the periods of depression, Sonya noticed what she felt like were improvements, where she would have an excess of energy and productivity, sometimes staying awake for days at a time. Sonya felt like she spent considerably more time feeling "down" and the periods of excess energy never lasted more than four or five days at a time.

One of Sonya's hypomanic episodes (periods of high activity, but still in touch with reality) was followed by a depressive episode (periods of inertia and lack of motivation) resulting in hospitalization. Sonya received medical attention and was diagnosed with bipolar disorder II. She was discharged home with a medication management routine, including lithium, and regularly scheduled therapy appointments.

Following her diagnosis of bipolar disorder II, Sonya has consistently attended therapy sessions and followed a medication routine. With the recent news of her pregnancy, Sonya learned a few of her current medications could potentially be harmful for her baby. Sonya's priority is to ensure she keeps her baby healthy throughout pregnancy, but also fears changes in her medication may lead to more hypomanic and depressive episodes. Sonya wants to establish a plan for how to continue to care for her mental health, Lina and Mikey, and baby throughout pregnancy.

Box 15.2   Learning activity

Discussion topics for small groups:

1. After reading about Sonya, what more would you want to know about her diagnosis?
2. What additional information about Sonya are you curious to learn more about?

Before continuing in your reading of this chapter, discuss the following questions to highlight the information you already know.

Box 15.3   Learning activity

1. What do you know about the brain and how it processes and regulates emotion?
2. How does neurotransmission occur in the brain? How is this system regulated?
3. How can participating in the role of a parent lead to mood fluctuations in daily life?

Neuroscience information to guide your thinking about Sonya.

Bipolar disorder is a group of diagnoses typically characterized by mood disturbances, including mania, hypomania, and depression. While fluctuations in mood during day-to-day life is common, especially in response to difficult or exciting situations, bipolar disorder characterizes abnormal elevated or depressed fluctuations in mood. The broader term bipolar disorder contains several diagnoses; this chapter focuses on the three most prevalent: bipolar I, bipolar II, and cyclothymic disorder (American Psychiatric Association, 2022). In addition to those three classifications, the Diagnostic and Statistical Manual-V

(DSM-V) includes several more general categories for individuals who may not meet the criteria for specific bipolar disorder diagnoses.

Prior to exploring the specific diagnosis, let's first learn generally about bipolar disorders. As mentioned, bipolar disorders are characterized by mood disturbances, which can include depressive or manic symptoms. The average age of onset is around 25 years old, and up to 1.5 percent of the population will have a diagnosis of one of the types of bipolar disorder (Merikangas et al., 2011). Bipolar disorder is strongly correlated with genetic factors, but environmental factors are also a strong predictor of the onset. Individuals who have experienced abuse in childhood or those with chronic stress are up to two times as likely to be diagnosed with bipolar disorder (Etain et al., 2008).

Bipolar I disorder

Bipolar I disorder is characterized by an individual having at least one manic episode that cannot be otherwise explained by a differing diagnosis, such as schizoaffective disorder or schizophrenia, or related to substance use or abuse. Over 90% of individuals with bipolar I disorder will experience more than one manic episode. While depressive episodes are not required for a bipolar I diagnosis, the majority of individuals diagnosed with bipolar I will experience depressive symptoms at some point throughout their lifespan that often follow a manic episode (American Psychiatric Association, 2022).

Manic episodes are characterized by periods of elevated or irritable mood that persists throughout the day for the course of one week or longer. In order to receive a diagnosis of mania, individuals must have three or more mania-related symptoms; individuals with irritable mood rather than elevated mood must have four symptoms to qualify (American Psychiatric Association, 2022). Mania includes, but is not limited to, the following symptoms: grandiosity or elevated thoughts of self, increased verbal output or pressured speech, racing thoughts, lack of sleep, and possibly involvement in risky or unsafe behaviors. The disturbances to mood will impair participation in daily occupations and social participation; individuals may necessitate hospitalization if they are at risk for harming themselves or others (American Psychiatric Association, 2022).

Bipolar II disorder

Bipolar II disorder is characterized by the individual experiencing a hypomanic episode, in addition to a major depressive episode. While only one episode of each is required for a diagnosis of bipolar II, around 50% of individuals with bipolar II will experience more than one episode within their first year of diagnosis (Radua et al., 2017). Hypomanic episodes are characterized by similar behavior to the previously stated manic episodes (lack of sleep, grandiosity, distractibility), elevated mood and increased energy, but differ in the required time frame of four days or more. Additionally, while the symptoms are relatively similar, individuals experiencing a hypomanic episode do not experience a significant impact on occupational performance, social interaction, or require hospitalization for symptoms (American Psychiatric Association, 2022).

The second requirement for a diagnosis of bipolar II disorder is the presence of a major depressive episode lasting at least two weeks, comprising five or more symptoms, two of which must include loss of interest and depressed mood. Symptoms include thoughts of death or suicidal ideation, weight loss or weight gain, loss of pleasure in most daily activities, decreased mood, feelings of worthlessness or guilt, difficulty focusing, and fatigue throughout the day (American Psychiatric Association, 2022).

The severity of the depressive symptoms impact participation in daily occupations and social interaction. Although functional performance may return to baseline following the depressive episode, some individuals experience lasting effects from symptomatology, negatively impacting occupational performance and cognitive functioning long-term (American Psychiatric Association, 2022; Bora et al., 2011). Individuals with bipolar II are more likely to seek medical attention following a depressive episode, rather than periods of hypomania. Additionally, up to 40% of individuals experiencing a depressive episode will complete self-harm, with around 5–8% of individuals completing suicide (Nordentoft, Mortensen, & Pedersen, 2011; Novick, Swartz, & Frank, 2010).

Cyclothymic disorder

Cyclothymic disorder is characterized by a shifting in mood, including both depressive symptoms and hypomania symptoms. For these individuals, the symptoms do not meet the number or severity criteria for mania, hypomania or major depression, but do persist for two years or longer in adults, with individuals not being symptom free for periods of two months or longer. Additionally, the symptoms cannot be explained by other diagnosis, such as schizophrenia or delusion disorder, or medication-related (American Psychiatric Association, 2022). The symptoms cause impairment in social engagement and occupational performance. Individuals diagnosed with cyclothymic disorder have up to a 50% chance of developing bipolar I or bipolar II disorder within their lifetime (American Psychiatric Association, 2022; Van Meter & Youngstrom, 2012).

While the three diagnoses have many overlapping similarities, it may be easiest to categorize them broadly in the following ways:

- **Bipolar I disorder:** Individual must have at least one manic episode. Depressive symptoms and hypomanic episodes may be present but are not required for a diagnosis.
- **Bipolar II disorder:** Individual must have a least one hypomanic episode and one major depressive episode.
- **Cyclothymic disorder:** Individual experiences hypomanic and depressive symptoms over the course of two-years, but symptoms do not meet criteria of mania, hypomania, or major depression.

The 5th edition of the DSM was released in 2013, but their most recent edition is the DSM-5-TR, including revisions to a few of the diagnostic criteria. For more information on the remaining bipolar diagnosis categories, or for information about prevalence, development, and risk factors for bipolar disorders, readers can find that information in the DSM-5 or DSM-5-TR.

Box 15.4   Learning activity

Sonya has bipolar II, meaning she has experienced at least one hypomanic episode and at least one major depressive episode.

1. Looking back through the case, what symptoms did Sonya experience that corresponds with a hypomanic episode?

2. What symptoms did Sonya experience that indicate a major depressive episode?
3. Why would Sonya not be diagnosed with bipolar I disorder?

Like the majority of individuals with bipolar disorder, Sonya first sought out medical attention after a depressive episode.

4. Why is it more common to seek medical care after a depressive episode than during a hypomanic episode?

Changes in neurotransmitters

Heritability and genetics

Bipolar disorders are heritable, meaning there is correlation between immediate family members and their children developing the condition. One study found that a child of individual with bipolar disorder has 10 times the risk of developing bipolar disorder when compared with the general population, with several identified genes and networks that can be inherited (Craddock & Skylar, 2013). While much of our knowledge about neurotransmission and bipolar disorder is continuing to evolve, this portion of the chapter will explore in further depth the current scientific understanding surrounding this topic.

Role of calcium

Calcium is an important substance that fosters neuronal signaling; scientists believe that calcium is dysregulated in persons with bipolar disorder. Studies have found an increase in calcium signaling channels in individuals with bipolar disorder, regardless of the person's current mood (Berridge, 2014; Warsh, Andreopoulos, & Li, 2004). Calcium channels are important for regulation of neurotransmitters and the excitability of neurons, so an increase in calcium signaling could have implications for the processes of neurotransmission (the chemical and electrical process of sending messages within the nervous system) in the brain (Reith, 2000).

Dopaminergic system

For more information on dopamine and substantia nigra, refer to Chapters 16 on Substance Abuse and Chapter 23 on Parkinson's disease.

The involvement of dopamine in bipolar disorder has been suspected since the 1970s, with a variety of research to support this hypothesis (Singh, 1970). Dopamine is a neurotransmitter that originates in hypothalamus and midbrain, more specifically the ventral tegmental area and the substantia nigra. Dopamine's primary responsibility is to signal and respond to rewards, but dopamine is associated with other important behaviors, including sleep, motivation, working memory and cognition, and inhibition (Juárez Olguín et al., 2016; Calabresi et al., 2007). Individuals with bipolar disorder experiencing mania may demonstrate a decreased need for sleep and increased mood or pleasure-seeking behaviors, which in part may be caused by increased dopamine neurotransmission (Cousins, Butts, & Young, 2009). Prior imaging and pharmacological studies have shown that elevation and hyperactivity of the dopamine receptor likely underlies mania and depressive symptoms of bipolar (Ashok et al., 2017).

Noradrenergic system

In addition to the dopaminergic system involvement, there is ongoing research to support the involvement of the noradrenergic system, or the system that regulates and releases norepinephrine. Norepinephrine is important for regulation of sleep and wakefulness, memory, and function of the endocrine system (Atzori et al., 2016). A study comparing healthy controls to individuals with bipolar disorder post mortem found lower levels of norepinephrine in those with bipolar disorder, suggesting disruption to the noradrenergic system (Wiste et al., 2008).

Serotonergic system

Serotonin is a neurotransmitter that works to regulate mood, sleep, hunger signals, and cognition. Lower levels of serotonin are associated with depressive symptoms and suicidality (Lv & Liu, 2017). Individuals with mood disturbances, including those diagnosed with bipolar disorder, have decreased serotonin transmission. A study looking at the implications of decreased serotonin binding in the brain found that the effects were widespread occurring in the amygdala, midbrain, hippocampus, and thalamus (Oquendo, Hastings & Huang, 2007). One possible cause of the decreased levels of neurotransmission is difficulty with the binding of serotonin which in part is regulated by norepinephrine (Oquendo, Hastings & Huang, 2007; Adell et al., 2002).

Box 15.5   Learning activity

Based on what you've learned so far in the chapter, discuss the following:

1. Discuss what you know about the heritability of bipolar disorders. While heritability is not a modifiable factor, take a moment to research what environmental factors can be controlled to decrease the likelihood of developing bipolar disorders.
2. Describe what was happening with dopamine transmission when Sonya was awake for several days at a time.

Prefrontal cortex

Role of the prefrontal cortex

The prefrontal cortex (PFC) is a portion of the frontal lobe, located anterior to the motor cortex (Carlson & Birkett, 2021). The PFC is highly connected to other regions of the brain, creating a complex network supporting emotional and cognitive regulation (Arnsten, 2009). The main responsibilities of the prefrontal cortex include initiating purposeful action, monitoring behaviors and thoughts, and housing our executive functioning skills (Goldman-Rakic, 1995, 1996). See Table 15.1 for information on the regions of the prefrontal cortex.

Table 15.1 Regions of the prefrontal cortex and their functionality

Region of prefrontal cortex	Connections to other brain regions and function
Dorsolateral PFC	Connections to the motor and sensory regions in the brain. Its primary function is to control attention and action; this portion of the PFC is considered to control executive functioning skills and cognition (Goldman-Rakic, 1987; Koenigs & Grafman, 2009).
Right inferior PFC	Primary role is inhibition of unnecessary motor response (Aron, Robbins & Poldrack, 2004).
Ventromedial PFC	Maintains connectivity with subcortical structures, which include the hypothalamus and amygdala. This portion of the PFC is thought to assist with regulating emotions (Koenigs & Grafman, 2009).
Dorsomedial PFC	Responsibility is to monitor errors (Modirrousta & Fellows, 2008).

Note: This table includes the different regions of the prefrontal cortex, their connectedness to other brain regions, and functionality.

These regions of the prefrontal cortex work in tandem to regulate and process thoughts, emotions, and action. During non-stressful situations and decisions, the brain maintains a top-down approach, in which the prefrontal cortex leads our behaviors and emotions. Periods of stress or new stimuli can shift to our subcortical structures, including our amygdala, managing our emotional responses and reactions (Arnsten, 2009). When psychological stress occurs, the amygdala communicates with the brainstem and hypothalamus to stimulate the stress pathways, releasing an increase in dopamine and noradrenaline. The release of these neurotransmitters strengthens the response from the amygdala, further dampening the response of the prefrontal cortex (Arnsten, 2009).

Box 15.6   Learning activity

Using internet or book resources, locate a picture of the prefrontal cortex and the subcortical structures in the brain. First, point to the part of the brain that guides decisions and emotional responses during non-stressful and routine events. Next, point to the part of the brain that takes over during stressful events or with new stimuli.
   Discuss the following:

1. What is happening with neurotransmission during stressful or new events?
2. Based on what we've covered earlier in the chapter, what do we know about those neurotransmitters and how they relate to bipolar disorders?

Keywords: prefrontal cortex, subcortical structures

Prefrontal cortex in bipolar disorder

Bipolar disorder can involve both manic and depressive episodes, so it is important to consider potential changes in the brain depending on the current mood disturbance. The following paragraphs will explore how the brain reacts and responds in both elevated and depressed mood states.

Manic and hypomania

Mania and hypomania are hallmark features of bipolar disorder, occurring in both Bipolar I and Bipolar II. Periods of mania are characterized by irritable mood, distractibility and possible engagement in risky behaviors. With the prefrontal cortex being intricately involved with executive functioning skills and emotional regulation, a clear connection exists between changes in the prefrontal cortex and manic episodes. One longitudinal study found that over the period of six years, individuals who experienced manic episodes had decreased cortical volume in their prefrontal lobe, specifically the dorsolateral and interior cortexes (Abé et al., 2015). Another study evaluating grey matter changes in the brain found that individuals with bipolar disorder had reduced grey matter in their prefrontal cortex, along with their temporal lobe (Selvaraj et al., 2012). These changes in the prefrontal cortex may lead to cognitive changes over time, involving fluctuating or worsening functional cognition in daily activities (Cardoso et al., 2015).

Depression

Several studies examine the role of the prefrontal cortex in depressive episodes. Consistently, research has found that individual's experiencing depression have an abnormal amount of activity in their ventromedial PFC, the portion of the PFC responsibility for managing emotions (see Table 15.1). In correlation with the increased activity in the ventromedial PFC, decreased activity has been shown in the dorsolateral PFC in individuals with depression, the portion of the PFC responsible for control executive functioning (Koenigs & Grafman, 2009). In individual's who recovered from their depressive episode, increase activity to the dorsolateral PFC returned with a decrease in the ventromedial PFC (Koenigs & Grafman).

   One treatment utilized for treatment-resistant depression is deep brain stimulation of a medial region of the prefrontal cortex to decrease the activity, resulting in increased activity in other areas of the prefrontal cortex (Mayberg et al., 2005). A decrease in activity in this medial region of the prefrontal cortex is associated with diminishing depressive symptoms, likely due to its connectivity with other brain regions controlling emotion. One of the key roles of the prefrontal cortex is to inhibit the amygdala from fear responses; by reducing the activity of the medial region of the prefrontal cortex, decreased messaging and connectivity occurs to the amygdala, reducing negative emotional responses (Mayberg et al., 2005; Carlson & Birkett, 2021).

Bipolar disorder and functional cognition

Due to the involvement of the prefrontal cortex, cognitive functioning is impacted for individuals with bipolar disorder. While the emotional and mood disturbances are often considered, it is important that cognitive implications be evaluated and treated. Individuals with bipolar disorder have impaired executive functioning skills, verbal memory, and attention (Cardoso et al., 2015; Sachs et al., 2020). Additionally, individuals with bipolar disorder have decreased activation in the dorsolateral PFC during a task, when compared with a control population. This finding demonstrates the implication that bipolar disorder has on cognitive functioning (Townsend et al., 2010). Increased cognitive impairment in individuals with bipolar disorder correlates with worsening performance in daily life, highlighting the importance for addressing cognitive changes to promote occupational engagement and participation (Sachs et al., 2020).

Drug actions in the brain

There are several different drugs and treatments utilized to treat bipolar disorders. This portion of the chapter we will explore the most used drugs and their implications for brain functioning. Thinking back to our case, Sonya is currently managing her Bipolar II with lithium.

Lithium

Lithium is a commonly utilized drug to treat bipolar disorder, working to stabilize one's mood (Malhi et al., 2013). Once the manic phases are treated, the individual is less likely to experience depression (Soares & Gershon, 1998). Lithium does not suppress typical emotional responses, such as happiness and sadness, but it does work to regulate unwanted severity of emotional responses (Fieve, 1979). Although it is well-tolerated in the majority of individuals with bipolar disorder, there are potential side effects, including weight gain, thirst, and tremors (Carlson & Birkett, 2021). Careful monitoring of lithium levels in the system due to low therapeutic index is important for ensuring an overdose does not occur (Carlson & Birkett, 2021).

Lithium has been used for many decades, but the effects the drug has on the brain are still being understood. Research has found that lithium works to preserve the volume of the brain in the hippocampus, amygdala, and prefrontal cortex. On a neuronal level, lithium works to diminish neurotransmitter activity by reducing dopamine and glutamate excitatory activity, while also increasing inhibitory GABA activity (Malhi et al., 2013). While the entire mechanism for how this occurs is unknown, ultimately lithium leads to mood stabilization (Malhi et al., 2013). Lithium also has neuroprotective and neurotrophic effects on the brain, including prevention of cell death and enhancing cell growth and regeneration (Machado-Vieira, 2018).

Anticonvulsants

While lithium often remains the primary drug for first-line defense against bipolar disorder, other classes of drugs, including anticonvulsants are used to treat bipolar disorder. Anticonvulsants, which can be used to treat other conditions such as epilepsy, can be effective in treating depressive symptoms and rapid-cycling between mania and depression (Wang et al., 2003; Kaufman, 2011). Many individuals with psychiatric diseases have lower levels of Gamma-aminobutyric acid (GABA), which is linked to mood instability (Allen, Sabir & Sharma, 2023). Anticonvulsant drugs, such as depakote (valproic acid) work to increase the GABA concentration with the goal of mood stabilization (Rahman & Nguyen, 2022; Allen, Sabir & Sharma, 2023).

Antipsychotics

Antipsychotic medications are another class of drug that can be utilized to treat bipolar disorder. Most commonly, antipsychotic medication is utilized for maintenance or adjunctive treatment (Lindström et al., 2017). Antipsychotic drugs such as haloperidol, are effective in managing manic episodes. One mechanism that antipsychotic drugs target is an antagonist or blocking of the dopamine receptors (Reynolds, 2011). Earlier in the chapter we discussed how individuals experiencing mania have increased dopamine receptor activity. Antipsychotic drugs can effectively alleviate manic symptoms by blocking dopamine receptors in the brain (Reynolds, 2011).

Daily life routine: parenting and caring for children

Parenting is often thought to be one of the hardest, yet most rewarding parts of life for individuals who choose to participate in that role. For Sonya and other individuals in her life stage, this phase in life is defined by balancing the demands of work, managing health conditions, and taking care of children. From birth through childhood, into the adolescent and teenage years, parenting is a full-time endeavor. For many, this involves daily tasks such as changing diapers, taking children to school, preparing balanced meals, and attending extracurricular events. Through the ups and downs of parenting, Sonya's story serves as a reminder of how caring for children is a key motivation for persistence through fluctuations in mood that accompany daily life.

Back to the person's life: Sonya wants to have a routine for caring for her children.

Now that we have learned about neurotransmitters, the prefrontal cortex, and drug actions in the brain for individuals with bipolar disorder, let's revisit Sonya and her story. How can we utilize what we've learned in this chapter about neuroscience to support Sonya and her primary goal of caring for her children?

Box 15.7   Learning activity

A retrospective study found that up to 23% of pregnant women experiences worsening bipolar symptoms while pregnant, and up to 52% during the postpartum period. Certain medications used to treat bipolar disorder may cause teratogenicity, or neurodevelopmental delay to the child prenatally (Sharma & Pope, 2012). Studies have shown an association between lithium exposure in the first trimester with increased risks of congenital malformations (Poels et al., 2018). Additionally, some medications may be contraindicated during certain trimesters and into the breast-feeding period (Sharma & Pope, 2012).

1. How may this knowledge impact Sonya and the medication choices she makes as a birthing individual?
2. What considerations and conversations need to take place between Sonya and her healthcare team about medical and therapeutic management of her bipolar disorder?
3. How does our knowledge of neuroscience help us to support Sonya in continuing to care for her children?

What do we know about ourselves and the population at large from this brain condition and this family story?

From this chapter, we have learned about the various aspects of mood that accompany a diagnosis of bipolar disorder. Many of us understand feelings of sadness and discouragement that attend the ebbs and flows of daily living. We can also resonate with emotions of happiness or elation when something positive occurs, like learning to ride a bike, getting married, or getting the dream job. While we may not experience these emotions to the same degree as someone with bipolar disorder, human emotion is a fundamental part of life that unifies us all. Now you can understand that your emotional states are outward manifestations of excitation and inhibitory control within your brain to regulate your moods and responses.

This chapter highlighted the different types of bipolar disorder, neurotransmission in the brain, the role of the prefrontal cortex, and how drugs impact brain functioning. For additional learning opportunities related to bipolar disorders, please refer to the list of resources under Further Reading.

Box 15.8   Learning activity

With your small group, complete the table in the Appendix about the integration of Sonya's needs to manage her manic and depressive symptoms to be a good parent in her family.

Further reading

American Psychiatric Association. (2022). Bipolar disorders. In *Diagnostic and statistical manual of mental disorders* (5th ed., text rev.). Washington, DC: American Psychiatric Association.
Jamison, Kay R. (1996). *An unquiet mind*. New York: Vintage Books
Lowe, J. (2017). *Mental: Lithium, love, and losing my mind*. Blue Rider Press.

References

Abé, C., Ekman, C. J., Sellgren, C., Petrovic, P., Ingvar, M., & Landén, M. (2015). Manic episodes are related to changes in frontal cortex: a longitudinal neuroimaging study of bipolar disorder 1. *Brain: A Journal of Neurology, 138*(Pt 11), 3440–3448. https://doi.org/10.1093/brain/awv266
Adell, A., Celada, P., Abellán, M. T., & Artigas, F. (2002). Origin and functional role of the extracellular serotonin in the midbrain raphe nuclei. *Brain Research Reviews, 39*(2–3), 154–180.
Allen, M. J., Sabir, S., & Sharma, S. (2023). GABA receptor. StatPearls Publishing.
American Psychiatric Association. (2022). Bipolar disorders. In *Diagnostic and statistical manual of mental disorders* (5th ed., text rev.).
Arnsten A. F. (2009). Stress signalling pathways that impair prefrontal cortex structure and function. *Nature reviews. Neuroscience, 10*(6), 410–422. https://doi.org/10.1038/nrn2648
Aron, A. R., Robbins, T. W., & Poldrack, R. A. (2004). Inhibition and the right inferior frontal cortex. *Trends in Cognitive Sciences, 8*(4), 170–177. https://doi.org/10.1016/j.tics.2004.02.010
Ashok, A. H., Marques, T. R., Jauhar, S., Nour, M. M., Goodwin, G. M., Young, A. H., & Howes, O. D. (2017). The dopamine hypothesis of bipolar affective disorder: the state of the art and implications for treatment. *Molecular Psychiatry, 22*(5), 666–679. https://doi.org/10.1038/mp.2017.16
Atzori, M., Cuevas-Olguin, R., Esquivel-Rendon, E., Garcia-Oscos, F., Salgado-Delgado, R. C., Saderi, N., Miranda-Morales, M., Treviño, M., Pineda, J. C., & Salgado, H. (2016). Locus ceruleus norepinephrine release: A central regulator of CNS spatio-temporal activation? *Frontiers in Synaptic Neuroscience, 8*, 25. https://doi.org/10.3389/fnsyn.2016.00025
Berridge M. J. (2014). Calcium signalling and psychiatric disease: bipolar disorder and schizophrenia. *Cell and Tissue Research, 357*(2), 477–492. https://doi.org/10.1007/s00441-014-1806-z
Bora, E., Yücel, M., Pantelis, C., & Berk, M. (2011). Meta-analytic review of neurocognition in bipolar II disorder. *Acta Psychiatrica Scandinavica, 123*(3), 165–174. https://doi.org/10.1111/j.1600-0447.2010.01638.x
Calabresi, P., Picconi, B., Tozzi, A., & Di Filippo, M. (2007). Dopamine-mediated regulation of corticostriatal synaptic plasticity. *Trends in Neurosciences, 30*(5), 211–219. https://doi.org/10.1016/j.tins.2007.03.001

Cardoso, T., Bauer, I. E., Meyer, T. D., Kapczinski, F., & Soares, J. C. (2015). Neuroprogression and cognitive functioning in bipolar disorder: A systematic review. *Current Psychiatry Reports, 17*(9), 75. https://doi.org/10.1007/s11920-015-0605-x

Carlson, N. R. & Birkett, M. A. (2021). *Physiology of behavior*. 13th ed. Boston, MA: Pearson Higher Ed.

Cousins, D. A., Butts, K., & Young, A. H. (2009). The role of dopamine in bipolar disorder. *Bipolar Disorders, 11*(8), 787–806. https://doi.org/10.1111/j.1399-5618.2009.00760.x

Craddock, N. and Sklar, P. (2013) Genetics of bipolar disorder. *Lancet* 381, 1654–1662

Etain, B., Henry, C., Bellivier, F., Mathieu, F., & Leboyer, M. (2008). Beyond genetics: childhood affective trauma in bipolar disorder. *Bipolar Disorders, 10*(8), 867–876. https://doi.org/10.1111/j.1399-5618.2008.00635.x

Fieve, R.R. (1979). The clinic effects of lithium treatment. *Trends in Neurosciences*, 2, 66–68

Goldman-Rakic, PS. (1987). In: *Handbook of physiology, The nervous system, higher functions of the brain*. Plum F, editor. Vol. V. Bethesda: American Physiological Society. pp. 373–417.

Goldman-Rakic P. S. (1996). The prefrontal landscape: implications of functional architecture for understanding human mentation and the central executive. *Philosophical transactions of the Royal Society of London. Series B, Biological Sciences, 351*(1346), 1445–1453. https://doi.org/10.1098/rstb.1996.0129

Goldman-Rakic P. S. (1995). Cellular basis of working memory. *Neuron, 14*(3), 477–485. https://doi.org/10.1016/0896-6273(95)90304-6

Juárez Olguín, H., Calderón Guzmán, D., Hernández García, E., & Barragán Mejía, G. (2016). The role of dopamine and its dysfunction as a consequence of oxidative stress. *Oxidative Medicine and Cellular Longevity, 2016*, 9730467. https://doi.org/10.1155/2016/9730467

Kaufman K. R. (2011). Antiepileptic drugs in the treatment of psychiatric disorders. *Epilepsy & behavior: E&B, 21*(1), 1–11. https://doi.org/10.1016/j.yebeh.2011.03.011

Koenigs, M., & Grafman, J. (2009). The functional neuroanatomy of depression: distinct roles for ventromedial and dorsolateral prefrontal cortex. *Behavioural Brain Research, 201*(2), 239–243.

Lindström, L., Lindström, E., Nilsson, M., & Höistad, M. (2017). Maintenance therapy with second generation antipsychotics for bipolar disorder—A systematic review and meta-analysis. *Journal of Affective Disorders, 213*, 138–150. https://doi.org/10.1016/j.jad.2017.02.012

Lv, J., & Liu, F. (2017). The role of serotonin beyond the central nervous system during embryogenesis. *Frontiers in Cellular Neuroscience, 11*, 74. https://doi.org/10.3389/fncel.2017.00074

Machado-Vieira R. (2018). Lithium, stress, and resilience in bipolar disorder: Deciphering this key homeostatic synaptic plasticity regulator. *Journal of Affective Disorders, 233*, 92–99. https://doi.org/10.1016/j.jad.2017.12.026

Malhi, G. S., Tanious, M., Das, P., Coulston, C. M., & Berk, M. (2013). Potential mechanisms of action of lithium in bipolar disorder. Current understanding. *CNS Drugs, 27*(2), 135–153. https://doi.org/10.1007/s40263-013-0039-0

Mayberg, H. S., Lozano, A. M., Voon, V., McNeely, H. E., Seminowicz, D., Hamani, C., Schwalb, J. M., & Kennedy, S. H. (2005). Deep brain stimulation for treatment-resistant depression. *Neuron, 45*(5), 651–660. https://doi.org/10.1016/j.neuron.2005.02.014

Merikangas, K. R., Jin, R., He, J. P., Kessler, R. C., Lee, S., Sampson, N. A., Viana, M. C., Andrade, L. H., Hu, C., Karam, E. G., Ladea, M., Medina-Mora, M. E., Ono, Y., Posada-Villa, J., Sagar, R., Wells, J. E., & Zarkov, Z. (2011). Prevalence and correlates of bipolar spectrum disorder in the world mental health survey initiative. *Archives of General Psychiatry, 68*(3), 241–251. https://doi.org/10.1001/archgenpsychiatry.2011.12

Modirrousta M, Fellows LK. Dorsal medial prefrontal cortex plays a necessary role in rapid error prediction in humans. *J. Neurosci.* 2008;28:14000–14005.

Nordentoft, M., Mortensen, P. B., & Pedersen, C. B. (2011). Absolute risk of suicide after first hospital contact in mental disorder. *Archives of General Psychiatry, 68*(10), 1058–1064. https://doi.org/10.1001/archgenpsychiatry.2011.113

Novick, D. M., Swartz, H. A., & Frank, E. (2010). Suicide attempts in bipolar I and bipolar II disorder: a review and meta-analysis of the evidence. *Bipolar Disorders, 12*(1), 1–9. https://doi.org/10.1111/j.1399-5618.2009.00786.x

Oquendo, M. A., Hastings, R. S., Huang, Y. Y., Simpson, N., Ogden, R. T., Hu, X. Z., Goldman, D., Arango, V., Van Heertum, R. L., Mann, J. J., & Parsey, R. V. (2007). Brain serotonin transporter binding in depressed patients with bipolar disorder using positron emission tomography. *Archives of General Psychiatry, 64*(2), 201–208. https://doi.org/10.1001/archpsyc.64.2.201

Poels, E. M. P., Bijma, H. H., Galbally, M., & Bergink, V. (2018). Lithium during pregnancy and after delivery: a review. *International Journal of Bipolar Disorders, 6*(1), 26. https://doi.org/10.1186/s40345-018-0135-7

Radua, J., Grunze, H., & Amann, B. L. (2017). Meta-analysis of the risk of subsequent mood episodes in bipolar disorder. *Psychotherapy and Psychosomatics, 86*(2), 90–98. https://doi.org/10.1159/000449417

Rahman, M., & Nguyen, H. (2022). Valproic acid. StatPearls Publishing.

Reith, M. E. (Ed.). (2000). *Cerebral signal transduction: From first to fourth messengers*. Springer Science & Business Media.

Reynolds G. P. (2011). Receptor mechanisms of antipsychotic drug action in bipolar disorder—focus on asenapine. *Therapeutic Advances in Psychopharmacology, 1*(6), 197–204. https://doi.org/10.1177/2045125311430112

Sachs, G., Berg, A., Jagsch, R., Lenz, G., & Erfurth, A. (2020). Predictors of functional outcome in patients with bipolar disorder: Effects of cognitive psychoeducational group therapy after 12 months. *Frontiers in Psychiatry, 11*, 530026. https://doi.org/10.3389/fpsyt.2020.530026

Sharma, V., & Pope, C. J. (2012). Pregnancy and bipolar disorder: a systematic review. *The Journal of Clinical Psychiatry, 73*(11), 1447–1455. https://doi.org/10.4088/JCP.11r07499

Selvaraj, S., Arnone, D., Job, D., Stanfield, A., Farrow, T. F., Nugent, A. C., Scherk, H., Gruber, O., Chen, X., Sachdev, P. S., Dickstein, D. P., Malhi, G. S., Ha, T. H., Ha, K., Phillips, M. L., & McIntosh, A. M. (2012). Grey matter differences in bipolar disorder: a meta-analysis of voxel-based morphometry studies. *Bipolar Disorders, 14*(2), 135–145. https://doi.org/10.1111/j.1399-5618.2012.01000.x

Singh M. M. (1970). A unifying hypothesis on the biochemical basis of affective disorder. *The Psychiatric Quarterly, 44*(4), 706–724. https://doi.org/10.1007/BF01563010

Soares, J. C., & Gershon, S. (1998). The lithium ion: a foundation for psychopharmacological specificity. *Neuropsychopharmacology: official publication of the American College of Neuropsychopharmacology, 19*(3), 167–182. https://doi.org/10.1016/S0893-133X(98)00022-0

Townsend, J., Bookheimer, S. Y., Foland-Ross, L. C., Sugar, C. A., & Altshuler, L. L. (2010). fMRI abnormalities in dorsolateral prefrontal cortex during a working memory task in manic, euthymic and depressed bipolar subjects. *Psychiatry Research, 182*(1), 22–29. https://doi.org/10.1016/j.pscychresns.2009.11.010

Van Meter, A. R., Youngstrom, E. A., & Findling, R. L. (2012). Cyclothymic disorder: a critical review. *Clinical Psychology Review, 32*(4), 229–243. https://doi.org/10.1016/j.cpr.2012.02.001

Wang, P. W., Ketter, T. A., Becker, O. V., & Nowakowska, C. (2003). New anticonvulsant medication uses in bipolar disorder. *CNS Spectrums, 8*(12), 930–947. https://doi.org/10.1017/s1092852900028704

Warsh, J. J., Andreopoulos, S., & Li, P. P. (2004). Role of intracellular calcium signaling in the pathophysiology and pharmacotherapy of bipolar disorder: current status. *Clinical Neuroscience Research, 4*(3–4), 201–213.

Wiste, A. K., Arango, V., Ellis, S. P., Mann, J. J., & Underwood, M. D. (2008). Norepinephrine and serotonin imbalance in the locus coeruleus in bipolar disorder. *Bipolar Disorders, 10*(3), 349–359. https://doi.org/10.1111/j.1399-5618.2007.00528.x

16 Preston wants to reconnect with his children and is in recovery from addiction

Neuroscience facilitates our understanding of family dynamics

Sally Wasmuth

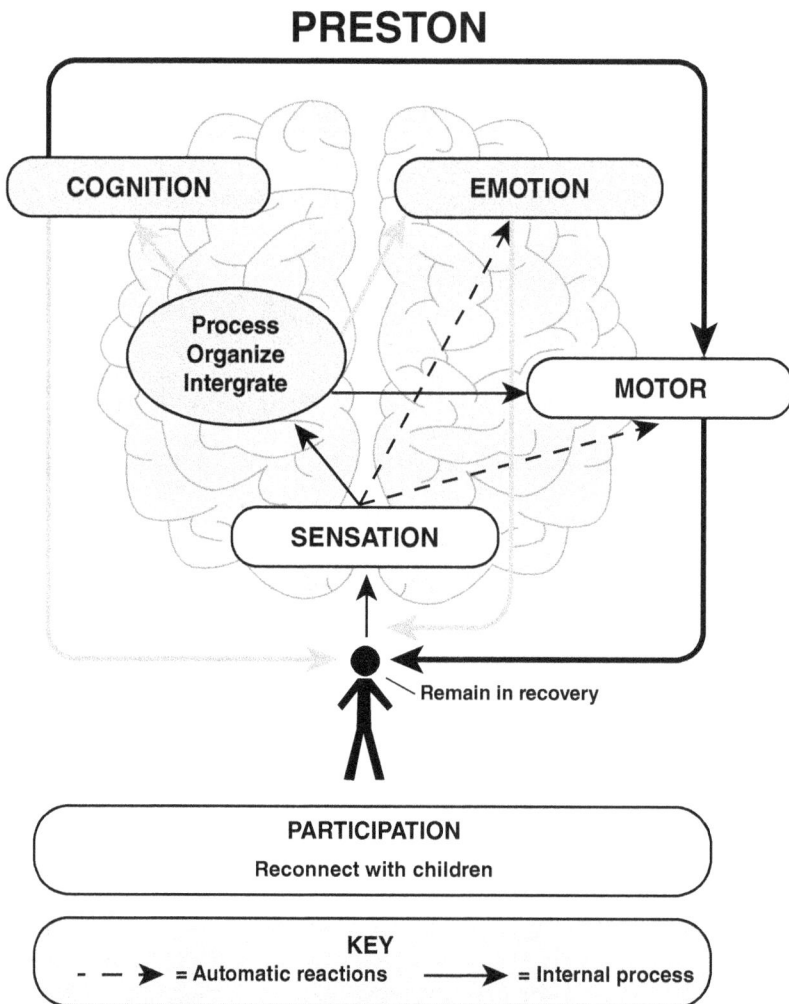

Figure 16.1 Preston brain figure

DOI: 10.4324/9781003524380-19

Purpose of this chapter

The purpose of this chapter is to discover how Preston, a father who is in recovery related to substance use, can reconnect with his children. People with substance use disorders and/or addictive behaviors demonstrate distinct, recognizable participation patterns with corresponding, identifiable neurological changes that, in turn, foster the continuation of "addictive" occupational participation. People in recovery from substance abuse can have full lives with their daily routines, relationships, work, and leisure, but may require modifications for function.

The key neuroscience concepts we will explore in this chapter include: the neuroscience underpinnings of substance use, the neurotransmitters that are involved, and drug actions to mediate differences in brain processing. A person's participation and neurobiology affect one another, resulting in recognizable patterns of occupational engagement with distinct neurobiological underpinnings. The occupations we engage in both shape and are shaped by our nervous system. What we do from day-to-day contributes to the flow of neurotransmitters, the shaping of synaptic pathways, and the connectivity within various regions of the brain. As with all chapters, these components of the nervous system work with other systems to support overall human function. Let's examine Preston's story to better understand how substance use disorders and addictive behaviors shape participation and neurobiology.

Keywords for this chapter are listed in the box below. Be sure you learn what these key features are so you can get the most out of the chapter.

Keywords for this chapter

12 step meetings	heroin	phencyclidine (PCP)
alcohol	lateral prefrontal cortex	reward center
amphetamines	medial prefrontal cortex	temporal discounting
anterior cingulate	morphine	ventral hippocampus
cocaine	nicotine	ventral prefrontal cortex
disinhibited	nucleus accumbens (NA)	ventral tegmental area
dopamine	opioid peptides	(VTA)

Box 16.1   Learning activity

Prior to reading the case:

1. How do you think substance use will affect Preston's ability to connect with his children?
2. Why is it important for an occupational therapy practitioner to understand the neurology of substance use?

Preston, a man who wants to reconnect with his children

Preston is a 28-year-old cis-gender, divorced man who currently resides in a residential facility for men recovering from alcoholism and drug addiction. Preston's ex-wife (Emily) and twin boys (age 5) live in an apartment in the same city. Preston also has an older brother, age 35, that he has not spoken to in over ten years. Preston's mother is deceased, and he never had a relationship with his dad. He has no other family or close friends.

Preston began drinking and smoking marijuana in high school with friends. Most of his friends drank and smoked marijuana like he did, but many times he would wake up in a "black out" at a party or find himself at home without remembering how he got there. His friends did not seem to have similar experiences. After high school, Preston got a job bussing tables at Chili's. He was eventually promoted to server and then bartender. Preston worked most evenings until 11 or 12 at night and then drank with co-workers at the bar next door to the restaurant. He would wake up around 1 p.m. each day, watch football, play video games, and then shower and go to work. He ate at the restaurant, so he had little need for instrumental activities of daily living such as grocery shopping or cooking.

Preston met Emily at work—she worked as a server while she finished her degree in art history. They dated for two years, and when Emily graduated, Preston proposed. They got married and moved into an apartment shortly after Emily got her first job as a docent and assistant manager at the local museum. She worked long hours, beginning at 8 a.m. and often not returning home until after 7 p.m. Emily gave birth to the twins within the first year of marriage, and Preston left his job at the restaurant to be a stay-at-home dad.

Preston and Emily did not consider Preston's drinking a problem until he tried to stop. The couple had hired a sleep coach to help with the twins at night so that Emily and Preston could get some sleep and feel better prepared for the day, but Preston was unable to sleep and felt irritable and restless at night. During the day, he loved his new role as a father and enjoyed feeding the twins and playing with them. He had a double stroller and enjoyed taking them for walks to the nearby park. However, within the first week, Preston began having panic attacks and acute anxiety. He began experiencing delusions related to his own and the twins' safety. He experienced bouts of intense sadness and fatigue. When the twins were napping, Preston began drinking to relieve his stress. He never drove after having a drink, so he did not view his drinking as a problem. At times, Preston found he had to drink more than usual to calm his nerves. Sometimes he would fall asleep and, upon waking, feel like he did not want to get out of bed or go on living.

After sharing his feelings with Emily, they agreed he needed to seek treatment. He spent 5 days in an acute psychiatric hospital to address his suicidal ideation, depression, and anxiety. When he was discharged from the hospital, Preston began drinking around the clock. When Emily confronted him about smelling of alcohol, he denied it. Preston feared that he could not fulfill his roles and responsibilities without alcohol. He knew that others would not approve, so he went to great lengths to keep his drinking a secret until one day, Emily found him passed out at home with the twins crying in their cribs. Shortly after that, she filed for a separation and eventually filed for divorce.

Preston continued to drink heavily and began smoking marijuana again. Late one night at the bar down the street from his apartment, a friend from high school offered Preston some cocaine, saying it would help him stay awake and be able to drink longer. Preston loved the feeling that cocaine gave him. He played pool with his friend all night at the bar. The next day, Preston called his friend and bought some cocaine. He continued to use cocaine daily for just under a year. During this time, Emily stopped visiting him with the twins. There were blankets over the windows of his apartment, serving as curtains to keep the sunlight out. Preston had lost several pounds and rarely ate more than ramen noodles and dry cereal. Emily did not want the twins to see their father in his current condition and did not feel it was a safe place to visit. Emily told Preston he could see the twins at her house, or they could meet in public places; however, Preston was too depressed and lacked the energy or motivation to contact her, so he ceased seeing the twins altogether.

Preston no longer took interest in playing video games or watching sports. Most of his time was spent sleeping and going to the bar down the street to drink and do cocaine in the bathroom. Sometimes he would stay in his apartment all day if he had enough cocaine. Using cocaine never gave him the euphoric high that he experienced the first time he tried it, but he continued to use it without much thought or reflection about it. He began smoking cigarettes, so his daily routine centered on contacting dealers, using cocaine, maybe eating, walking to the gas station for cigarettes, smoking, using more cocaine, smoking more, drinking, getting sick in the bathroom, and eventually maybe going to the bar to use cocaine and drink with friends.

On one of his trips to the gas station, Emily happened to be driving by and saw how much weight he had lost and how unwell he appeared. The twins were at preschool, so she stopped the car and asked him to get in. She pleaded with him to seek help, and he agreed. After a few phone calls, Emily took him to the Progress House, where he attended his first 12 step meeting, and where he would live for the next 13 months.

Box 16.2   Learning activity

Before reading the next section about the neurobiology of substance use and addictive disorders, discuss in your small group some salient characteristics you noticed about Preston's occupational patterns.

1. What strengths did you notice about Preston?
2. How did Preston's occupational patterns change over time?
3. How did Preston's social support networks change over time?

Neuroscience information to guide your thinking about Preston

The Diagnostic and Statistical Manual of Mental Disorders, Fifth Edition (DSM-5) describes "substance-related and addictive disorders" as a list of behaviors that share specific behavioral and neurobiological characteristics. Within this definition are the several types of substance use disorders (SUDs), such as alcohol use disorder, opioid use disorder, and cocaine use disorder, as well as addictive behaviors such as gambling.

Box 16.3   Learning activity

Pause here and discuss in a small group what you think each of these SUDs and non-substance-related activities have in common, both behaviorally and neurologically. Here are some questions to guide your thinking:

1. What is different about recreational substance use and a substance use disorder? What characteristics distinguish problematic versus unproblematic substance use?

2. How do societal norms impact how we understand substance use and its consequences?
3. What are some possible consequences of addictive behaviors that do not involve substances? How might these have consequences that resemble those of substance use disorders?
4. How does stigma play into the harms of substance use and/or the definitions of substance use disorders?
5. What social, cultural, historical and/or contextual factors might influence people's experiences and interpretations of substance use?

Temporal discounting and competing neural systems

Decades ago, Bechara (2005) suggested the theory of competing neural systems to help understand the neurobiology of addictive behaviors. Shortly thereafter, Bickel and colleagues illustrated that people with a wide variety of conditions—including all substance use disorders—preferred immediate but small rewards over larger rewards that were not available until later in the future. This temporal discounting, the tendency to devalue rewards that are not received until far into the future. Showed up at the behavioral and neurological level. In a behavioral study, Bickel and his team provided the following prompt to research participants: "After awakening, Bill began to think about his future. In general, he expected to …" Thirty-four heroin-addicted participants and 59 healthy control participants were asked to generate the ending of the story in any way they wished, and to give an approximation of the time in which the story took place. The healthy control participants' stories took place an average of 4.7 years in the future. The heroin-addicted participants' stories took place an average of nine days in the future, illustrating the different ways in which addicted and non-addicted people view and experience temporal structure (Bickel et al., 2017).

Box 16.4 Learning activity

What are some ways that you and your family/friends/peers/colleagues seek and gratify immediate desires?

1. What aspects of society support or incentivize immediate gratification?
2. What are some common, "binge-worthy" rewards that are frequently enjoyed in modern society?

A preference for smaller, immediate rewards over larger but more delayed rewards is not, in itself, pathological. This tendency toward instant gratification is, in fact, quite common in modern society. However, temporal discounting becomes problematic if it interferes with more long-term, desired pursuits. For example, pursuing a graduate degree allows for some short-term rewards and gratifications such as taking a night off from studying to binge-watch a new Netflix series. However, if a person continually chooses watching Netflix at the expense of completing required coursework, this preference for immediate rewards becomes problematic in the context of the person's life. While studying, attending classes, and performing clinical educational duties may be more cognitively demanding and provide less immediate gratification to the impulsive reward center of the brain, over time, the rewards that result, such as sense of accomplishment and/or a promising career are much larger, sustained, and potentially more satisfying. If a person lacks the capacity to sustain their attention and delay immediate gratification to pursue such long-term rewards, their lives and their neurobiology are impacted.

At the neurological level, people with substance use disorders demonstrate neurological changes that are associated with temporal discounting, including the highly reinforced dopamine transmission in the reward center brain (i.e., the limbic system; see also Chapter 17) and diminished prefrontal cortex processing (see also Chapter 12).

Box 16.5   Learning activity

Find images of the limbic system and prefrontal cortex so you have a sense about where these structures are in the brain. Take a moment with your group to discuss what you already know about the reward center and the prefrontal cortex.

1. What cognitive functions is the prefrontal cortex known for?
2. What would diminished processing in the prefrontal cortex look like?
3. What functions are associated with the reward center?
4. What behaviors might result from reinforced reward center processing?

Keywords: limbic system, mesolimbic pathway, reward pathway, dopamine pathway

---

According to Bechara's competing neural systems theory, the impulsive reward center is in constant competition with the more reflective and executive functions housed in the prefrontal cortex. Both vie for control over our behaviors. Adaptive occupational engagement requires that these systems are in balance with individual occupational needs and wants, given a person's context(s), values, capacities, and goals.

The prefrontal cortex has been conceptualized as having three functionally distinct but overlapping areas—the medial, lateral, and ventral prefrontal cortex. Each of these works together to temper our instinctual drives, rooted in and reinforced by the pleasure that is processed via dopamine transmission in the reward center. The lateral prefrontal cortex has been linked to goal-directed behavior—it is involved in working memory tasks in which we must sustain our attention and hold various sources of information in our minds while evaluating options and making choices. The medial prefrontal cortex has been described as the area that allows us to perceive others' emotions, evaluate our own emotions, and attach emotional thoughts and experiences to pleasure. The ventral prefrontal cortex is most known for its role in social behavior. It allows us to evaluate socially appropriate responses by observing and learning from feedback to various actions. It also gives us a sense of the motives and trustworthiness of others.

Box 16.6   Learning activity

Take a moment to consider how a lesion to each of these areas of the prefrontal cortex might show up in the context of a person's life. What areas of occupation may be affected and how?

The reward center (also called the limbic system) is an evolutionarily older region of the brain than the prefrontal cortex. The reward center is activated by and facilitates experiences of pleasure. It is part of the limbic system; some have referred to this area as the "lizard brain"—highlighting its role in more basic, animalistic drives rooted in pleasure, such as eating and reproduction. However, the reward center in human brains is highly interconnected to several evolutionarily newer structures related to memory, emotion, and decision making, including the prefrontal cortices. The reward center is part of the cognitive basal ganglia connections including parts of the thalamus, several areas of the cortex, the hippocampus, and the amygdala (see also Chapter 23).

Box 16.7   Learning activity

Take a moment to search for images of these structures and their locations in the brain in relation to one another. List the main functions of each of these neural areas. Search for an image of the cognitive basal ganglia and sketch a diagram of how these areas project to one another in the cognitive basal ganglia loop.

Keywords: thalamus, hippocampus, basal ganglia-thalamo-cortical circuits, amygdala, reward-based learning, ventral striatum, midbrain dopamine neurons, ventral midbrain

---

Two key structures involved in reward center processing include the ventral tegmental area (VTA) and the nucleus accumbens (NA). The NA contains medium spiny neurons modulated by dopamine from the VTA, which is a dopamine-rich nucleus in the ventral midbrain. The VTA is the main source of dopamine input for reward center processing. The NA also receives input from areas of the brain involved with memory (ventral hippocampus) and emotion (anterior cingulate, amygdala, ventral and medial prefrontal cortices). By integrating these excitatory inputs, people register and learn from how various activities feel (was it pleasurable? uneventful? scary?). The reward center directs attention toward activities that are pleasurable or unpredictable.

Box 16.8   Learning activity

Take a look at the following open-access article to learn more about how/why activities that elicit uncertainty or unpredictability capture the "attention" of the reward system:

Floresco, S. B. (2015). The nucleus accumbens: An interface between cognition, emotion, and action. *Annual Review of Psychology, 66*, 25–52. https://doi.org/10.1146/annurev-psych-010213-115159

Dopamine transmission

Potentiation is a term in neuroscience that can refer to connectivity between neurons. The phrase "use it or lose it" suggests that when neural pathways are reinforced (through repeated experiences or actions) they become more robust/more engrained. This is how habits form, neurologically, and these robust connections can make behavior change (or perceptual change) more challenging. Potentiation between the VTA and NA via do-pamine transmission is central to addiction at the neurological level. Under "normal" conditions, dopaminergic neurons in the VTA transmit dopamine to the NA. When a person engages in an activity such as drug use, that results in continuous action potentials producing bursts of dopamine to the NA. Medium spiny neurons in the NA become much more responsive to excitatory input from the amygdala and orbital medial prefrontal cor-tex. This excitation produces a "go" signal to repeat the activity in question. The VTA also projects directly to the cortex to reinforce this motivation to engage in the activity in ques-tion (Purves & Platt, 2017).

Drug actions

The drugs that are included in the SUD diagnostic classification affect dopamine trans-mission between the VTA and NA. For example, amphetamines promote the release of dopamine from the VTA. Cocaine blocks the reuptake of dopamine released from the VTA to allow more time for the NA to respond to the drug. Heroin and morphine block the release of inhibitory transmitters such as gamma-aminobutyric acid (GABA) to the VTA— when the system blocks GABAergic neurotransmission, the VTA becomes disinhibited. In other words, the VTA releases more dopamine than it otherwise would have because it is less inhibited by GABA. Nicotine enhances excitatory input to the VTA and NA to increase dopamine transmission between the two. Phencyclidine (PCP) enhances excita-tory input to the NA, causing it to be more affected by dopamine input. Finally, alcohol increases the release of dopamine, opioid peptides, and GABA. GABA reduces social inhibition and motor control. However, excessive alcohol consumption causes decreased release of the same chemicals and also releases corticotropin-releasing factor (CRF). This release of CRF activates the amygdala and produces the experience of stress. People then drink more alcohol to relieve the stress that is paradoxically induced by heavy drinking in the first place (Purves & Platt, 2017).

Box 16.9   Learning activity

Based on what was described here about the effects of different substances, how would you describe what is happening with Preston at the neurological level?

Drugs of abuse and sociocultural/historical/contextual factors

We can learn a lot about substance use disorders and addictive behaviors from neuro-logical and behavioral phenomena; but we must also consider our interpretations within sociocultural and historical contexts. Historical, social, and cultural structures influenced what behaviors were acceptable versus unacceptable and what substance was considered illicit or addictive. As Acker wrote over a decade ago:

> to treat scientific findings as a neutral lens through which to view historical evidence avoids important questions. A burgeoning literature in the history, sociology and anthropology of science has shown that the laboratory, far from being an isolated and impermeable space, is intimately linked with the social world around it. Influence flows in both directions.
>
> (Acker, 2010, p. 71)

Acker goes on to illuminate the history of legal attitudes toward substance use linked to the activities of marginalized racial groups that were viewed through the lenses of stigma, racism, and ethnocentrism that have pervaded US history. Acker explains:

> Most of the psychoactive drugs that the US government has declared unfit for non-medical use first aroused concerns because of their associations with marginal racial groups. Images of opium-smoking Chinese in the late nineteenth century, cocaine-maddened African Americans in the early twentieth century and marijuana-puffing Mexicans in the 1930s fueled movements that culminated in passage of the Harrison Narcotic Act in 1914 and the Marijuana Tax Act in 1937. Moral entrepreneurs … cast drug use as a threat to the national fabric; these attitudes, hardened into law, became the basis of American drug policy—which, as noted, has been tightly linked to addiction research. Given the intertwined nature of addiction research, public policy, media coverage and public attitudes, taking science seriously means engaging it critically.
>
> (Acker, 2010, p. 73)

Thirteen years later, how do changing laws and policies surrounding drug use influence the degree to which people experience harm in the contexts of their occupational lives? Think, for instance, about two marijuana users engaged in a plethora of meaningful occupations—one lives in a state where the substance is legal and decriminalized; the other lives in a state where it is illegal. The latter suffers recurring consequences related to legal difficulties; they are referred to SUD treatment centers and are ostracized by friends and family; they experience isolation, disapproval, and rejection. These experiences are due not to substance use itself, nor are they due to the substance's impact on their ability to function in the context of their daily occupations but rather, are due to stigma and policy related to the substance—stigma that influences how people treat the substance user. The former user who lives in a state where marijuana is legal and decriminalized may in fact be using in a way that is more detrimental to their occupational life but suffers fewer negative consequences because they are not ostracized or criminalized.

Box 16.10   Learning activity

Take a moment to consider other ways in which stigma may impact a substance using person. Think about law enforcement, access to care, and societal reactions to drug users.

**Daily life routine: Reestablishing family connections
when they have been broken**

During Preston's first week at the Progress House, he attended two 12-step meetings a day. His morning meeting involved listening to a speaker talk about his own experience using drugs and alcohol, what happened that caused him to stop using drugs and alcohol, and what his life is like now. The speakers often spoke about their drug use beginning in high school in seemingly unproblematic ways. Some of the speakers were arrested and served time in prison. Others spent time in psychiatric institutions, and others experienced weeks, months, or years of homelessness. Preston noticed some parts of speakers' stories that he could not relate to, such as being in jail, but other parts of each story sounded very similar to his own. He identified with feeling like he needed alcohol to be able to do his everyday occupations. He could relate to experiencing disapproval from friends and family who didn't understand his need for alcohol, and the estrangement of spouses and children. While Preston had never been homeless, he could easily imagine losing his apartment. He was nearly out of money, he didn't have a job, and he lacked the motivation to find work. He did not have family members or friends who would provide financial support, and if Emily hadn't encouraged him to find help, he was certain that homelessness would have been imminent. Preston's decline in motivation for activities other than drug and alcohol use is a hallmark symptom of neurological changes associated with SUD. At this time in his life, dopamine processing in the reward center was fine-tuned to respond to dopamine surges produced by drug and alcohol use. The dopamine produced by every day meaningful activities was no longer strong enough to capture Preston's attention or to stimulate his motivation. Moreover, he was likely drinking to relieve stress, paradoxically induced by his alcohol use activating the amygdala by producing increased stress hormones such as CRF.

Preston's evening 12-step meetings involved reading literature on the 12 steps and sharing personal experiences about trying to implement the first of the 12 steps in life. Preston did not like to share during meetings because he didn't understand the 12 steps or how they worked, and he did not believe in God or a higher power, nor did he want to. He was not interested in being religiously converted, and at times, he was suspicious that the 12-step meetings were led by the church he so adamantly rejected. However, the people in the meetings never tried to push religion. They only suggested to Preston that he accept his lack of power to stop drinking and using drugs despite negative consequences. If he accepted this fact, they said, his willingness to seek help would naturally follow. Preston's regular engagement in reading literature and engaging in conversation with other recovering people engaged his executive neurological systems. As previously described, strengthening executive functioning can help to rewire the neuropathology of SUD, as it is the executive systems that inhibit the impulsivity associated with reward center processing. By abstaining from the substances that reinforced Preston's reward center and simultaneously engaging the executive systems, Preston started to see progress in his recovery.

After several weeks without access to drugs and alcohol and attending 12-step meetings, Preston noticed that the desire for drugs and alcohol was no longer persistent. He began to enjoy attending meetings, and he began to think about things he would like to do, which included spending time with his children. He recalled his interest in watching football and began to watch games with other men in the Progress House. One of the men, Marcus, shared he was in an adult flag football team and invited Preston to join.

Preston began playing flag football weekly. He became close friends with Marcus, and they often shared "war stories" about their substance using histories. Marcus did not like to attend the 12-step meetings, but he enjoyed working closely with a therapist and engaging in leisure and work occupations to improve his physical and mental health. Both men respected their different approaches to recovery. Engaging in physical activity was particularly helpful in Preston's recovery journey. From a neurological perspective, exercise enhances reward center processing. When Preston abstains from drugs and loses the expected jolts of dopamine, exercise makes up for this by replacing dopamine transmission in the reward center (Heijnen et al., 2016). However, the dopamine transmission fueled by exercise differs from that of drug use in important ways. Consistent aerobic exercise reinforces reward center dopamine while also improving attention, working memory, and inhibition of impulses (Mandolesi et al., 2018).

Back to the person's life: Preston finding ways to reconnect with his children

After a few months passed, Preston decided to invite Emily to bring the twins to one of the football games. She agreed, and after the game, they all went for ice cream. Preston began seeing the twins every Saturday. At first, they went for ice cream each week, but as time passed, Preston would think of new fun things to do with the kids, and they expanded their activities to going to parks, pools, playgrounds, and other restaurants.

Eventually, Preston felt that living in the recovery house did not match his life stage and his recovery needs. To have the ability to live on his own, he began applying for jobs in local diners that did not serve alcohol. He was able to get a regular daytime schedule as a server and was soon able to afford the deposit on a small apartment. He continues to attend daily 12-step meetings, go to work, and play with his children. He and Emily have a positive co-parenting relationship. Preston is not sure what he sees for his future, but he continues to think about and envision possible future goals.

What do we know about ourselves and the population at large from this brain condition and this family story?

Regardless of whether we can identify with Preston's use of alcohol, marijuana, and eventually cocaine, all humans have in common that the brain's reward center is inextricably linked to pleasurable and/or captivating experiences of occupational engagement. We can likely relate to the desire for engaging in occupations that provide immediate gratification, and we may have activities in our lives that tempt us to draw away from more long-term endeavors. Some of us may greatly benefit from these miniature retreats from life, while others may have trouble balancing our long-term pursuits and the temptations of more immediate pleasure.

Understanding the effects of occupations on the brain's reward center and dopamine processing allows us to determine whether an occupation facilitates or inhibits meaningful and engaging participation. It can also help us understand substance use disorders and addictive behaviors in occupational terms; their underlying neuroscience is similar to that of any occupation. We can see in Preston's story how drug and alcohol use may have initially been a meaningful form of social engagement and a way to relax. However, alongside neurological changes, Preston's drug and alcohol use progressed to a restrictive and harmful endeavor that interfered with his ability to engage in life and connect with and care for the people he loved.

Finally, we can understand others' experiences by examining sociopolitical, cultural, and historical contexts. Is the substance or activity in question truly harmful to a person's occupational life? Is it being viewed as harmful solely because of external factors designated to marginalize groups? We can use our knowledge and expertise as occupational therapists to analyze how occupations facilitate or restrict health and affect a person in the context of their own, unique lived experience. When activities such as substance use are deemed harmful in individuals' life contexts, occupational therapists can use their vast knowledge of the interrelationships between the person, occupations, and contexts to promote health and wellbeing.

Box 16.11   Learning activity

With your small group, complete the table in the Appendix about the integration of Preston's needs to find long-term success staying connected with his children.

Further reading

If interested in further reading about substance use disorders and addictive behaviors:

Mattila, A., Santacecilia, G., & Lacroix, R. (2022). Perceptions and knowledge of substance use disorders and the role of OT: A national survey. *The American Journal of Occupational Therapy*, 76(Supplement_1), 7610510156p1. https://doi.org/10.5014/ajot.2022.76S1-PO156

Rawat, H., Petzer, S. L., & Gurayah, T. (2021). Effects of substance use disorder on women's roles and occupational participation. *South African Journal of Occupational Therapy*, 51(1), 54–62. http://dx.doi.org/10.17159/2310-3833/2021/vol51n1a8

Wasmuth, S., Brandon-Friedman, R. A., & Olesek, K. (2016). A grounded theory of veterans' experiences of addiction-as-occupation. *Journal of Occupational Science*, 23(1), 128–141. https://doi.org/10.1080/14427591.2015.1070782

Wasmuth, S., Crabtree, J. L., & Scott, P. J. (2014). Exploring addiction-as-occupation. *British Journal of Occupational Therapy*, 77(12), 605–613. https://doi.org/10.4276/030802214X14176260335264

Wasmuth, S. L., Outcalt, J., Buck, K., Leonhardt, B. L., Vohs, J., & Lysaker, P. H. (2015). Metacognition in persons with substance abuse: Findings and implications for occupational therapists; La métacognition chez les personnes toxicomanes: Résultats et conséquences pour les ergothérapeutes. *Canadian Journal of Occupational Therapy*, 82(3), 150–159. https://doi.org/10.1177/0008417414564865

Wasmuth, S., Pritchard, K., & Kaneshiro, K. (2016). Occupation-based intervention for addictive disorders: A systematic review. *Journal of Substance Abuse Treatment*, 62, 1–9. https://doi.org/10.1016/j.jsat.2015.11.011

References

Acker, C. J. (2010). How crack found a niche in the American ghetto: The historical epidemiology of drug-related harm. *BioSocieties*, 5, 70–88. https://doi.org/10.1057/biosoc.2009.1

American Psychiatric Association. (2013). *Diagnostic and statistical manual of mental disorders* (5th ed.). Washington, DC: American Psychiatric Association. https://doi.org/10.1176/appi.books.9780890425596

Bechara, A. (2005). Decision making, impulse control and loss of willpower to resist drugs: A neurocognitive perspective. *Nature Neuroscience*, 8(11), 1458–1463. https://doi.org/10.1038/nn1584

Bickel, W. K., Stein, J. S., Moody, L. N., Snider, S. E., Mellis, A. M., & Quisenberry, A.J. (2017). Toward narrative theory: Interventions for reinforcer pathology in health behavior. In J. Stevens (Ed.), *Impulsivity. Nebraska Symposium on Motivation, 64*. Cham: Springer. https://doi.org/10.1007/978-3-319-51721-6_8

Floresco, S. B. (2015). The nucleus accumbens: An interface between cognition, emotion, and action. *Annual Review of Psychology, 66*, 25–52. https://doi.org/10.1146/annurev-psych-010213-115159

Heijnen, S., Hommel, B., Kibele, A., & Colzato, L. S. (2016). Neuromodulation of aerobic exercise—A review. *Frontiers in Psychology, 6*(1890). https://doi.org/10.3389/fpsyg.2015.01890

Mandolesi, L., Polverino, A., Montuori, S., Foti, F., Ferraioli, G., Sorrentino, P., & Sorrentino, G. (2018). Effects of physical exercise on cognitive functioning and wellbeing: Biological and psychological benefits. *Frontiers in Psychology, 9*(509). https://doi.org/10.3389/fpsyg.2018.00509

Purves, D. & Platt, M. (2017). Emotion. In Purves, D., Augustine, G. J., Fitzpatrick, D., Hall, W. C., LaMantia, A. S., Mooney, R. D., Platt, M. L., & White, L. E. (Eds.). (2017). *Neuroscience* (6th ed.). Oxford: Oxford University Press.

Unit III
Cognitive systems

17 Peter wants to build a playhouse for his siblings and has ADHD

Neuroscience facilitates our understanding of task completion

Timothy Dionne

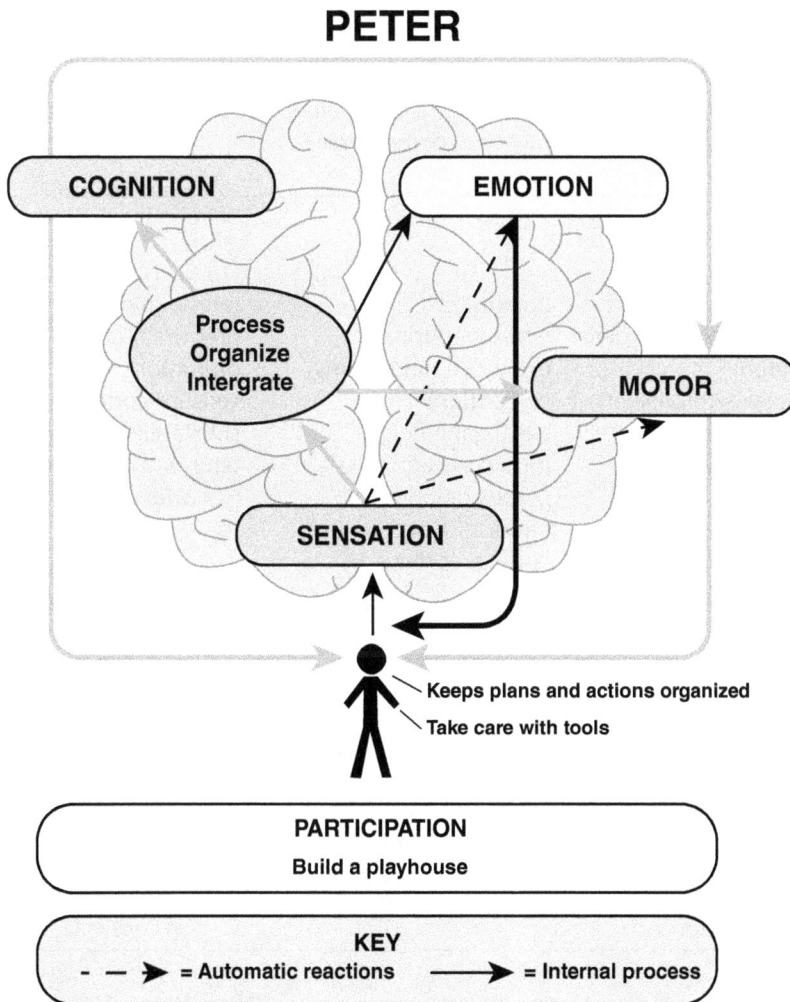

Figure 17.1 Peter brain figure

DOI: 10.4324/9781003524380-21

Purpose of this chapter

The purpose of this chapter is to explore how Peter, an 11-year-old who has attention deficit and hyperactivity disorder (ADHD), can find ways to finish tasks he starts. ADHD is a condition that changes how the brain processes information, remains motivated and engaged and tracks task components to complete projects. Children and adults with ADHD can have full lives with their daily routines, relationships, work and leisure, but may require modifications to function.

Following the example of the previous chapters, we will learn how neurological processes affect motivation, engagement, and participation in leisure activities. ADHD is the most common neurodevelopment disorder that exists on a spectrum with varied combinations of inattention to hyperactivity (Solanta, et al., 2001). The combination and presentation often has a significant impact in the development of personal, social, academic, and occupational functioning (Konopka, 2014). As with all the chapters, these components of the nervous system work with other systems to support overall human function.

Keywords for this chapter are listed in the box below. Be sure you learn what these key features are so you can get the most out of the chapter.

Keywords for this chapter

attention deficit and hyperactivity disorder (ADHD)	dopamine	temporal cortex
	norepinephrine	prefrontal cortex
	executive functioning	premotor cortex
hyperactivity/impulsivity subtype of ADHD	cerebellum	sensory cortex
	basal ganglia	substantia nigra
inattention subtype of ADHD	limbic system	temporal association cortex
	globus pallidus	
bottom-up attention	motor cortex	
top-down attention	parietal cortex	

Box 17.1   Learning activity

Prior to reading the case:

1. How do you think the ADHD symptoms of will affect Peter's occupational performance of designing and building the playhouse?
2. Why is it important for an occupational therapy practitioner to understand the nervous system of someone with ADHD?

Let's find out about Peter, his family, and his dreams of building a playhouse for his siblings, so that we can understand his nervous system processes while Peter completes the desired occupations.

**Peter, an 11-year-old boy, who wants to build a
playhouse for his younger siblings**

Peter is the oldest child in a household of three children. Peter loves being the big brother, even though he knows he does not always set the best example for his younger brother (5 years old) and sister (3 years old). Peter enjoys playing with friends in the neighborhood and on the soccer team. Peter's dad even convinced him to join Cub Scouts in Kindergarten. Now in fifth grade, Peter has grown quite a bit from those early days, and is now ready to lead the younger scouts in nature walks, camping, and fire safety—his favorite topics. Peter really enjoys immersing himself in nature, dad notices that it is one of few times he is calm and focused. Although if you asked his dad about his attention and focus, he would not be able to overstate Peter's energy and extreme difficulty completing specific complicated tasks. Peter's room is full of wall to wall of half-finished projects. If mom or dad asks Peter about finishing a specific project, Peter suddenly remembers that he really did want to finish that marble run or snap circuit, or erector set he got as a birthday gift five months ago.

Despite his love for the outdoors, STEM-themed projects, and being a big brother, he often spends his time alternating between video games and internet videos about video games. Sometimes Peter's parents catch him doing both at the same time, alone in the dark. Peter has difficulty discontinuing engagement with those activities, even with often excessive parental prompting, protesting very enthusiastically. Once Peter gets "forced" to go outside, he suddenly remembers how great it is outside to run, jump, and play with friends.

At school, Peter is in fifth grade. Peter does really well in math and science. He expresses dislike for reading and writing, even though his verbal vocabulary is well beyond a fifth grader. He's usually the first to finish anything, often speeding through the assignments, although with some coaching from his teacher this year, he's gotten a lot better at taking his time. Early in his primary education, his first-grade teacher noticed he was really uncomfortable and squirming a lot in his seat, especially when he was supposed to be listening and not talking. School administration and Peter's parents met to discuss some accommodations at his desk, they decided to let Peter use a Bouncy Band (large rubber band) around his chair and a fidget toy. Upon starting fifth grade, Peter expressed that he didn't want the Bouncy Band anymore. He felt that it made him "look like a weird kid." During teacher-parent conference this year, he received glowing marks except with bringing back completed homework. Peter has never had this problem in previous school years, so his parents are concerned. In response, they have set up structured homework time. Peter is not doing well with the new external structure, the attraction of STEM-projects in his room, games in the backyard, and video games are too strong for him to even focus. His family wants to address Peter's ability to engage and complete activities he begins. They know he enjoys all the activities he begins, but his ability to plan and execute disrupts their completion.

Box 17.2   Learning activity

Discuss with your peers:

1. What aspects of Peter's story sparks your interest?
2. What information do you already know?
3. What more information would you like to know?
4. What are some potential pitfalls you can anticipate with Peter's Story?

Box 17.3   Learning activity

Stop here and work in a small group to discuss Peter's story.

1. How would it help if you understood the neurological basis for Peter's challenges?
2. What components of the brain address attention, emotional regulation, and filtering external stimuli?

Neuroscience information to guide your thinking about Peter

Attention deficit hyperactivity disorder (ADHD) is a neurodevelopmental disorder characterized by inattention, hyperactivity, and impulsivity (Solanto, Arnsten, & Castellanos, 2001). ADHD is considered a neurodevelopmental disorder due to the significance of an individual's neurological development as they age, presenting as a delay in brain regions compared to age-appropriate maturation (Konopka, 2014; Rakic, 1995). Symptoms of ADHD can have a significant impact on an individual's ability to function in daily life that can interfere with academic, social, and professional success. ADHD is commonly divided into two subtypes: inattention and hyperactivity/impulsivity (Konopka, 2014).

The neuroscience of ADHD is complex and involves multiple brain regions and systems. Research has identified several brain areas that have reduced in activity in individuals with ADHD, including the prefrontal cortex, basal ganglia, limbic system, and cerebellum (Cortese, Kelly, Chabernaud, Proal, Di Martino, Milham, Castellanos, 2012; Rubia, 2018). These brain regions are important for executive functioning (Friedman & Robbins, 2022), which includes skills such as planning, organizing, and problem-solving; emotional regulation; integration of sensory stimuli and knowledge. Research has also shown that in individuals with ADHD, the neurotransmitter systems that regulate attention function differently than expected, including dopamine and norepinephrine (Solanto, Arnsten, & Castellanos, 2001; Friedman & Robbins, 2022). In addition, research suggests that individuals with ADHD have variations in these regions processing sensory information differently (Solanto, Arnsten, & Castellanos, 2001), which can impact the ability to filter out distractions and focus on relevant stimuli.

Behavior of individuals with inattention subtype of ADHD are characterized by difficulty paying attention, following instructions, and completing tasks (Solanto, Arnsten, & Castellanos, 2001; Konopka, 2014; Rakic, 1995). This subtype is associated with variations in function of the prefrontal cortex and basal ganglia, which are important for executive functioning and decision-making. Behavior of individuals with hyperactivity/impulsivity subtype of ADHD are characterized by higher levels of activity and impulsivity (Friedman & Robbins, 2022). This subtype is often associated with variations the basal ganglia and cerebellum, which are important for movement control and impulse regulation (Friedman & Robbins, 2022). Often individuals with ADHD will display a complex integration of some or all of the challenges previously mentioned, providing us with a small picture of the complex beauty of brain processing.

Box 17.4   Learning activity

In small groups, discuss the following:

1. What challenges and opportunities does someone with the Inattentive subtype of ADHD face?
2. What challenges and opportunities would Peter face, when planning and designing the playhouse, with the inattentive subtype?
3. What challenges and opportunities does someone with the hyperactivity/ impulsivity subtype of ADHD face?
4. What challenges and opportunities would Peter face, when planning and designing the playhouse, with hyperactivity/impulsivity subtype?

Prefrontal cortex

The prefrontal cortex (PFC) controls behavior of an individual through its connections to sensory and motor cortices, as well as the important motor and emotional circuits in the limbic system and the cerebellum. The PFC registers a reduced response in functional imaging studies of individuals with ADHD while they are trying to regulate attention and behavior (Solanto, Arnsten, & Castellanos, 2001). Since the PFC functions through the use of dopamine and norepinephrine, and a reduced amount of these neurotransmitters results in blunted regulation. Notably, studies have found discrepancies in the genes associated with this specific neurotransmitter production among those with ADHD.

The PFC is located in the frontal lobe anterior to the premotor cortex (motor planning) and the motor cortex (voluntary motor control).

Box 17.5   Learning activity

Find some images of the frontal and prefrontal cortex to orient yourself to the brain regions of interest in this discussion.

Keywords: frontal lobe, prefrontal lobe, schematic

The specific areas of interest lie along the dorsal and lateral aspects of the PFC, and they are of the last areas of the brain to fully mature, typically maturing in late adolescence (Konopka, 2014). The PFC functions as a top-down attention or goal-directed attention. This essentially means that the PFC can be influenced by our wants and desires, this is why those with ADHD seem to be much better during intrinsically motivating activities, tricking parents, teachers, and caregivers into thinking they have more control in their attention than it often seems.

Box 17.6   Learning activity

1. How do you relate to the lack of top-down control?
2. What situations make it easier or harder to sustain your attention to things that you find boring?
3. How would you handle a situation where you want to read your current fiction novel about a murder mystery and the slow burn is about to turn into a raging fire of prose, but you have to read a research article for school? Which item would you prefer to read? How would you structure your reading so you complete the necessary task versus the preferred leisure task?
4. How can you adapt the strategies to a clinical setting working with children with ADHD?

In an individual with ADHD, Bottom-up attention may contradict their intended focus. Bottom-up attention stems from the sensory areas in the parietal and temporal cortices of the brain. They process sensory information, presenting the most salient input to consciousness. In other words, when Peter begins to plan the playhouse, his desire to focus on selecting a design can be countermanded by online video content with cool turrets and nerf-gun fights. The brain region responsible for identifying what we see (i.e., processing and perceiving visual stimuli) is the temporal association cortex. The parietal cortex helps identify the visual input's location and its spatial relationship, often in the right hemisphere. Peter's motivation driven attention to design the playhouse becomes second to attention grabbing elements—like nerf-guns.

Basal ganglia and limbic system

The basal ganglia and the limbic system are situated in the inner portions of the brain; the limbic system creates the border separating these inner structures and the cerebral cortex. The basal ganglia are a group of structures (the striatum, globus pallidus, substantia nigra and subthalamic nucleus) deep to the frontal cortex responsible for helping to regulating movement, emotions, and behavior.

Box 17.7   Learning activity

1. Find images of the brain that show where the basal ganglia and limbic system structure are located. Note their relationships with the cortex and the brain stem.
2. Find images that mark the globus pallidus, substantia nigra and subthalamic nucleus within the basal ganglia system.
3. Find images that mark the hippocampus, amygdala and cingulate gyrus within the limbic system.

Keywords: basal ganglia, limbic system, cortex, brain stem, substantia nigra, subthalamus, hippocampus, amygdala, cingulate gyrus

Medical imaging studies conflict in those with ADHD some noting varied or delayed maturation while others noting overdeveloped structures on one side of the brain (Friedman, & Rapoport, 2015). The understanding of what structures are responsible for what functions, particularly in those with ADHD are constantly evolving. This is especially true with the limbic system, which is full of controversy. Consisting of several structures, including the hippocampus, amygdala, and cingulate gyrus; the limbic system. Many modern neuroscientists believe that emotions are much more complicated than just one system, which is evidenced by the numerous structures mentioned in this chapter. The components of the limbic system play a role in emotions, motivation and memory associations with emotions. The amygdala is connected to the hippocampus, and it is associated with encoding memories based on emotional states, particularly anxiety or fear-based emotions. The cingulate gyrus is associated with focusing attention to events based on emotional salience. The hippocampus is associated with forming memories and their long-term storage.

Cerebellum

The cerebellum's primary function is to modulate motor signals based on sensory input from many places in the body, allowing for precise and coordinated movement. The cerebellum connects to the basal ganglia and the limbic system. For Peter and others with ADHD, the cerebellum is implicated in either providing too much motor regulation or not enough.

Box 17.8   Learning activity

1. Find images of the cerebellum that show where the cerebellum is located related to the cortex.
2. Find images showing the inner surfaces of the cerebellum. Read about the specialized Purkinje cells that facilitate motor regulation.
3. Discuss your findings with peers.

Keywords: cerebellum, Purkinje cells

Understanding the neuroscience behind ADHD is complex and a rapidly evolving field. More research is needed to definitively identify the brain mechanisms. However, current research has provided important insights into the brain regions and systems involved in ADHD. These findings have not only helped with pharmacological and non-pharmacological treatment, but also our understanding in how occupational therapy practitioners can support individuals with ADHD.

Daily life routine: finding ways to complete tasks in a timely manner

Timely and successful task completion requires a command on executive control balancing sensory and cognitive demands. The internal motivation, especially at Peter's age, may not be a strong enough to drive him to maintain task engagement to complete it. This is where external structure provides the foundation for success. Looking to adults for examples of supports, they include chore lists, calendar reminders, and task-priority lists. External structure can provide additional stimuli to engage areas of the brain such as the prefrontal cortex to provide more motivation and awareness to the task at hand. Additionally, allowing for ample time to complete activities and being realistic in the time it requires to complete a given task is crucial. Time management from an external source via technology is possible. Technology provides an abundance of external motivation and time management supports, but can also provide easy distractions to the desired task at hand. Managing technology use can be so daunting, to the point that apps exist to block out all but productivity-related ones. Timing apps where time can be visualized, allowing for multi-sensory input, can be very helpful. All of these strategies reinforce motivation via external means, which reinforce internal motivations directing engagement and awareness. Another supportive activity that can help provide focus during activity is a method of negating disruptive sensory input. A common example includes listening to white noise while working (eliminating auditory input) or sitting in a cubicle to work (eliminating visual input). This filters out specific sensory inputs to allow for more focus on the desired activity. It is important to experiment with which strategies are a match for Peter.

Back to the person's life: Peter planning his playhouse construction

So now that you understand more about the neurological underpinnings of ADHD symptoms, how can we use scientific reasoning to support Peter in planning to build a playhouse? How do we leverage Peter's ability to hyper-focus or motivation-driven attention in the plan of the playhouse?

Box 17.9   Learning activity

In your class or small groups, discuss what accommodations Peter's parents can provide to help successful completion of the playhouse construction. Use neuroscience and what you know about Peter to guide your idea generation.

What do we know about ourselves and the population at large from this brain condition and this family story?

We learned a lot about people with ADHD, and they face many challenges when compared to neuro-typical children in their academic, social, and occupational life. But with care and understanding of appropriate supports children with ADHD can shine and grow into successful adults. It's important to remember that challenges faced in childhood can influence who that child grows up to be. We often hear people saying they "feel ADHD right now!" Or "I'm so scatterbrained!" disparaging their attention span or current behavior, often to the chagrin of people with ADHD. Everyone can have experiences just like those described in this chapter about ADHD, the difference is how often they experience them. Dealing with competing stimuli for attention is a common human experience; people with ADHD have these experiences so frequently, they can interfere with even highly desired activities. We can develop empathy through our experiences with distractibility and inattention (the same brain mechanisms are working when we have these moments);

we must also remain respectful that for people with ADHD, these occurrences are quite frequent.

Peter wants to build a playhouse (i.e., his inner drive is high), yet immediate sensory events (e.g., seeing his gaming program on his computer, hearing others playing nearby, smelling dinner being prepared) can activate neural systems for immediate attention, dampening his frontal and prefrontal lobes from a more internal planning process. By understanding Peter's nervous system, we can make adjustments to support him to finish the playhouse; along the way, he will learn strategies he can apply in future endeavors.

Box 17.10   Learning activity

With your small group, complete the table in the Appendix about the integration of Peter's needs to build a playhouse for his siblings.

Further reading

If interested in further reading about ADHD:

Barkley, R. A. (Ed.). (2018). *Attention-deficit hyperactivity disorder, fourth edition: A handbook for diagnosis and treatment* (4th ed.). Guilford Publications.
Chandler, C. (2011). *The science of ADHD: A guide for parents and professionals.* John Wiley & Sons.

References

Cortese, S., Kelly, C., Chabernaud, C., Proal, E., Di Martino, A., Milham, M. P., & Castellanos, F. X. (2012). Toward systems neuroscience of ADHD: a meta-analysis of 55 fMRI studies. *American Journal of Psychiatry*, 169(10), 1038–1055.
Friedman, L. A., & Rapoport, J. L. (2015). Brain development in ADHD. *Current Opinion in Neurobiology*, 30, 106–111.
Friedman, N. P., & Robbins, T. W. (2022). The role of prefrontal cortex in cognitive control and executive function. *Neuropsychopharmacology*, 47(1), 72–89.
Konopka, L. M. (2014). Understanding attention deficit disorder: a neuroscience prospective. *Croatian Medical Journal*, 55(2), 174.
Rakic, P. (1995). The development of the frontal lobe: a view from the rear of the brain. Discussion. *Advances in Neurology*, 66, 1–8.
Rubia, K. (2018). Cognitive neuroscience of attention deficit hyperactivity disorder (ADHD) and its clinical translation. *Frontiers in Human Neuroscience*, 12, 100.
Solanto, M. V., Arnsten, A. F. T., & Castellanos, F. X. (Eds.). (2001). *Stimulant drugs and ADHD: Basic and clinical neuroscience.* New York: Oxford University Press.

18 Marcus wants to interact with friends via social media and has developmental language disorder

Neuroscience facilitates our understanding of social media use

Caroline Larson

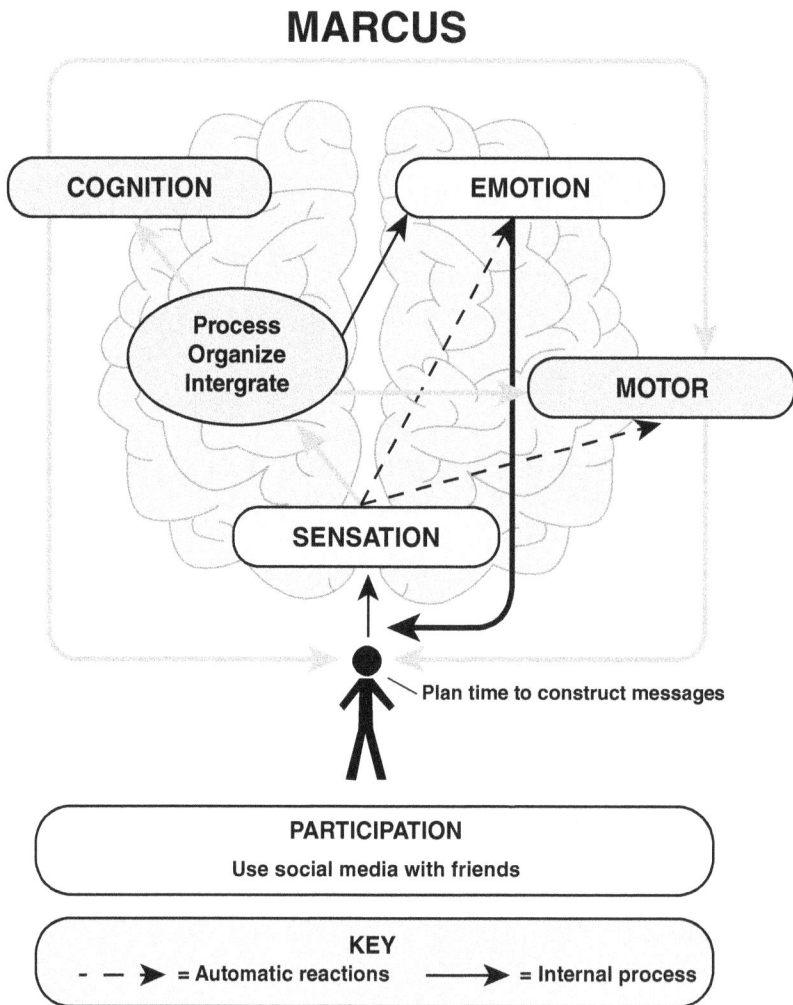

Figure 18.1 Marcus brain figure

DOI: 10.4324/9781003524380-22

Purpose of this chapter

This chapter will show how Marcus, a 19-year-old who wants to interact with friends through social media might be affected by having a developmental language disorder (DLD), a condition affecting his language skills. This will show how the neuroscience of language is relevant to our everyday lives and everyday interactions with others. We will learn about this relevancy through the eyes of someone who experiences difficulty with using and understanding language, a young adult with developmental language disorder (DLD). Individuals with DLD have trouble putting words together to make sentences, understanding what they read, and keeping up in conversations with friends, even though they have relative strengths with non-linguistic information, such as solving complex puzzles and perceiving others' emotions. We will explore how brain function underpins the strengths and challenges individuals with DLD experience and how these neural underpinnings manifest in daily life through the eyes of Marcus, a young man who wants to use social and visual media to make his transition to college more accessible.

The key neuroscience concepts we will explore in this chapter include neural specialization, functions of left hemisphere brain regions, neural networks, and the dual-stream model of spoken language processing.

Keywords for this chapter are listed in the box below. Be sure to learn what these key features are so you can get the most out of the chapter.

Keywords for this chapter

developmental language disorder	language-related brain activation	neural networks
		neural specialization

Marcus, a 19-year-old who wants to interact with friends using social media

Marcus has recently started his freshman year of college, studying graphic design at a state university about two hours from his hometown. He is excited to join a club related to his major, and maybe participate in a club sport, as long as they aren't too competitive and time consuming—he always enjoyed tennis but was never the star player. Marcus has always enjoyed problem solving. He plays Tetris (a puzzle solving game) whenever he has free time during car rides or between classes, and he and his friends are avid gamers, particularly enjoying Portal, but also well-designed, old-school games, like Super Mario. He also enjoys tennis for the spatial beauty of tennis strategy—the sharp angles, deep-in-the-court shots followed by droppers, and the changing spin of the ball. Marcus is really hoping that his difficulty with spoken language and reading don't affect his ability to pursue his visual design and problem solving interests in college. He is also hoping that he can use his skills in these areas to make new friends and participate in new social circles. Even though he isn't far from home, only a couple of his friends, and neither of his best friends, are attending the same college as him and he is worried that his language challenges will affect his ability to make new friends.

Marcus has DLD, a neurodevelopmental condition that presents in early childhood and that affects someone throughout their life (another lifelong neurodevelopmental condition is autism spectrum disorder, though autism has different diagnostic features than DLD, see Chapter 11). When he was a toddler, Marcus's mom noticed that he started saying words, like "milk" and "ball," and putting words together to make sentences, like "bye doggy," "me up," and "open book," at a later age than his cousins. She wasn't too concerned though because his pediatrician said his language skills would likely catch up over the next couple of years. When Marcus started kindergarten, however, his mom noticed that he was behind his peers in his spoken language and in his early literacy skills, such as pointing to named letters and rhyming simple words. His teacher also noticed that he was quieter than his peers, preferring to *point* and *show* his new friends how to play with a toy or go through the tunnel on the playground than to use *spoken words* to describe these activities.

Marcus was evaluated by a speech-language pathologist after a couple of months in kindergarten who determined that he needed specialized services addressing his spoken language skills, particularly his ability to produce (e.g., "I play ball" vs. "I played with the ball") and understand (e.g., "Do you like playing with the ball?" vs. "What game did you play with the ball today?") spoken sentences of increasing complexity. Marcus was seen by the speech-language pathologist consistently during his grade school years, but only for 30-minutes a week and sometimes in groups of 2–3 other children, and his specialized services were no longer available in middle and high school. Though he was able to get by in school, language-based education and reading were never a strength of his, and he always benefitted from accommodations, like extra time on tests, using graphics for classroom presentations, and teachers using visual cues during lectures. Relying in part on his strengths in non-linguistic areas and help from teachers, family, and friends with his application, he was able to get into college—a great achievement!

Now that Marcus is in college, the language demands of the classroom are much higher and he receives even fewer accommodations because his speech-language services were discontinued after elementary school. Marcus now wants to figure out how to use visual media to better access the college classroom in ways that work well for him and bypass some of his language difficulties. It is also effortful for Marcus to make new friends since he has essentially had the same friends since kindergarten until now. Social media plays a *huge* role in establishing and maintaining friendships for college-age young adults, and Marcus is hoping to capitalize on social media to make new friends. He might be in luck, other students who are majoring in graphic design may share his interest in using more visual, or *graphical*, means to communicate, like emojis and animations. But not all of Marcus's new friends are as *into* graphic design as he is, namely his dormmates and tennis friends.

Box 18.1   Learning activity

1. Having read the narrative, what are you curious about?
2. What do you need to know more about?

Now discuss the following questions with a small group and see what you know, as well as what you might learn more about from this chapter.

Box 18.2   Learning activity

1. How can the study of brain function, or neuroscience, shed more light on your thinking?
2. What brain regions might be responsible for language production and comprehension?
3. What do Marcus's accommodations in the classroom tell you about brain regions that might support language function beyond those that are typically or more narrowly responsible for language?
4. How might additional or different brain regions support language in the context of social media? Or in the context of graphics and social media?

Here are some resources for seeing these relationships:

Larson, C., Thomas, H. R., Crutcher, J., Stevens, M. C., & Eigsti, I. M. (2023). Language Networks in Autism Spectrum Disorder: A systematic review of connectivity-based fMRI studies. *Review Journal of Autism and Developmental Disorders*, 0123456789. https://doi.org/10.1007/s40489-023-00382-6

Friederici, A. D., & Gierhan, S. M. E. (2013). The language network. *Current Opinion in Neurobiology*, *23*(2), 250–254. https://doi.org/10.1016/j.conb.2012.10.002

We now turn to neuroscience to build on this thinking and to better understand what demands are placed on the brain when Marcus uses language versus visual and social media during his college experiences.

Neuroscience information to guide your thinking about Marcus

Clinical neuroscience, psychology, and the speech, language, and hearing sciences have led to a strong understanding of DLD, though much more research needs to be done. We will first focus on brain development as it relates to language, and then how this development may differ in individuals with DLD. Thereafter, we will ground this information will be in real-world situations that Marcus may experience.

Language and brain development. Early in infancy, many brain regions and both brain hemispheres are equally involved language function. Both hemispheres show substantial brain activity in response to hearing and using language, such as when parents are naming objects and talking about actions during play (e.g., *that's a horse*, *bounce the ball*). Across development, as children learn more words, sentences, and complex language, left hemisphere brain regions become increasingly responsible for language function due to neural specialization. Neural specialization is the process by which some neural pathways become strengthened and others become weakened, or pruned away. Neural pathways that are strengthened form structurally (e.g., brain volume, white matter connections) and functionally (e.g., brain activity, communication among brain regions) specified brain networks whereas neural pathways that are weakened become dormant.

This developmental process results in brain organization, or brain networks, that reflect the specialized, functional roles of brain regions and neural pathways that connect these brain regions, allowing them to communicate. In the case of language, left hemisphere brain regions become specialized for language function with nearly no involvement of right hemisphere brain regions by early adulthood. There is an image in Larson et al.

(2023) that illustrates these networks (see also Box 18.2 for resources). This highly special-ized brain network for language allows us to acquire highly complex language, progress-ing from speaking single words and short phrases as children to speaking and writing narratives with embedded clauses and intricately organized ideas as college students, for instance. One prominent model of spoken language processing, the dual-stream model (see Hicock & Poeppel, 2007), describes connections between language-related brain regions and the specific functions of these connections, referred to as *streams* (i.e., path-ways for information to flow).

This model proposes a ventral stream and a dorsal stream. The ventral stream is a more anterior, or frontal, set of connections and the dorsal stream is the more posterior set of connections. The ventral stream involves connections between the anterior and posterior portions of the middle temporal gyrus and inferior temporal sulcus. The ventral stream is re-sponsible for mapping sound to meaning, such as word recognition and spoken language comprehension. The dorsal stream involves connections of the Sylvian fissure at the meeting point of the parietal and temporal lobes (including the posterior superior temporal gyrus, also referred to as Wernicke's area) with the posterior inferior frontal gyrus (also referred to as Broca's area), premotor cortex, and anterior insula. The dorsal stream is responsible for mapping sound to action, such as linking speech perception and spoken language features with frontal lobe articulatory function. More recently, the dual-stream model has been expanded to include a hierarchical semantic-syntactic stream that involves connections of the posterior middle temporal gyrus and posterior inferior frontal gyrus (Broca's area) with both the dorsal and ventral streams. The semantic-syntactic stream is responsible for comprehension and production of semantic and syntactic meanings, such as understand-ing the meaning of complex sentences and producing verb tense morphology (e.g., past tense -*ed*). Whereas the dorsal and semantic-syntactic streams are predominantly evident in the left hemisphere, the ventral stream is evident in the left *and* right hemisphere. Thus, the ventral stream is associated with parallel processing functions, suggesting that speech is processed simultaneously in both hemispheres to some extent. This parallel processing might support spoken language recognition when the signal is degraded or when there are competing signals, such as when listening to speech in background noise.

For individuals with DLD, like Marcus, who struggle to learn and understand language, the neural specialization process might look quite different and result in a language network that *functions* quite differently from those who do not struggle to learn and un-derstand language.

Box 18.3   Learning activity

1. Find another picture of the brain. Match up regions depicted in Figure 18.1 with left hemisphere and right hemisphere homologue regions in the new brain picture.
2. Trace connections (e.g., with your finger) of the ventral, dorsal, and semantic-syntactic streams on Figure 1 and on the picture of the brain that you have found.
3. Do you notice any challenges or discrepancies between brain images? Why might that be? Discuss with your neighbor.

Keywords: brain, cortex, structure

Language-related brain function in individuals with language impairments

Though this area of research is relatively new and there are few research studies on which to draw upon, there is some evidence shedding light on the language-related brain function of individuals with language impairments. Individuals with DLD show less of the *expected* language-related brain activation in the left hemisphere, yet more *unexpected* language-related brain activation in the right hemisphere than same-age peers who do not have DLD. These patterns are particularly evident in regions of the brain most closely associated with language function, such as Broca's and Wernicke's areas, in the left hemisphere (Figure 18.1) and corresponding regions in the right hemisphere (known as right hemisphere homologue regions). Relative to neurotypical peers, individuals with DLD also show more language-related brain activation in regions that are not associated with language in typical development and that do not represent right hemisphere homologues, such as the caudate nucleus and the insula. Although research studies vary in their specific findings, the collective evidence suggests differences in brain organization in DLD, and, therefore, a different developmental trajectory of neural specialization for language. The neural specialization process in DLD may result in a language network involving more widespread regions (i.e., a less-specialized language network) and heightened, or stronger, activation in at least some brain regions than what is observed in neurotypical peers. The brain appears to be working harder to learn, understand, and produce language in DLD than in peers without language impairments.

For Marcus, this functional brain organization means that his ability to learn, understand, and produce language may be inefficient and may require supportive, or compensatory, processes, such as relying on attention and visual skills and corresponding brain regions. Because Marcus engages a more widespread brain network, it may take him longer to transition from understanding and producing single words to understanding and producing sentences. It may also take him longer to process and produce sentences or more complex written language than his peers. He cannot rely on quick, effective communication among highly specialized language-related brain regions. Instead, he must rely on brain regions that *he uses* during language function, but that are not necessarily *built for* language function.

Placing Marcus's brain function in the context of the dual-stream model, we might expect the semantic-syntactic stream to be most affected given that morphosyntax is an area of particular weakness in DLD. Specifically, the functions of the middle temporal gyrus and posterior inferior frontal gyrus may be distributed to other brain regions associated with language function uniquely in DLD, such as right hemisphere homologues, the caudate nucleus, and the insula. The connections of the posterior inferior temporal gyrus and middle temporal gyrus with the dorsal and ventral streams may, therefore, be weaker than in NT peers or also distributed to other brain regions; patterns which would reflect the global language challenges observed in DLD, as well as disproportionate challenges in morphosyntax. When Marcus hears or reads complex sentences (e.g., *the dog who wasn't on a leash chased three rabbits down the street*), the speech sounds are mapped to meaning through the parallel processing in the left and right hemisphere by the ventral stream. This mapping will interface with the semantic-syntactic stream, yet these connections and overall activation may be weaker and distributed to more widespread regions in DLD relative to NT peers, resulting in inefficiency. For instance, Marcus may be slower to understand the sentence or may miss key information, such as it was the dog who *wasn't on a leash* rather than *another dog present* that chased the rabbits, or the rabbits were chased *down the street* rather than *into the neighbor's yard*. The less efficient signal will also interface with the dorsal stream to map sound to action, resulting inefficient production in addition to inefficient comprehension. As a result, there may be parallel processing, analogous that associated with the ventral stream, associated with semantic-syntactic and dorsal stream function in DLD that is not evident in neurotypical peers. When Marcus hears a complex question to which he must respond, this inefficient neural function for comprehension and production may result in him missing key information in the question and producing a response that is both inaccurate *and* involving simplified sentence structure.

Daily life routine: Marcus and his college experiences

Clearly, this less specialized and less efficient language network has real-world consequences for Marcus. The language of college classrooms is highly complex and often presented with few non-linguistic visual supports (e.g., videos, figures) and few repetitions. Moreover, the college classroom requires complex language-based thinking and writing to learn and demonstrate learning. These contextual demands do not play into Marcus's strengths, like spatial problem solving and depicting information graphically, nor do they engage brain regions involved in these visual and spatial functions, such as right hemisphere parietal and bilateral occipital regions. There are barriers to making friends that Marcus faces as a result an inefficient language network as well. Given that Marcus made most of his friends starting on the playground in elementary school—a context that did not place significant demands on language—he has not experienced the high reliance on language-based communication that making friends as a young adult requires. In college, many friends are made through conversations over meals, on walks to class, during shared schoolwork, and through group exchanges via text or social media. Once again, many of these contexts do not play into Marcus's strengths because these potential friends are not familiar with his communication style and these interactions do not allow Marcus to offload communication to more visual-spatial processes and brain regions.

Back to Marcus's life: Neuroscience-informed supports for Marcus

Fortunately for Marcus, there are an increasing number of ways that digital platforms may engage a widespread brain network and reduce barriers that individuals with DLD face in effectively participating in the classroom and in social interactions. Most college courses involve a web-based platform and most courses are taught with the support of PowerPoints that are provided ahead of lectures. Marcus can use these tools to review what information may be discussed during class ahead of attending class, allowing him to process any language-based information at his own pace and providing multiple opportunities to process language-based content. These strategies accommodate his more widespread, somewhat inefficient language network and allow him to offload at least some linguistic information to other modalities and corresponding brain regions (e.g., visual processing in occipital regions). Particularly in the graphic design courses that Marcus will be taking, his instructor may *show* rather than primarily *tell* as a means of educating, and Marcus may be able to *show* instead of *tell* on his assignments. For instance, rather than verbally describing the steps involved in applying color-correcting filters to images, Marcus may be taught visually and walked through these steps using examples. He may also be tested by color-correcting images independently. These approaches to education and testing certainly allow Marcus to support his somewhat inefficient language processing and production with visual processing and production, drawing on brain regions involved in his broader language network and in networks of relative strength.

Social media offers similar advantages within the context of making friends. Social media use is primarily self-guided and often involves visual-spatial *and* language-based communication. Unlike spoken communication (e.g., conversation), which is rapid and fleeting, Marcus can process information at his own pace because he can re-read text or re-play videos, he can pause to Google information, or he can ask a clarifying question. He can also take breaks when the task drains his brain resources, a common experience for individuals with DLD, by simply closing an app or silencing his device. These strategies allow him to support his somewhat inefficient language network and engage brain regions associated with skills of relative strength, such as drawing on right *and* left hemisphere brain regions, all while participating in social interactions similarly to peers who do not have language impairments—an opportunity he does not necessarily have during spoken conversations on walks to class and over meals, for instance. Gestures represent the primary form of visual-spatial communication commonly used during conversation, yet images, emojis, gifs, and videos represent some of the vast visual-spatial communication commonly used during exchanges over social media. Thus, there are many more opportunities to use visual-spatial communication that taps into a more widespread brain network via social media than during conversation. Marcus can capitalize on these features to communicate in a manner that draws upon this broader brain network without compromising his participation to the extent that he experiences in typical conversation (e.g., not understanding part of the conversation, disengaging when he becomes fatigued). Especially when interacting with other graphic design majors and with other tennis enthusiasts, discovering more interesting and nuanced ways to communicate using graphics may be a highly valued (and *fun*) interaction style. For instance, graphic design majors may enjoy the challenge of creating complex algorithms to develop animated videos, and tennis enthusiasts may appreciate the advantage of seeing visuals that depict where an opponent's serve typically lands in the service box. Taken together, visual and social media may unlock access to brain regions and networks of relative strength for Marcus and others with DLD that are not otherwise possible when relying solely on his inefficient language-related brain network.

Box 18.4 Learning activity

List five ways you use visual, digital, and social media in the classroom and when interacting with your friends. How might the ways you are already using media in these contexts offload language function to other areas, like visual and spatial skills?

What do we know about ourselves and the population at large from this brain condition and from Marcus?

DLD is a lifelong condition that affects how individuals learn and use language. It leads to widespread challenges, such as in learning to read and communicating with friends, that can affect lifelong happiness and wellbeing. We have seen how some of these challenges manifest in everyday life through Marcus, though it is important to recognize that others with DLD may have quite different experiences and challenges. Moreover, everyone has unique profiles of strengths and challenges which may help us understand the experiences of individuals with neurodevelopmental conditions like DLD, as well as help us better understand ourselves.

Differences in brain function related to DLD manifest in everyday behavior and experiences. In Marcus's case, his brain is organized differently than individuals his age who have relatively strong language skills. This brain organization, likely reflecting less neural specialization for language across development, means that individuals with DLD may rely on other, non-linguistic skills and corresponding brain regions, like regions associated with visual and spatial processing, to use and understand language. It also means that individuals with DLD may take more time to use language effectively, such as during conversations with friends and to understand a classroom lecture. Social and visual media represent excellent supports individuals with DLD because they can engage relative strengths in visuospatial skills, and because they allow for more processing time and self-paced interactions. For instance, when Marcus is able to use written language and emojis to text with friends, he can *show* the message he is trying to convey in addition to *telling* the message using language. These supports allow engagement of brain regions and networks that support and, perhaps, bypass regions and networks that are less efficiently and effectively specialized for language function in DLD. It is beneficial to understand the unique experiences of neurodiverse individuals, like Marcus and others with DLD, because it broadens our perspective on, as well as our sensitivity to, how strengths and challenges manifest in everyday life.

Box 18.5 Learning activity

With your small group, complete the table in the Appendix about how Marcus can interact with friends through social media while managing his developmental language disorder.

Further reading

If interested in further reading about the lived experiences of individuals with DLD:

Ekström, A., Sahlén, B., & Samuelsson, C. (2023). "It depends on who I'm with": How young people with developmental language disorder describe their experiences of language and communication in school. *International Journal of Language and Communication Disorders, 58*(4), 1168–1181. https://doi.org/10.1111/1460-6984.12850

Hobson, H. M., & Lee, A. (2022). Camouflaging in developmental language disorder: The views of speech and language pathologists and parents. *Communication Disorders Quarterly, 44*(4). https://doi.org/10.1177/15257401221120937

Lieser, A. M., Van der Voort, D., & Spaulding, T. J. (2019). You have the right to remain silent: The ability of adolescents with developmental language disorder to understand their legal rights. *Journal of Communication Disorders, 82*(June), 105920. https://doi.org/10.1016/j.jcomdis.2019.105920

McGregor, K. K., Ohlmann, N., Eden, N., Arbisi-Kelm, T., & Young, A. (2023). Abilities and disabilities among children with developmental language disorder. *Language, Speech, and Hearing Services in Schools, 54*(July), 1–25. https://doi.org/10.1044/2023_lshss-22-00070

Orrego, P. M., McGregor, K. K., & Reyes, S. M. (2023). A First-Person Account of Developmental Language Disorder. *American Journal of Speech-Language Pathology, 32*(July), 1–14. https://doi.org/10.1044/2023_ajslp-22-00247

See also these references about the condition:

Abbott, N., & Love, T. (2023). Bridging the divide: Brain and behavior in developmental language disorder. *Brain Sciences*, *13*, 1–39.

Briggs, R. G., Conner, A. K., Baker, C. M., Burks, J. D., Glenn, C. A., Sali, G., Battiste, J. D., O'Donoghue, D. L., & Sughrue, M. E. (2018). A connectomic atlas of the human cerebrum-Chapter 18: The connectional anatomy of human brain networks. *Operative Neurosurgery* (Hagerstown, Md.), *15*(1), S470–S480. https://doi.org/10.1093/ons/opy272

Larson, C., Rivera-Figueroa, K., Thomas, H. R., Fein, D., Stevens, M. C., & Eigsti, I.-M. (2022). Structural language impairment in autism spectrum disorder versus loss of autism diagnosis: Behavioral and neural characteristics. *NeuroImage. Clinical*, *34*, 103043. https://doi.org/10.1016/j.nicl.2022.103043

Matchin, W., & Hickock, G. (2020). The cortical organization of syntax. *Cerebral Cortex*, *30*, 1481–1498. https://doi.org/10.1093/cercor/bhz180

Olulade, O. A., Seydell-Greenwald, A., Chambers, C. E., Turkeltaub, P. E., Dromerick, A. W., Berl, M. M., Gaillard, W. D., & Newport, E. L. (2020). The neural basis of language development: Changes in lateralization over age. *Proceedings of the National Academy of Sciences of the United States of America*, *117*(38), 23,477–23,483. https://doi.org/10.1073/pnas.1905590117

Or visit the following advocacy group websites:

- Raising Awareness of Developmental Language Disorder: https://radld.org/
- DLD and Me: Spreading the word about Developmental Language Disorder: https://dldandme.org/

References

Hicock, G., & Poeppel, D. (2007). The cortical organization of speech processing. *Nature reviews: Neuroscience*, *8*, 393–402. https://doi.org/10.1038/nrn2113

Larson, C., Mathée-Scott, J., Kaplan, D., & Ellis, S. (2023). Cognitive processes associated with working memory in children with developmental language disorder. *Journal of Experimental Child Psychology*, *234*, 105709. https://doi.org/10.1016/j.jecp.2023.105709

19 Paul wants to participate in his routine at home and has Alzheimer's disease

Neuroscience facilitates our understanding of place and routines

Melanie Morriss Tkach

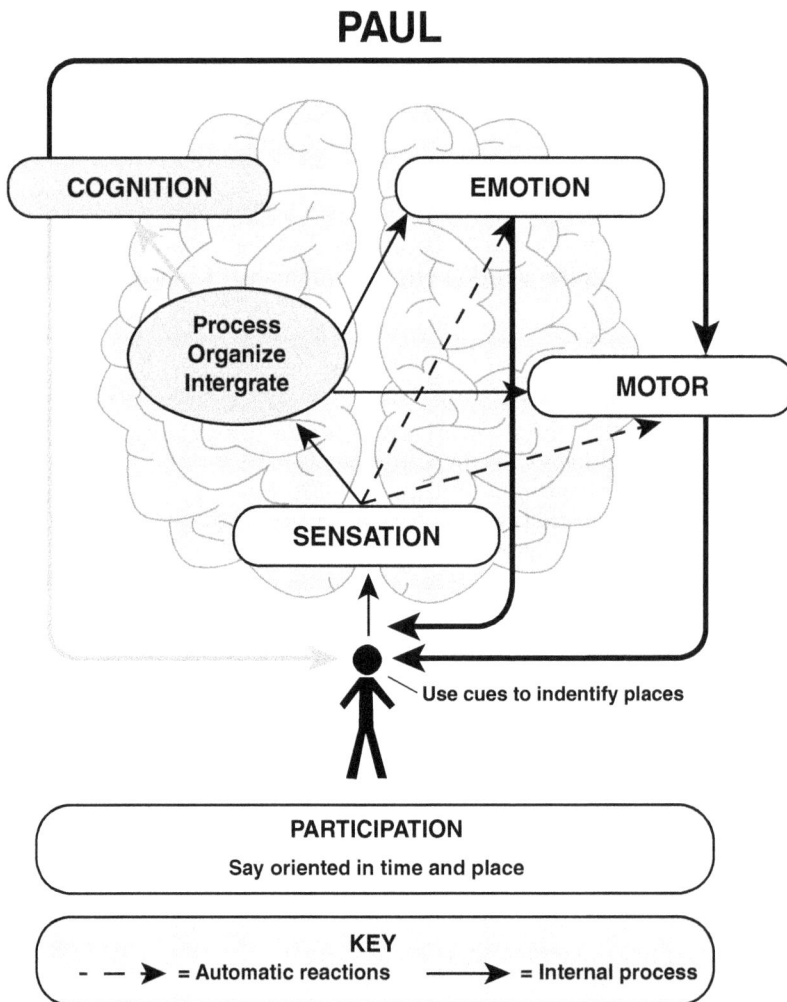

PAUL

COGNITION

EMOTION

Process
Organize
Intergrate

MOTOR

SENSATION

Use cues to indentify places

PARTICIPATION
Say oriented in time and place

KEY
- — ▶ = Automatic reactions   ⟶ = Internal process

Figure 19.1 Paul brain figure

DOI: 10.4324/9781003524380-23

Purpose of this chapter

The purpose of this chapter is to explore the neuroscience behind memory and participation in daily routines to inform our clinical reasoning. We will learn from people with Alzheimer's disease (AD) who benefit from routines to stay active and provide structure for meaningful engagement in everyday life. We will meet Paul and learn about his lived experience with AD so that we have a framework for thinking about how progressive nervous system damage impacts human performance and participation.

Keywords for this chapter are listed in the box below. Be sure to learn what these key features are so you can get the most out of the chapter.

Keywords for this chapter

Alzheimer's disease	hippocampus	posterior multimodal association area
amygdala	long-term memory	prefrontal cortex
amyloid plaques	long-term potentiation	short-term memory
	neurofibrillary tangles	working memory

Paul, a retiree who wants to participate in meaningful routines in his home environment

Paul is a 79-year-old retired radiologist who lives at home with his wife of 50 years. He and his wife have two adult children and four grandchildren who live nearby. Paul enjoys playing golf and participating in community service projects with a local men's organization. Paul is very proud of his family, and his pride shines through in the home videos he makes to document family events. While Paul and his wife like to travel, they have not been able to go on any trips this year because Paul has trouble navigating uneven surfaces and becomes forgetful in unfamiliar environments. Paul and his family found out that he has AD three years ago. He has been under the direct supervision of his primary care doctor and a neurologist since that time.

On a typical day, Paul wakes up and gets himself dressed. Then, he eats breakfast and runs small errands to the grocery store or bank. In the afternoon, Paul likes to drink an ice-cold soda on the porch while supervising yardwork or other neighborhood activities. Paul and his wife primarily spend their evenings at home unless attending grandkids' ballgames or concerts. Paul gets himself ready for bed and usually falls asleep quickly. However, he has recently experienced more frequent night wakings requiring assistance from his wife to reorient to person and place.

Paul reports that errands are the most important activity in his day because they give him a chance to help his wife take care of their home and finances. However, Paul has recently taken a break from community outings at the request of his family. Paul's wife and children are concerned that Paul frequently misplaces his keys and cannot retrace his steps to find them; he was also at fault for a small fender bender in the grocery store parking lot last month. Paul has become withdrawn and spends more time watching television in his recliner now that he cannot run errands.

Paul and his wife live in a two-story home. Paul is familiar with his surroundings and comfortable in his home after residing there for the past 40 years. However, Paul fell twice last year while climbing stairs to his second story bedroom. On one occasion, Paul bumped his head on tile flooring and was taken to the emergency room for stitches. Paul's family moved his bed downstairs into one of the main living spaces, and they added a walk-in shower to the downstairs bathroom to reduce the likelihood of falls. While these home modifications improve home safety, Paul's wife has noticed that he is more confused, struggles to find items needed for self-care tasks, and requires more assistance to complete daily routines.

Because of AD progression and changes in functional status, Paul's medical team consulted home occupational and physical therapy. Paul's family and care team want to find ways to structure daily routines and the home environment so that Paul can continue to live at home and contribute to the household in meaningful, life-giving ways.

Box 19.1   Learning activity

Discuss the following questions with your peers:

1. What piques your interest about Paul and his family?
2. What do you need to know more about to support Paul in his daily life?

Box 19.2   Learning activity

Before you continue to read this chapter, discuss what you may already know.

1. How can neuroscience concepts inform your thinking?
2. What parts of the brain are involved in memory?
3. How does a person make and use memories during daily routines?
4. How can the home context impact memory during daily routines?

Great thinking! Now, let's consider the neuroscience behind memory to better understand how we participate in daily routines.

Neuroscience information to guide your thinking about Paul.

Basic research on neural activity, biomarkers, and brain lesions helps us understand AD better. We will focus on the neuroscience of memory and AD and then weave that information together with what we know about natural contexts and participation in daily routines.

Alzheimer's disease

Alzheimer's disease (AD) is a progressive brain condition that impairs memory, thinking, and the ability to perform daily activities. People with AD often struggle to create new memories, retrieve existing memories, and use information to make decisions (Centers for Disease Control and Prevention, 2020; National Institute on Aging, 2017). As a result, people with AD may forget appointments, mishandle money, or get lost and wander away from home. People with AD may also experience changes in balance and functional mobility that begin early in the disease process and deteriorate more rapidly over time than healthy older adults (Fujisawa et al., 2017; Suttanon et al., 2013). Physical differences, combined with cognitive impairment, increase the risk and occurrence of falls in people with AD compared to healthy older adults and can result in less physical activity over time (Cedervall et al., 2015; Suttanon et al., 2013).

Box 19.3   Learning activity

Find a list of the seven clinical stages of AD so that you can understand how symptoms progress over time as you read.

Keywords: Alzheimer's stages, Alzheimer's progression

Early in the disease process, people with AD may not show overt symptoms, or they may present with mild memory loss that passes as acceptable forgetfulness. As the disease progresses, people with AD develop mild cognitive impairment, which may be characterized by problems finding the right word in conversation, and advance to more significant short-term memory impairments such as forgetting important more recent experiences. In later stages of the disease, people with AD may need constant supervision for safety and help to complete daily activities. Additionally, they may forget family members and friends. The final stage of AD is marked by significant communication, self-feeding, and continence challenges.

AD symptoms are the direct result of several important brain changes that begin long before symptoms appear. Specifically, people with AD develop amyloid plaques and neurofibrillary tangles throughout the brain, and the brain shrinks in size. We will discuss these brain changes more in the next section.

Box 19.4   Learning activity

Find pictures of amyloid plaques and neurofibrillary tangles so that you can visualize key brain changes in AD as you read. Find a picture that compares healthy brains to brains with AD.

Keywords: Alzheimer's plaques and tangles, amyloid plaques, neurofibrillary tangles, Alzheimer's vs. typical brain, normal brain vs. Alzheimer's

---

Amyloid plaques and neurofibrillary tangles

In AD, two naturally occurring proteins disrupt brain function. Beta-amyloid proteins and other molecules stick together forming plaques in the space between neurons. These amyloid plaques disrupt communication between the neurons and trigger an immune response that destroys neurons (Alzheimer's Association, 2023; National Institute on Aging, 2017). Additionally, tau protein collects inside neurons creating neurofibrillary tangles. Neurofibrillary tangles disrupt processes inside the neuron and, as a result, interfere with communication between neurons (Alzheimer's Association, 2023; National Institute on Aging, 2017).

Amyloid plaques and neurofibrillary tangles spread throughout the brain as AD progresses. In the early and middle stages of AD, plaques and tangles form in the hippocampus, an area important for learning and memory (Alzheimer's Association, 2023). Then, the plaques and tangles spread to the frontal lobe, language centers of the temporal lobe, and parietal lobe affecting thinking and planning, communication, and sensory and spatial relationships respectively. In the late stages of AD, amyloid plaques and neurofibrillary tangles cause widespread cell death in the cortex, and the brain shrinks in size (Alzheimer's Association, 2023). Refer to the Introductory chapter for more detailed information on the lobes of the brain and their functions.

Progressive memory loss and functional decline

Initially, the brain changes associated with AD affect short-term memory (STM), or the ability to remember people we meet and experiences that happen as recently as one hour ago or less. The effects of AD extend to working-memory, an element of STM that gives us the ability to temporarily store, retrieve, and use information during daily activities. As a result, a person with AD may forget the date and time of a doctor's appointment that they recently scheduled or the steps to make cookies when they are no longer looking at a recipe. In contrast, people with AD typically retain long-term memory (LTM), or more permanent information about facts, experiences, and automatic processes during the early and middle stages of the disease process. Thus, people with AD may continue to recall past events like pranks they pulled at summer camp with conscious thought as well as the sequence of steps for activities like tying shoes that happen without conscious thought.

Box 19.5   Learning activity

Discuss the following questions in small groups:

1. What activities require the following types of memory?

   a. Working memory
   b. Short term
   c. Long term
   d. Procedural memory

2. How would your behavior change if you could not create or store new memories?
3. How would your changed behavior affect others?
4. How would you complete daily routines if you could only rely on LTM?

From a neuroscience perspective, we know that memory depends on integrated neural networks that involve the hippocampus, cortex, and select subcortical structures (Brodal, 2004; Gutman, 2016; Kitamura et al., 2017; McBean & Van Wijck, 2012). These neural networks help us create, store, and retrieve memories during daily routines. However, amyloid plaques and neurofibrillary tangles disrupt neural networks and memory processes in AD.

For Paul, we are most interested in the following parts of the neural network for memories (Brodal, 2004; Gutman, 2016; McBean & Van Wijck, 2012):

- The **hippocampus** makes connections between new and existing knowledge. It helps transition memories to long-term storage.
- The **prefrontal cortex** temporarily stores new information, converts new information to long-term storage, and helps with memory retrieval.
- The **cerebral cortex** permanently stores long-term memories.
- The **amygdala** attaches emotional significance to memories.
- The **basal ganglia** processes automatic learning and memory.
- The **cerebellum** processes automatic learning, motor learning, and memory.

Box 19.6   Learning activity

Find pictures of the hippocampus, cerebral cortex, amygdala, basal ganglia, and cerebellum as well as the neural pathways that connect these brain structures. The images you find will help you visualize the complex connections that support our memory processes as you continue to read.

Keywords: hippocampus, cerebral cortex, amygdala, basal ganglia, cerebellum, hippocampal network, hippocampal-prefrontal interactions

---

Hippocampal function

The hippocampus, located deep in the medial temporal lobe, is one of the first brain areas impacted by AD. It plays a crucial role in the memory of everyday experiences (i.e., episodic memory) and our ability to remember and navigate everyday environments (i.e., spatial memory). The hippocampus supports the creation, storage, and retrieval of memories through reciprocal connections with the cerebral cortex and subcortical structures like the amygdala (Brodal, 2004; Carlson & Birkett, 2021; Kitamura et al., 2017).

When we participate in an activity, the hippocampus receives complex sensory, motor, and spatial information related to our experiences from the entorhinal cortex as well as subcortical structures like the amygdala and basal ganglia (Brodal, 2004; Carlson & Birkett, 2021). Additionally, special hippocampal place cells respond to information about our location in space during everyday experiences and create a map within the hippocampus that helps us navigate our environments successfully as we perform everyday routines (Brodal, 2004; Moser et al., 2015). The hippocampus compares incoming information to what we already know or have already experienced and then works with the amygdala and prefrontal cortex to make meaningful connections between new input and existing knowledge. The hippocampus and amygdala work together to create memories associated with strong emotions, whereas the hippocampus and prefrontal cortex work together to convert memories from short- to long-term store and retrieve memories later (Carlson & Birkett, 2021; Gutman, 2016; Kitamura et al., 2017).

How does the hippocampus support successful learning and memory processes in the brain? On a macro level, the hippocampus stores traces of a memory and its details rather than the memory itself, and its connections with other brain regions help convert the memories to long-term storage (Carlson & Birkett, 2021; Kitamura et al., 2017). On a micro level, neurons in the hippocampus and related brain regions respond together creating a neural network that processes specific experiences or locations in everyday life. The more we use that neural network to think or talk about our everyday experiences and locations, the stronger the neural network and our memory becomes (Carlson & Birkett, 2021; Gutman, 2016). This process, called long-term potentiation (LTP), results in lasting changes to brain connections that improve the efficiency of memory processes over time.

Knowledge of hippocampal function helps us understand progressive memory loss in AD. Amyloid plaques and neurofibrillary tangles damage the hippocampus and disrupt communication within neural networks that involve the hippocampus. As a result, people with AD cannot create new short-term memories or move them to long-term storage. Let's take a closer look at some of the neural networks impacted by AD.

Neural networks for storing memories

Memory storage depends on an intricate neural network that supports communication between the hippocampus and cortex. Initially, memory cells in the hippocampus actively respond to new information, connect new and old knowledge, and support memory retrieval, whereas memory cells in the prefrontal cortex are present but inactive (Gutman, 2016; Kitamura et al., 2016). As we think and talk about our experiences, connections between the hippocampus, prefrontal cortex, and other cortical storage areas are strengthened. As a result, memory cells in the cortex become more active, and the cortex takes over responsibility for our memories with support from the hippocampus (Kitamura et al., 2017). Therefore, LTP creates lasting changes in the connections between the hippocampus and the cerebral cortex, and those changes represent the conversion of memories to long-term storage.

Neural networks for retrieving memories

Cues from our external and internal environments trigger memory retrieval processes in the brain. Retrieval cues help us draw on the associations that we made between certain features of the environment or our internal emotions and sensations when we formed the memory (Gutman, 2016; Frankland et al., 2019). So, you are more likely to perform better on a neuroscience exam when tested in the room where you learned the material, and people with AD are more likely to perform daily routines better in familiar, home environments that makes them feel safe compared to a hospital room or rehabilitation facility. You are also more likely to remember information or experiences that are emotionally meaningful to you, which means that memories associated with strong emotions like excitement, joy, fear, or sadness come to mind more readily than others.

Memory retrieval occurs through a variety of neural structures and networks. Neurons in the prefrontal cortex retrieve and send sensory information related to our memories from long-term storage across the cerebral cortex to the posterior multimodal association area in the parietal cortex (Gutman, 2016; Frankland et al., 2019). The posterior multimodal association area combines a variety of sensory information to reconstruct memories of our everyday experiences and environments. The retrieval process is dependent on LTP, so the more we retrieve a memory the more likely we are to recall that memory in the future (Carlson & Birkett, 2021; Gutman, 2016). As memories grow stronger, we rely less on the posterior multimodal association area and more on the direct connections between cerebral cortices for memory retrieval.

Procedural memory for activities with a specific sequence of steps like riding a bike or tying shoes, relies on the basal ganglia and cerebellum (Carlson & Birkett, 2021;

McBean & Van Wijck, 2012; Saywell & Taylor, 2008). When activity sequences are repeated over and over again, the basal ganglia takes on responsibility for the activity so that the cortex is free to participate in more complicated cognitive processes. The basal ganglia monitors sensory and motor activity and then sends that information to the frontal lobe where movements are planned (e.g., premotor and supplementary motor cortex) and executed (e.g., primary motor cortex; Carlson & Birkett, 2021; McBean & Van Wijck, 2012). The cerebellum coordinates movements and may play a role in the automation of movement patterns. You can read more about motor learning and the automaticity of movement in the first section of the book.

The neuroscience of memory retrieval helps us understand why LTMs including procedural memory are preserved in the early stages of AD. Memory retrieval bypasses the damaged hippocampus and draws on intact cortical and subcortical structures, so people with AD can remember facts and experiences they learned long ago or brush their teeth without conscious thought. The key to memory retrieval is finding the right cue in the external or internal environment to trigger the memory. In the late stages of AD, plaques and tangles will damage the cerebral cortex and disrupt LTM as well.

Daily life routine: keeping track of where one is and who is there to help

Late adulthood is characterized by retirement, aging, and changes in a person's social context. Many adults transition from work responsibilities and schedules to unstructured personal time. Some adults participate in part-time or volunteer work, whereas others prioritize leisure pursuits and family time. Regardless of the activity, adults rely on existing habits, routines, and their social support system to create a new schedule that gives life meaning and purpose.

The aging process can impact how adults choose to spend their time. Some adults experience good physical and mental health that supports participation in everyday life, whereas others experience physical or cognitive decline that limits participation. When facing physical or cognitive decline, adults must identify activities that match their abilities and values to live a meaningful, satisfying life. Adults navigate and interact with complex home or community environments to complete those activities. Some adults rely on familiarity with an environment, whereas others use maps, navigational systems, or cues and strategies to participate.

The people adults spend time with during daily routines changes over time. When close loved ones pass away, adults grieve, grapple with their own mortality, and restructure their daily routines. Some adults become socially isolated, whereas others intentionally seek out new friendships and companionship.

In sum, people in late adulthood create daily life routines that allow them to live out their values with the people who mean the most to them. Adults modify their daily routines as their physical and cognitive abilities change and update their social support network as loved ones pass away or they establish new friendships.

Box 19.7   Learning activity

With your small group, complete the table in the Appendix about Paul's daily life routines and the neuroscience that affects his participation.

Back to the person's life: Paul wants to feel comfortable in his home with his wife.

When we met Paul earlier in the chapter, he was three years into his AD diagnosis. Paul's most significant symptoms at that time were intermittent episodes of forgetfulness in familiar and unfamiliar environments as well as challenges with problem solving, judgment, and safety during everyday activities like driving. He had fallen twice indicating changes in his ability to balance and mobilize during daily activities. As the disease progressed, Paul began to forget important information about his loved ones like where they lived, the jobs they worked, and, eventually, that people who made up his social context, like his parents, had passed away. He also struggled to follow and participate in conversations at family gatherings. Paul became restless during downtime, and he often appeared disinterested in activities that normally brought him joy. Paul's physical condition continued to decline as well. He transitioned from a cane to a walker and then a manual wheelchair for functional mobility and required increasing levels of assistance from his wife to eat, bathe, and get dressed. Approximately eight years after diagnosis, Paul passed away from complications related to recurrent pneumonia. At the time of his death, Paul only recognized his wife, and he required total assistance for all of his daily activities.

You have learned a lot about brain function in people with AD and how the disease progresses over time. How can we use this scientific understanding to support Paul and other people with AD in their daily routines as the disease progresses? While future courses will explore more details about rehabilitation for people with AD and their families, a strong foundation in the neuroscience of memory and AD will enhance your ability to select interventions that meet client needs and help them reach their goals for participation in daily routines.

Box 19.8   Learning activity

In class or small groups, discuss what activity or home modifications Paul's family and/or therapy team can make to support his success in daily routines at home. Use your neuroscience knowledge and what you know about Paul and his memory to guide your thinking. Consider how your answer may change at different stages of AD.

What do we know about ourselves and the population at large from this brain condition and this family story?

While we primarily learned about memory loss in people with AD, it's important to remember that their brains created, stored, and retrieved memories well for many years. Furthermore, all people in the general population occasionally forget important information that impacts their daily lives. We may misplace our wallet, struggle to recall the name of a new coworker, or forget to pick up milk on the way home from work. Moments of forgetfulness are a common experience that we share with people who have AD albeit for different reasons. The way we feel and how we want to be treated when we experience a memory lapse should inform how we interact with people who have AD whether they are conscious of their memory lapses or not.

Additionally, people in the general population experience decreases in memory over time, especially as we age. Our memories become fuzzy and the number of cues that help us retrieve a memory dwindles. So, we adopt strategies that help us remember important information. For example, we might use checklists to remember everything we need from the grocery store or phone reminders to remember important meetings or appointments. The same types of strategies that we use to help us remember everyday facts, experiences, and procedural memories can trigger participation in people with AD as well. Since people with AD experience more extreme and progressive memory loss, they have helped us identify various types of retrieval cues that can trigger memory and use that information to develop strategies that help people participate successfully in everyday life.

Further reading

If interested in further reading about the lived experience of AD or caring for someone with AD:

Beebe, J. (2022, May 24). What dementia feels like. AARP. www.aarp.org/health/dementia/info-2022/living-with-dementia.html

Doucette, C. (Host). (2018–2019). Caregiver storyteller: About Alzheimer's and dementia caregiving [Audio podcast]. CaringKind. www.caringkindnyc.org/podcast/

Górska, S., Forsyth, K., & Maciver, D. (2018). Living with dementia: A meta-synthesis of qualitative research on the lived experience. *The Gerontologist*, 58(3), e180–e196. https://doi.org/10.1093/geront/gnw195

Peacock, S., Duggleby, W., & Koop, P. (2014). The lived experience of family caregivers who provided end-of-life care to persons with advanced dementia. *Palliative & supportive care*, 12(2), 117–126. https://doi.org/ 10.1017/S1478951512001034

VPM News. (2016, November 11). Alzheimer's: The caregiver's perspective [Video]. YouTube. www.youtube.com/watch?v=CcBH077AEm8

Wolverson, E. L., Clarke, C., & Moniz-Cook, E. D. (2016). Living positively with dementia: A systematic review and synthesis of the qualitative literature. *Aging & Mental Health*, 20(7), 676–699.

References

Alzheimer's Association. (2023). Inside the brain—A tour of how the mind works: Part 2—Alzheimer's effect. www.alz.org/alzheimers-dementia/what-is-alzheimers/brain_tour_part_2

Brodal, P. (2004). *The central nervous system: Structure and function*. Oxford University Press.

Carlson, N. R., & Birkett, M. A. (2021). *Physiology of behavior*. Pearson Higher Ed.

Cedervall, Y., Torres, S., & Åberg, A. C. (2015). Maintaining well-being and selfhood through physical activity: experiences of people with mild Alzheimer's disease. *Aging & Mental Health*, 19(8), 679–688. https://doi.org/10.1080/13607863.2014.962004

Centers for Disease Control and Prevention. (2020). Alzheimer's disease and related dementias. www.cdc.gov/aging/aginginfo/alzheimers.htm

Frankland, P. W., Josselyn, S. A., & Köhler, S. (2019). The neurobiological foundation of memory retrieval. *Nature Neuroscience*, 22(10), 1576–1585. https://doi.org/10.1038/s41593-019-0493-1

Fujisawa, C., Umegaki, H., Okamoto, K., Nakashima, H., Kuzuya, M., Toba, K., & Sakurai, T. (2017). Physical function differences between the stages from normal cognition to moderate Alzheimer disease. *Journal of the American Medical Directors Association*, 18(4), 368-e9. https://doi.org/10.1016/j.jamda.2016.12.079

Gutman, S. A. (2016). *Quick reference neuroscience for rehabilitation professionals: The essential neurologic principles underlying rehabilitation practice*. (3rd ed.). Routledge.

Kitamura, T., Ogawa, S. K., Roy, D. S., Okuyama, T., Morrissey, M. D., Smith, L. M.,... & Tonegawa, S. (2017). Engrams and circuits crucial for systems consolidation of a memory. *Science*, 356(6333), 73–78. https://doi.org/10.1126/science.aam6808

McBean, D., & Van Wijck, F. (Eds.). (2012). *Applied neurosciences for the allied health professions*. Elsevier Health Sciences.

Moser, M.-B., Rowland, D. C., & Moser, E. I. (2015). Place cells, grid cells, and memory. *Cold Spring Harbor Perspectives in Biology*, 7(2), a021808. https://doi.org/10.1101/cshperspect.a021808

National Institute on Aging. (2017). What happens to the brain in Alzheimer's disease? www.nia. nih.gov/health/what-happens-brain-alzheimers-disease

Saywell, N., & Taylor, D. (2008). The role of the cerebellum in procedural learning—Are there implications for physiotherapists' clinical practice? *Physiotherapy Theory and Practice*, 24(5), 321–328. https://doi.org/10.1080/09593980701884832

Suttanon, P., Hill, K. D., Said, C. M., & Dodd, K. J. (2013). A longitudinal study of change in falls risk and balance and mobility in healthy older people and people with Alzheimer disease. *American Journal of Physical Medicine & Rehabilitation*, 92(8), 676–685. https://doi.org/10.1097/PHM.0b013e318278dcb3

20 Louise wants to organize her schedule and routines and has breast cancer

Neuroscience facilitates our understanding of life organization

Bridget Kraus and Timothy J. Wolf

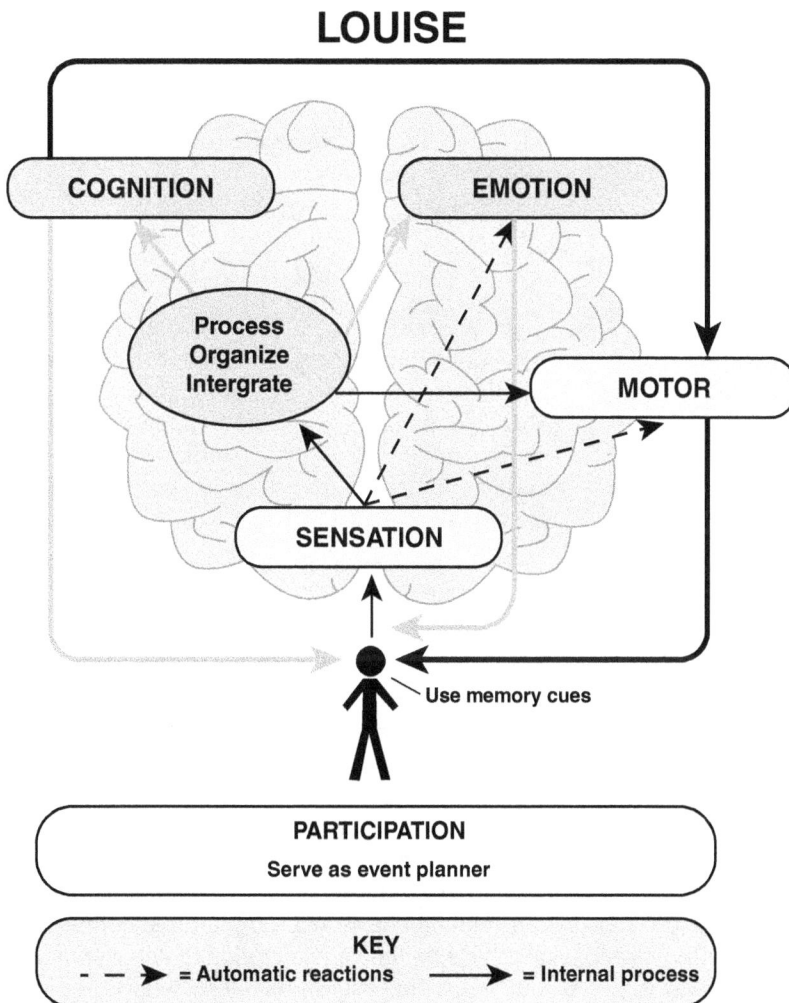

Figure 20.1 Louise brain figure

DOI: 10.4324/9781003524380-24

Purpose of this chapter

The purpose of this chapter is to understand how the ability of a working middle-aged mother, Louise, to engage in and organize robust schedules and routines is impacted by the neurological changes of breast cancer. For many, our weekly schedules can become habitual, and navigating what we need and want can feel like minimal effort. For people who have breast cancer, managing the complexities of daily schedules and responsibilities can dramatically shift because of the impact of diagnosis and treatment on the brain. Let's meet Louise and her family to gain more understanding of how our neurological systems impact our ability to successfully establish and carry out organized weekly routines.

The key neuroscience concepts we will explore in this chapter include a phenomenon referred to as cancer related cognitive impairment and other brain changes, like neurotoxicity, due to breast cancer and treatment. We will also learn about the neural networks required to access established routines, mechanisms related to fatigue, frontal and parietal lobe support for organization, and self-monitoring pathways. As with all the chapters, these components of the nervous system work with other systems to support overall human function.

Keywords for this chapter are listed in the box below. Be sure to learn what these key features are so you can get the most out of the chapter.

Keywords for this chapter

adenocarcinoma	dopamine system	metastasis
benign	functional connectivity	neuroinflammation
cancer related cognitive	functional MRI	nulliparity
impairment	hormone therapy	radiation therapy
chemotherapy	malignant	serotonin
acute/ chronic fatigue	mastectomy	task switching
cognitive flexibility	menarche	TNM system

Louise is a 42-year-old mom who runs an event planning business

Louise is a busy mom of two children and runs a small event planning business for which she organizes weddings, graduations, and other special occasions for people in her community. Her partner, Sam, is a nurse and works the evening shift in the emergency department. Her two children are in middle and high school and are both involved in activities like sports and theater club. Louise spends a lot of her evenings driving her children to and from practices while conducting phone calls and emails with vendors and clients. Due to the nature of her event planning business her working hours vary a lot, and no day or week often looks the same. While it can be hectic, she loves connecting with her customers and finds pride in taking the extra time and attention to detail to make an event.

Louise often jokes that she could "put out fires" in her sleep. Louise is direct but personable and well-liked by her peers and clients. She has quick decision-making skills and is great at problem-solving and executing a plan, which is critical to throwing a large event. She often acts as a liaison between vendors and clients juggling flower deliveries, payment schedules, decorations, event timelines, menus, and more. Change agility and organization are her strong suits, it is why she is one of the top event planners in the town- and why her event calendar is always booked.

Several months ago, Louise dropped off her children at basketball and drama club before getting ready for a client's wedding. While she was changing, she felt a lump on her right breast and some swelling of her underarm. She had never noticed it before and decided to make an appointment with her doctor the next morning. After meeting with her doctor and having a biopsy performed, Louise was diagnosed with Stage 2 breast cancer that had spread to her lymph nodes. Her tumor was also triple-negative, meaning it has low levels of the HER2 protein and no estrogen or progesterone receptors. Triple-negative breast cancer cells typically grow and spread faster than most other types of breast cancer and are not treatable with hormone therapy. For Louise, this meant that a mastectomy, radiation, and chemotherapy were her best options for treatment for remission and to reduce the risk of recurrent cancer.

Box 20.1   Learning activity

1. Now that you've met Louise, what roles and routines are important to her?
2. Is there anything you need or want to know more about?

Present day

Since her mastectomy surgery, Louise has been having a lot of pain and fatigue. She notices she doesn't have the energy to do it all like she did before. She doesn't even know *how* she did it all before. When she has been mustering up the energy to try and handle her home responsibilities, she finds that she doesn't know where to start. The house is in disarray, dishes and laundry are piling up. She will often go to start a load of laundry and finds a stale and musty load in the washing machine that she forgot to put in the dryer. She can't remember what nights her children have events. Her children have been trying to be patient, but they keep running late and don't have clean jerseys or costumes to wear. Louise's forgetfulness is causing a lot of tension in her household. She finds herself getting irritable and losing her temper more easily. Her partner wants to help, but they are unavailable in the evenings because of their work schedule. It doesn't help that Louise hasn't been sleeping well due to persistent nausea and headaches.

At work, Louise is also having difficulties. Her clients and vendors are getting frustrated, and she keeps getting voicemails from clients about things that she forgot to do. Her events were scheduled months ago. Therefore, she can't back out now because venues have been booked and she and vendors have already accepted payment. However, her clients are noticing, and just this week she had two clients pull out from future events and one vendor terminate a contract. Even when she tries to explain or talk with her clients about what is going on, she finds her thinking is slow, like walking through mud. She has a hard time concentrating and finding words. Overall, Louise is struggling to prioritize and organize her schedule and her energy to do what she needs to do to run her business.

What is breast cancer?

Genes provide the instructions for how the cells in our body work. Cancer is a disease that affects the genes which then give faulty information to the cells. When these genes malfunction it can cause the cells to grow, divide, and sustain themselves in ways that they shouldn't. These abnormal cells then can become cancer which grows uncontrollably and spreads to other parts of the body.

Box 20.2 Learning activity

1. What is a tumor?
2. If a person has a tumor, does that mean the person has cancer? How do they find out?

Tumors are classified as either benign or malignant. Benign tumors are non-cancerous cells which do not spread into nearby tissues and when removed often do not grow back. A cancerous tumor, however, can spread and invade other tissues all over the body through a process called metastasis. When cancer metastasizes to another part of the body, it is still considered cancer of the primary site. For example, if breast cancer metastasizes to the lungs, it is called "metastatic breast cancer" and not "lung cancer." Cancer is also categorized by the type of cell from which the cancer originates. Most breast cancers originate from epithelial cells which produce fluids or mucus and are called adenocarcinomas. In the breast, cancerous tissue is most commonly found in the lobules, ducts, or connective tissue.

Worldwide, Breast Cancer is the most common cancer occurring in women and accounts for approximately 25% of all cancers (Ghoncheh et al., 2016; Tao et al., 2015).

Box 20.3 Learning activity

1. How common is breast cancer? What is the current incidence and prevalence? *Hint: if you can't find any statistics for the current year, look at the most recent year for which you can find statistics.*
2. Do ethnic/racial/cultural factors influence the breast cancer, incidence, prevalence, and death rate
3. How likely are women to die of breast cancer in the U.S.?
4. Can men get breast cancer?
5. What do you think may be risk factors for breast cancer?

Keywords: incidence, mortality, risk factors

Risk factors

There are many risk factors for cancer. It is important to know that not all risk factors for cancer are controllable. For example, as we age our body's ability to sense and eliminate faulty cells diminishes, which is why the increased risk of developing cancer is associated with increased age. Other examples of non-controllable risk factors are gender, personal and familial history of breast cancer, and breast density. For women, the risk of breast cancer is much higher than men, and gender-specific non-controllable risk factors such as: early menarche, nulliparity, late age of first pregnancy, and late menopause also increase the risk of developing breast cancer. Controllable factors which increase breast cancer risk include smoking, alcohol consumption, obesity, and low physical activity.

Staging

Breast cancer severity is measured using a process called staging. The stage of cancer describes how much cancer is in the body and, helps determine best treatment, and prognosis. The lower the stage, the less cancer has spread and vice versa. The American Joint Committee on Cancer (AJCC) created the TNM System for staging breast cancer. Breast cancer is unique because it includes four additional factors which make staging more complex than other cancers.

Box 20.4   Learning activity

1. What is meant by "staging" for cancer?
2. What are the seven factors by which breast cancer is staged?

Keywords: staging, diagnostic process

Treatment

Treatment of breast cancer is usually dependent upon its stage. Also, an individual's overall health, menopause status, and personal preferences are important factors to consider. Women with breast cancer may get various types of treatments or a combination of treatments. Treatments are often considered either local or systemic. Local treatments include surgery, such as a lumpectomy or mastectomy, and external or internal radiation therapy. One type of systemic treatment is chemotherapy which uses anti-cancer drugs that are administered intravenously or by mouth. Chemotherapy drugs travel through the bloodstream to reach cancer cells throughout the body. Other systemic treatments include hormone therapy, targeted drug therapy, and immunotherapy. Not every one of these treatments will be appropriate for every person with breast cancer, which is why treatment may vary for each individual.

Common treatment approaches by stage

- **Stage 0:** Breast conservation surgery, followed by radiation therapy, and potentially hormone therapy if applicable.
- **Stages I–IV**: Surgery (lumpectomy or mastectomy), radiation, and systemic therapy/ies.

Triple-negative breast cancer: TNBC is not a good candidate for hormone therapy, so chemotherapy is the primary systemic treatment option. However, despite good initial response to treatment, TNBC is more likely to reoccur.

Box 20.5   Learning activity

1. Find an illustration of breast anatomy and locate the lobules, ducts, and connective tissues.
2. How are cancer cells different from normal cells? Find photos of cancer cells and compare it with healthy cells.
3. Look up internal and external radiation therapy techniques, hormone therapy, and targeted drug therapy for breast cancer treatment.

Keywords: breast anatomy, cells, radiation therapy, hormone therapy, targeted drug therapy

Now that you have had some time to think and discuss, let's consider some of the common effects of cancer treatment on the nervous system and how they may impact organization and execution of our weekly routines.

Neuroscience information to guide your thinking about Louise

Cognitive dysfunction is pervasive following treatment in breast cancer survivors (Collins et al., 2012; Falleti et al., 2005; van Dam et al., 1998). Up to 75% of patients with cancer experience such central nervous system (CNS) side effects. While some people only experience these cognitive problems during active cancer treatment, the symptoms and effects can continue long after treatment over. One study examining the long-term effects of chemotherapy reported survivors performed significantly poorer on neuropsychological tests 20 years after chemotherapy than age-matched controls (Koppelmans et al., 2012; Wolf et al., 2016).

Box 20.6   Learning activity

1. Knowing what you do about Louise, how might her roles and routines be impacted?
2. Consider Louise's experience: what are the common cognitive problems experienced by people who are undergoing or have undergone cancer treatment?
3. What parts Louise's brain support executive functions like organization and problem-solving?
4. What mechanisms in the nervous system promote error detection?
5. How does neuro-fatigue impact the ability to make decisions?
6. What areas of the brain are associated with word finding and speech?

Keywords: executive functioning, error detection, neuro-fatigue, language processing

Common symptoms reported by patients include but are not limited to memory, thinking clearly and concentrating (Falleti et al., 2005) and complex attention (Vardy, Rourke, & Tannock, 2007). Previously often referred to as "chemo brain," the associated cognitive dysfunction from cancer treatment is becoming more commonly referred to as cancer related cognitive impairment (CRCI) because it does not strictly affect only those who receive chemo treatment. There is no known way to prevent CRCI at this time as the direct causes are still unknown. However, it is hypothesized that breast cancer treatments, like chemotherapy, increase neuroinflammation which expedites the process of brain aging (Kovulchuk & Kolb, 2017). While specific causes are not well understood, there are several things that can make the likelihood of experiencing CRCI greater such as: polypharmacy, comorbid conditions like hypertension or diabetes, poor nutrition, mental health diagnoses like depression and anxiety, infections, substance use, and being post-menopausal. Mounting evidence suggests that neurotoxicity of the CNS may be involved.

Neurotoxicity

While cancer treatment agents, like chemotherapy, are toxic to cancer cells, they are also toxic to healthy cells in the body and CNS. Neurotoxicity as a result of cancer treatment is widely recognized (Stone & DeAngelis, 2016) and can affect both the CNS and peripheral nervous system (PNS). Neurotoxicity has no definitive test and is largely a diagnosis of exclusion. Toxicity can occur by either direct injury to neurons (cells in nervous system) and glia (support cells in the nervous system), or by way of a change in the local micro-environment which houses the neural cells. Neurotoxicity is mediated by several factors, including cancer treatment dosage, administration type, interactions with other drugs, presence of comorbid neural disease or damage, and individual vulnerability. However, many of these factors are not well understood (Stone & DeAngelis, 2016). The presence of neurotoxicity also impacts our energy levels, particularly, mental fatigue.

The neuroscience of fatigue

Fatigue is a concept that is intuitively well understood but is broadly applied and has different meanings depending upon the context. For individuals with diagnoses like breast cancer, fatigue often manifests both physically and mentally. It is estimated that about 33% of breast cancer survivors experience persistent fatigue up to ten years into survivorship (Bardwell & Ancoli-Israel, 2008). Although physical and mental fatigue have some overlap, there are specific characteristics of mental fatigue at the neural and brain level, such as inflammation due to neurotoxicity and neurotransmitter involvement which are unique (Bardwell & Ancoli-Israel, 2008; Kok, 2022).

Mental fatigue

Mental fatigue stems from prolonged periods of cognitive load or activity and can also result from loss of sleep. When under excessive cognitive load for an extended duration of time, mental fatigue can become chronic. Onset of chronic fatigue can drastically impact reward-based, or goal-based, decision making. By judging a goal or activity based on its mental effort, an individual determines if the cognitive effort required to complete a task is worth the reward (Kok, 2022). Mental fatigue can decrease one's willingness to exert this effort to reach goals, which in turn can impact their work, social participation, engagement in life, and productivity (Wolf et al., 2016). It is theorized that this effort-based decision-making stems from several areas in the brain including: the amygdala, basal ganglia, and the dopamine system (Kok, 2022). When fatigue becomes chronic, it cannot be remediated by rest alone, thus the mental effort required for tasks continually increases, while motivation and cognitive performance diminish.

The dopamine system and chronic fatigue

It is hypothesized that neurotransmitters are involved in both acute and chronic fatigue. Fatigue appears to be the result of these specific neurotransmitters presence and their ratios in neuronal synapses and their sensitivity to post-synaptic receptor binding (Kok, 2022).

Neurotransmitters like dopamine, noradrenalin, and serotonin, are involved in both acute and chronic mental fatigue. Chronic fatigue syndrome (CFS) is characterized by long term structural connectivity changes in the brain (Boissoneault et al., 2016; Kok, 2022). These changes, in turn, impact overall brain network connectivity and function which can negatively impacts cognitive and behavioral performance (Boissoneault et al., 2016; Kok, 2022; Qi et al., 2019).

Brain connectivity

An overview of brain structure function has been provided in other chapters of this text, e.g., primarily in the TBI chapter. It would be helpful to review this content as well in relation to this discussion on brain connectivity. In simple terms, following treatment for breast cancer, there are changes in white matter integrity. There are also abnormalities in gray matter volume (Bekele et al., 2021).

Functional MRI studies have also found abnormalities in brain regions related to task-based cognitive. functioning such as the frontal, temporal, and parietal brain regions (Bekele et al., 2021; Li & Caeyenberghs, 2018). These abnormalities impact the brain's ability to establish connectivity and functional networks between brain regions to combine and distribute relevant information during functional activities and tasks (Bekele et al., 2021).

Box 20.7   Learning activity

1. What is white matter and what is gray matter?
2. Look up the brain regions listed above. Can you find pictures of the networks that connect these areas?

Keywords: brain anatomy, neural networks

For many years prior to the advent of neuroimaging, brain activity was thought to be highly localized, i.e., one area of the brain was responsible for a specific function that another area would not be. As our knowledge of brain function has evolved, we now understand that while there is some degree of localization of function in the brain there is also a significant amount of connectivity between regions in the brain which are typically associated with more complex functions. Recently, studies have identified neural networks in the brain which include interconnected regions that are associated with complex activities, e.g., cognitive control (Marek & Dosenbach, 2018). fMRI is able to identify the strength of both passive (when the person is at rest) and active (when the person is doing a task) functional neural connectivity across neural networks. Functional connectivity is determined by how various neurons across the brain activate or don't activate in different types of behavior, including rest. Being able to evaluate changes in neural networks provides an opportunity to better investigate more subtle changes in neural communication that would not typically be identified by structural imaging (Rogers et al., 2007). These techniques have provided an opportunity to better explore neural mechanisms associated with "chemo brain" where there are observable changes in cognitive function but not necessarily a discernable structural change in the brain. Relatively recent research has been exploring changes in the frontal-parietal network, which is associated with cognitive control, associated with breast cancer treatment (Wolf et al., 2016). Ideally, a better understanding of these mechanisms may help provide insight into who may experience cognitive changes during and/or after cancer treatment and also to track recovery.

Box 20.8   Learning activity

1. What cognitive networks do we access to execute routines?
2. How might the behaviors associated with these networks impact occupational performance?
3. Look up information on the following:

   a. Default-mode network.
   b. Frontal parietal network.
   c. Dorsal attention network.
   d. Central executive network.
   e. Ventral attention network.

Keywords: cognitive networks (default-mode, frontal parietal, dorsal attention, central executive, ventral attention)

Box 20.9   Learning activity

For each of the following, discuss how they may be experienced by someone with breast cancer:

1. Physical and sensory pain.
2. Cognitive and emotional pain.
3. Social pain.

Explore how the brain processes each; does it differ based on the type of pain experienced?

Keywords: pain, pain receptors, spinal tracts

Daily life routine: Managing organization of daily life

For busy adults, managing schedules and routines is a precursor to successful participation in many meaningful roles and activities. It is an integral part of engaging in work and work-related tasks, from showing up on time to executing detailed to-do lists and processes. For parents like Louise, it can be especially tricky as they juggle their own schedule alongside their children's. It requires cognitive flexibility, task switching, prioritization, and conscious organization of parallel itineraries into a cohesive timeline that accomplishes necessary goals.

Box 20.10   Learning activity

With your small group, complete the table in the Appendix about the impacts of neuroscience on Louise's desire to organize and execute her weekly routines

---

Back to the person's life: Louise wants to feel competent in daily life organization

Now that you know more about the changes that happen to brain functioning as a result of breast cancer and treatment, how can we use this knowledge to support Louise in her organization of weekly routines? You have a good foundation of knowledge to determine interventions that will support Louise by understanding the neuroscience behind what is happening.

Box 20.11   Learning activity: application to the client

In class or small groups, discuss what strategies or intervention approaches you can use to help Louise organize and execute her weekly routines. Think about:

1. What are Louise's strengths and supports that may help her reach her goals?
2. What are possible barriers Louise may experience to reaching her goals?

Use what you already know about neuroscience and what you know about Louise to guide your treatment options.

What do we know about ourselves and the population at large from Louise and her experience with Breast Cancer?

Like Louise, many of us navigate complex routines and schedules throughout our week. For each of us, with or without a diagnosis like breast cancer, there is a load that managing these routines has on our brains and bodies, and each of us have a defined capacity to manage this load before it results in performance breakdown. We see time management and scheduling products and tools everywhere in our day-to-day life. Email notifications, calendars, timers, reminders, and more. People with and without neurological challenges can—and do!—benefit from using these strategies. It is important to remember that we all need help with things like managing our time and balancing our responsibilities, especially during times of busyness and stress.

We are each different in the amount of complexity or number of items that can be added to our routines before it becomes too much and there begins to be a breakdown in performance. This can happen from something as simple as a poor night's sleep before a busy day. Think about the last time you didn't sleep well. A day that would otherwise be "normal" for you may feel arduous, long, or particularly difficult because you're fatigued. You may notice that it takes you longer to get ready that morning, you forget things here and there, your thinking is slower, and you have difficulty concentrating. Keep moments and days like this in mind when you are working with someone who may have neuro fatigue and forgetfulness due to changes in their neurological function. Consider: What are other things that happen in your life that result in a performance breakdown?

Lastly, some people are better at error detection and recognizing when this performance breakdown occurs for them in their life. They may be able to recognize it, but not problem solve a solution, or they may even start to try and implement some strategies but struggle to remain consistent in their application. Noticing that something is different in our thinking and behavior can feel unsettling and can bring up a lot of emotions like sadness and frustration, these are normal, and are important to consider when selecting strategies to improve performance. None of us like to feel incompetent. Selecting strategies for ourselves or those we work with to be difficult, but manageable, is an important skill to build. We often call this a "just-right" challenge. Our chosen strategies should be challenging, but achievable. We want to build confidence and help motivate the person, whether it is a client, a friend, or even ourselves to continue working towards our goals. We take consistent, small steps to progress towards something we want to do. You may want to run a marathon one day- what is the first small step you might take to help you achieve your goal? If you don't run at all now, it's probably best to start with a run around the block rather than running a 10k and risking passing out on mile four. You probably won't feel incredibly confident or motivated to try again if that was your experience. Apply this same approach to thinking about interventions for people who struggle with managing complex routines. What is the first achievable step they could take that will advance them toward their goal?

Further reading

If interested in further reading about breast cancer, visit the following websites

- National Cancer Institute (NCI): www.cancer.gov
- American Cancer Society (ACS): www.cancer.org

Or read the following books:
Galgut, C. (2013). *Emotional support through breast cancer: The alternative handbook*. CRC Press.
Greenhalgh, T., & Riordan, L. (2018). *The complete guide to breast cancer: How to feel empowered and take control*. Random House UK.
Lourde, A. (1980). *The cancer journals*. Penguin Random House.
Marshall, J., & Marshall, L. (2021). *Off our chests*. Ideapress Publishing.
Miller, K., & Camp, M. (2021). *The breast cancer book*. Johns Hopkins Press.

References

Bardwell, W. A., & Ancoli-Israel, S. (2008). Breast cancer and fatigue. *Sleep Medicine Clinics*, *3*(1), 61–71.

Bekele, B. M., Luijendijk, M., Schagen, S. B., de Ruiter, M., & Douw, L. (2021). Fatigue and resting-state functional brain networks in breast cancer patients treated with chemotherapy. *Breast Cancer Research and Treatment*, *189*, 787–796.

Boissoneault, J., Letzen, J., Lai, S., O'Shea, A., Craggs, J., Robinson, M. E., & Staud, R. (2016). Abnormal resting state functional connectivity in patients with chronic fatigue syndrome: an arterial spin-labeling fMRI study. *Magnetic Resonance Imaging*, *34*(4), 603–608.

Collins, O., Dillon, S., Finucane, C., Lawlor, B., & Kenny, R. A. (2012). Parasympathetic autonomic dysfunction is common in mild cognitive impairment. *Neurobiology of Aging*, *33*(10), 2324–2333.

Falleti, M. G., Sanfilippo, A., Maruff, P., Weih, L., & Phillips, K.-A. (2005). The nature and severity of cognitive impairment associated with adjuvant chemotherapy in women with breast cancer: A meta-analysis of the current literature. *Brain and Cognition*, *59*(1), 60–70.

Ghoncheh, M., Pournamdar, Z., & Salehiniya, H. (2016). Incidence and mortality and epidemiology of breast cancer in the world. *Asian Pacific Journal of Cancer Prevention*, *17*(sup3), 43–46.

Kok, A. (2022). Cognitive control, motivation and fatigue: A cognitive neuroscience perspective. *Brain and Cognition*, *160*, 105880.

Koppelmans, V., Breteler, M., Boogerd, W., Seynaeve, C., Gundy, C., & Schagen, S. (2012). Neuropsychological performance in survivors of breast cancer more than 20 years after adjuvant chemotherapy. *Journal of Clinical Oncology*, *30*(10), 1080–1086.

Kovalchuk, A., & Kolb, B. (2017). Chemo brain: from discerning mechanisms to lifting the brain fog—an aging connection. *Cell Cycle*, *16*(14), 1345–1349.

Li, M., & Caeyenberghs, K. (2018). Longitudinal assessment of chemotherapy-induced changes in brain and cognitive functioning: A systematic review. *Neuroscience & Biobehavioral Reviews*, *92*, 304–317.

Marek, S., & Dosenbach, N. U. (2018). The frontoparietal network: Function, electrophysiology, and importance of individual precision mapping. *Dialogues in Clinical Neuroscience*, *20*(2), 133–140.

Qi, P., Ru, H., Gao, L., Zhang, X., Zhou, T., Tian, Y., Thakor, N., Bezerianos, A., Li, J., & Sun, Y. (2019). Neural mechanisms of mental fatigue revisited: New insights from the brain connectome. *Engineering*, *5*(2), 276–286.

Rogers, B. P., Morgan, V. L., Newton, A. T., & Gore, J. C. (2007). Assessing functional connectivity in the human brain by fMRI. *Magnetic Resonance Imaging*, *25*(10), 1347–1357.

Stone, J. B., & DeAngelis, L. M. (2016). Cancer-treatment-induced neurotoxicity—focus on newer treatments. *Nature Reviews Clinical Oncology*, *13*(2), 92–105.

Tao, Z., Shi, A., Lu, C., Song, T., Zhang, Z., & Zhao, J. (2015). Breast cancer: epidemiology and etiology. *Cell Biochemistry and Biophysics*, *72*, 333–338.

van Dam, F. S., Boogerd, W., Schagen, S. B., Muller, M. J., Droogleever Fortuyn, M. E., Wall, E., & Rodenhuis, S. (1998). Impairment of cognitive function in women receiving adjuvant treatment for high-risk breast cancer: High-dose versus standard-dose chemotherapy. *JNCI: Journal of the National Cancer Institute*, *90*(3), 210–218.

Vardy, J., Rourke, S., & Tannock, I. F. (2007). Evaluation of cognitive function associated with chemotherapy: A review of published studies and recommendations for future research. *Journal of Clinical Oncology*, *25*(17), 2455–2463.

Von Ah, D., Russell, K. M., Storniolo, A. M., & Carpenter, J. S. (2009). Cognitive dysfunction and its relationship to quality of life in breast cancer survivors. *ONF*, *36*(3), 326–336.

Wolf, T. J., Doherty, M., Kallogjeri, D., Coalson, R. S., Nicklaus, J., Ma, C. X., Schlaggar, B. L., & Piccirillo, J. (2016). The feasibility of using metacognitive strategy training to improve cognitive performance and neural connectivity in women with chemotherapy-induced cognitive impairment. *Oncology*, *91*(3), 143–152.

Unit IV

Integrated systems

21 Xavier wants to complete his personal hygiene by himself and has had a stroke

Neuroscience facilitates our understanding of daily routines

Anna Boone and Bridget Kraus

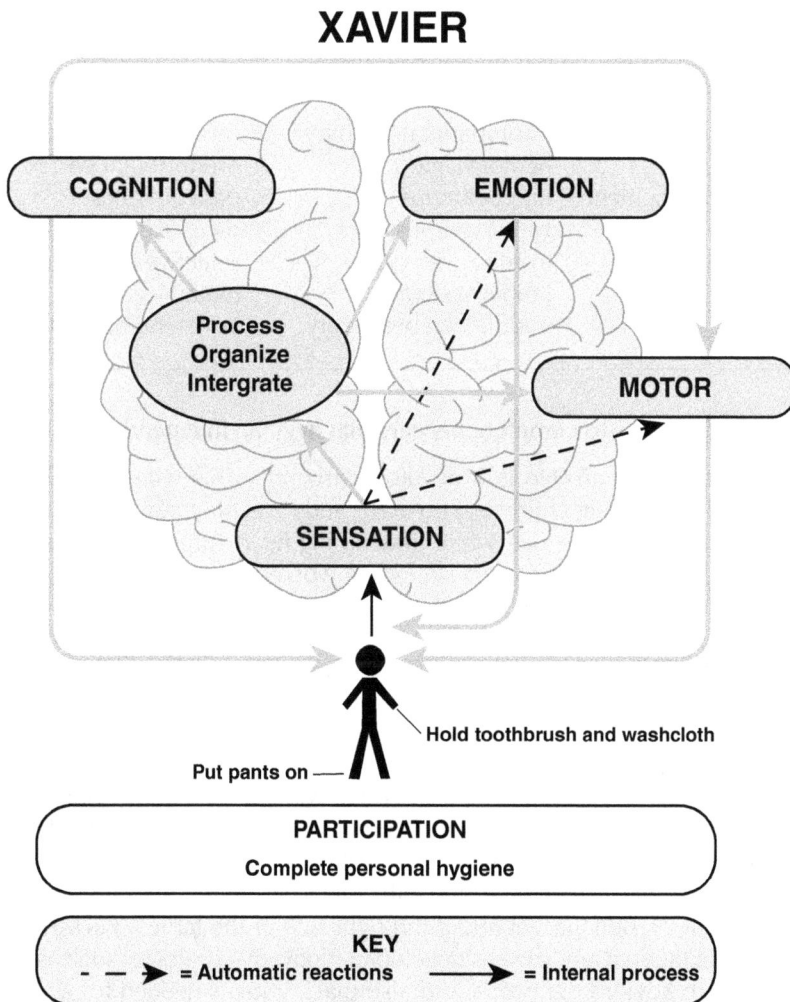

Figure 21.1 Xavier brain figure

DOI: 10.4324/9781003524380-26

Purpose of this chapter

The purpose of this chapter is to connect much of the information we have learned about neurological processes underlying everyday function with a new, broader lens of how we as humans integrate all these processes to fully engage in daily life. In keeping with the format of this textbook, we will accomplish this goal using a case study of an individual who has had a stroke. Due to the multifaceted nature of stroke and its potential wide-spread neural impact, the stroke population makes for an interesting choice to explore how humans can integrate all of these incredible processes. We will use Xavier, an adult who experienced a stroke, as the basis of this chapter to craft our expertise in understanding how neuroscience impacts participation in daily life routines.

Keywords for this chapter are listed in the box below. Be sure to learn what these key features are so you can get the most out of the chapter.

Keywords for this chapter

amygdala	frontoparietal circuitry	non-fluent aphasia
basal ganglia	hemorrhagic	orbitofrontal cortex
cerebrovascular accident	hippocampus	parietal lobes
(CVA)	hypothalamus	receptive aphasia
cingulate cortex	insula	selective attention
fluent aphasia	limbic system	thalamus
frontal lobe	middle cerebral artery	unilateral neglect

Xavier, a man who wants to complete his personal hygiene independently

Xavier is a 39-year-old man. He is a devoted husband to his wife, Madeline, and an engaged father of two young children who are 5 and 7 years of age. Xavier experienced a left middle cerebral artery stroke while undergoing heart surgery for a genetic condition about six months ago. Prior to his stroke, he worked long hours as a car mechanic on luxury cars. In addition to a lifelong interest in cars and mechanics, Xavier's personal interests include playing the banjo, reading historical non-fiction, and gardening. Xavier and Madeline typically share all household and parenting duties with each contributing more at times when the other spouse is particularly busy with work or other personal responsibilities.

After his stroke, Xavier received treatment at an inpatient rehabilitation facility before being discharged back to the community. Although coming back home took a bit of read-justment, he has settled into a routine and found alternate ways to fulfill his life roles. He can perceive all of his surroundings with cues to direct his attention towards anything oc-curring on his right side. Madeline occasionally will verbally remind him to look towards his right: "Hey, Xavier, don't forget about the right side of the table!" However, with the help of the rehabilitation team, she has developed innovative strategies such as an audible watch reminder on Xavier's right wrist and also placing items needed for a task towards the center or left side of Xavier's view if the focus is on completing the task.

Socially, Xavier understands what others are saying to him, but he continues to have some difficulty in articulating himself to others. For example, he often struggles to find the correct word for what he wants to express. He effectively communicates through word substitution but becomes frustrated when his speech is halting and consists of just a few words. Xavier has noticed that he excels at tasks where he can focus his attention on a single thing such as unloading the dishwasher, folding clothes, or listening to an audio-book. Physically, Xavier has progressed to WFL (within functional limits) motorically, and his balance is good with no assistive devices.

Xavier and his family are pleased with the progress he made during his acute care and inpatient rehabilitation stay and he continues to receive support through a day program consisting of OT, physical therapy (PT), and speech language pathology (SLP) services twice a week. Xavier set a goal with his OT team to become independent in his everyday self-care routine. Currently, Madeline sets up the items he needs to complete these tasks each morning and provides prompts to help him move from step to step. Xavier feels as if independence in self-care would allow him to take some strain off of his wife's daily responsibilities and give him a sense of accomplishment.

Box 21.1   Learning activity

Discuss with your peers:

1. What are the main occupations and life roles that are important to Xavier?
2. If you were meeting with Xavier as his OT, what other questions would you ask?
3. Given Xavier's current abilities and desires, what types of goals should he focus on first?

What do you already know about Xavier's case?

Box 21.2   Learning activity

Reflect on your own:

1. How does your ability to complete your self-care routine affect your mental state and quality of life?
2. What about being able to pay attention to your environment? How does this impact your self-care routine?
3. How can Xavier's home environment be modified to support his ability to perform his self-care routine?

Neuroscience information to guide your thinking about Xavier

Every person who has had a stroke experiences a slightly different presentation of motor, physical, cognitive, sensory, and psychosocial effects. The enormous variety in stroke presentation stems from exactly what neural structures are affected, to what extent they are affected, the influence of the individual's personal factors (e.g., age, IQ, personality predisposition), occupations, and life contexts (e.g. social support, built home environment, work environment). Strokes, or cerebrovascular accidents (CVA), are usually caused by a blood vessel blockage (i.e., ischemic stroke) during which cerebral blood flow is reduced to any brain area that is "downstream" (or in other words, branches) from that blood vessel. About 13% are hemorrhagic (bleeding) strokes that result from a weakened wall structure in blood vessels causing them to burst (Tsao et al., 2023). Any area that has reduced or absent blood flow because of a stroke will likely not be as effective at performing its normal functions. Because of the brain's interconnectivity between regions, it is important to remember that areas without blood flow disruptions could still be impacted because they network with an area that was.

Xavier experienced a blockage within his middle cerebral artery. The middle cerebral artery supplies much of the lateral surface of the cortex including large portions of the frontal, temporal, and parietal lobes; it also provides blood supply (and thus, oxygen) to deep, subcortical structures such as the basal ganglia (Navarro-Orozco & Sánchez-Manso, 2021; Shapiro et al., 2020; Tatu et al., 1998). Let's take a closer look at how alterations in any of these regions could impact Xavier's behavior and thus, how an individual participates in daily tasks.

The parietal lobes allow for humans to process incoming sensory information and work in concert with the frontal lobe on precisely where to direct our attention. Interestingly, the right parietal lobe appears to play a larger role in our perception of our body sensations (peripersonal) and space around us (extrapersonal) as compared to the left parietal lobe. The reason behind this lateralization of function is still debated in the literature (Corbetta & Schulman, 2011; de Schotten et al., 2011). The most widely held theory is that right parietal lobe processes sensory information from both the left and right left side of the world, while the left parietal lobe is less dominant and attends only to the right side of the world (Mesulam, 1981). Inattention (also known as unilateral neglect) presents in roughly half of those with a right-sided lesions and a third of those with left-sided lesions (Chen et al., 2015). It is important to note that inattention differs greatly from a visual field cut which results from a lesion along the visual pathway itself (see Chapter 3 on spinal cord injury for further discussion). Since neglect is an impairment of awareness, it is substantially more difficult to teach clients to compensate for it in daily life activities. Another consideration in daily activities is the motor impairments that can arise from an MCA stroke.

Box 21.3   Learning activity

With your peers, find a photo of the MCA:

1. What regions of the brain does the MCA supply? Label them.
2. Discuss what physical motor changes might you expect from a MCA stroke. Consider each of the following:

   a. Left versus right sided.
   b. Tone.
   c. Spasticity.
   d. Coordination.
   e. Balance.

2. Knowing what you do about neuroscience, why do you think CVA presentation is so variable?

Keywords: middle cerebral artery, brain arterial supply

Neural underpinnings of receptive and expressive language ability

Our first understandings of the neurological regions underlying the critical human ability to verbally convey and comprehend information came in the late 1800s from observing individuals who had sustained a stroke. Neurologists during this time (for whom Broca's and Wernicke's aphasia are named) observed that their clients had difficulty speaking or comprehending according to which neural areas were damaged most severely. The idea that a single region of the brain was solely responsible for a given function has fallen out of favor recently; the advent of neuroimaging has led to the understanding that although there are indeed key regions for certain functions, most rely upon distributed networks in the brain. Language ability is such a function.

Traditionally, aphasias have been distinguished as fluent or non-fluent. In fluent aphasia, the ability to speak or to produce language is retained; however, in non-fluent aphasia, a client has difficulty producing words. The second important feature of aphasia is whether the individual can understand the actual content or meaning of words. In Broca's aphasia, a subtype of non-fluent aphasia, clients speak in short, halting sentences or are only able to produce a word or two. In spite of this difficulty, the ability to understand word meaning is relatively intact; therefore, their speech is sensible and they are able to comprehend what others are saying. In contrast, Wernicke's aphasia, a type of fluent aphasia, consists of the ability to produce words and sentences, but these sentences have little to no meaning. This type of presentation is often referred to as "expressive aphasia." Individuals with Wernicke's aphasia do not understand word meaning and thus, do not understand what others are saying to them, referred to as "receptive aphasia." Individuals who cannot produce any speech, sensible speech, or understand speech have what is referred to as "global aphasia." See recommended readings for more detailed classifications of aphasia.

The regions that serve as "hubs" for these communication abilities are the (1) inferior frontal gyrus (i.e., Broca's region) and (2) posterior temporal region (i.e., Wernicke's region). Literature is building to support the notion that the complex function of language and communication results from a distributed network of both cortical and subcortical structures (Bonilha et al., 2009; Hillis et al., 2004). It is important to note that although these clean classifications of aphasia make discussion of them simpler, clinically there is a wide range of presentation and severity levels.

OT practitioners work closely with speech language pathologist colleagues to discover the most effective means of communication for our clients with aphasia. Because of the dependency of rehabilitation on communication to facilitate the learning process, clients with aphasia are at a higher risk of a longer length of stay, not being discharged to the home environment, and greater disability (Flowers et al., 2016). Specific to the realm of OT, clients with aphasia also have lower reported quality of life and daily life participation (Hilari, 2011; Wray & Clarke, 2017). OT interventions may be used to improve these important, real-world outcomes (Escher et al., 2022).

Box 21.4   Learning activity

Find a photo of the brain to label and discuss with your peers:

1. What areas of the brain are responsible for understanding and producing speech? Locate and label them on a picture of the brain.

2. Based upon Xavier's presentation, what words could we use to describe his language abilities?
   Impact on social connection/daily life?
3. What questions might we ask SLP?

Keywords: brain regions, neuroanatomy

Box 21.5   Learning activity

Xavier experienced a stroke in his MCA; however, strokes can occur in many places in the brain. For each of the following common CVA locations, identify a photo of the vasculature, label it, write down what regions of the brain would be affected, and a few side effects you may expect to see based on your understanding of neuroscience:

1. Anterior cerebral artery.
2. Posterior cerebral artery.
3. Cerebellar.
4. Brain stem.

Keywords: brain arterial supply, cerebral blood supply, cerebral arteries

---

Emotional networks in the brain

Individuals post-stroke may experience psychosocial effects resulting from neurophysiological changes and/or as a natural psychological response to a large health event and the associated functional changes. The most common post-stroke emotional changes are depression, apathy, and anxiety (Schöttke & Giabbiconi, 2015). These negative psychological constructs are associated with lower rates of engagement in rehabilitation, occupational performance, and life participation (Cooper et al., 2014; Schöttke et al. 2020; Skidmore et al 2010). Decreased social participation can in turn lead to poorer psychosocial functioning; therefore, recognition of these symptoms and timely intervention is necessary to diminish the cyclical process (Ayerbe et al., 2011, 2013). Clinical psychologists are often not a part of routine post-stroke care (Intercollegiate Stroke Working Party, 2015); therefore, occupational therapists may play a key role in formal and informal screening of psychological difficulties and referrals to mental health professionals. Positive psychological attributes such as happiness and adaptability may also be protective factors for post-stroke participation outcomes (Lee et al., 2021; Cooper et al., 2014).

Aligning with our understanding of other neural functions, the brain basis of emotion also lies within distributed networks of cortical and subcortical regions (Kragel & LaBar, 2016). In other words, a single emotion cannot be traced to a singular neurologic location, but a single neurologic location can assist in processing multiple emotions. Frontoparietal circuitry involved in executive functioning shows increased activation during conscious emotional regulation (Etkin et al., 2015). Key cortical regions involved in emotional processing include the orbitofrontal cortex, the cingulate cortex, and the insula. Subcortical regions, including the amygdala and basal ganglia, also play a major role in the generation of emotions (Baars & Gage, 2018; Chanes & Barrett, 2016).

Box 21.6   Learning activity

On your diagram of the brain label each of the following and list their primary functions. Use different colors for cortical regions versus subcortical regions:

1. Orbitofrontal cortex.
2. Cingulate cortex.
3. Insula.
4. Amygdala.
5. Basal ganglia.

The limbic system: Emotional regulation and behavior

The limbic system is comprised of four key components: the hypothalamus, amygdala, thalamus, and hippocampus. The limbic system serves many functions such as motivation, long-term memory, olfaction, and emotions and behavioral response to them. The limbic system drives human behavior until prefrontal networks develop in early adulthood which can override what would be initial behavioral responses to emotions. Consider how younger children often have a harder time controlling their behaviors in response to how they are feeling. This is because their prefrontal cortex does not yet have the ability to halt and alter their response to a big emotional feeling.

Box 21.7   Learning activity

1. On the diagram, find and label the four components of the limbic system.
2. How might a CVA impact a person's behaviors in response to their emotions?
3. What are some strategies we could use to manage their emotions and behaviors?

Daily life routine: completing tooth brushing, hand and face washing by himself

Completion of a morning self-care routine and other basic activities of daily living (ADLs) provides a sense of independence and can serve as the basis for developing self-efficacy in other more complex tasks. Completion of ADL tasks such as toothbrushing and hand and face washing requires integration of sensory, motor, and cognitive processes. Although there is considerable variability in how each person approaches these tasks, there is high consistency in how one approaches the task over time given the repetitive nature of the task. Basic everyday routines such as morning self-care generally require little conscious thought or problem-solving; however, the effects of stroke may make this once routine sequence of events novel as one must problem-solve new ways to complete the task. Many of us have had life experiences that may have mirrored this change from automaticity to requiring conscious thought, even if only temporary. For example, having a fractured bone in a cast, having a string of nights with difficult sleep, or even being further along in pregnancy may impact the ease or effectiveness of doing one's morning routine.

Back to the person's life: Xavier wants to get up and get himself ready on his own

Completing his morning routine without family assistance is the first goal that Xavier would like to accomplish. He reports that doing so would relieve stress on his wife during their family's hectic morning rush and be a huge step forward in regaining his functional independence.

Box 21.8   Learning activity

1. Make a list of Xavier's strengths and limitations. How would you expect each of these to impact his ability to perform these tasks?
2. What questions about Xavier's abilities might you want to ask to get a more well-rounded picture of his current task performance prior to observation? What would you want to know about his environment or task objects? Why is this information important?
3. What changes could Xavier make in how he completes the task to be more independent?
4. In what ways would reaching Xavier's goal impact his overall health?

What do we know about ourselves and the population at large from this brain condition and this family story?

Although this chapter has highlighted the clinical presentation of stroke, we all have differing levels of abilities in many of the same ways. Each of us learns to adapt to our own physical, cognitive, and sensory abilities over time. A stroke happens quickly and the abrupt, sometimes substantial, change in abilities can require additional time, support, and problem-solving to adapt. Consideration of our own strengths and areas where we stray from the "norm," can help provide insight and empathy towards our clients.

For example, humans are not able to consciously pay equal attention to everything that is occurring around them. A process of selective attention allows us to choose which aspects of our environment we pay attention to. Allocating our cognitive resources to only those environmental aspects deemed most important conserves energy for the task at hand. For example, while reading this textbook, you most likely have other visual stimuli that you are inattentive to (e.g., the task bar on a computer screen, a person sipping coffee at the table next to you in your visual periphery). A relative inattention to these irrelevant factors allows you to pay better attention to reading this text. Humans tend to overestimate our attentional capacities and our ability to detect meaningful changes in our environment. For examples of this, search "inattentional blindness" on Google or YouTube. There have been many intriguing scientific studies on this topic. *Be sure to get guidance from your instructor about how to find quality YouTube videos for this activity.*

Box 21.9   Learning activity

Discuss with your peers:

1. What factors determine how well you are able to pay attention?
2. What types of environments do you tend to function well in?
3. What types of activities require more of your attention? What about less? Does this differ from your peers?
4. What changes do you make when you need to improve your attention?

Along with the expansion of the prefrontal cortex, humans have improved our abilities to self-regulate our emotions and thus, to modify our behaviors to adapt to social norms. We each possess a different level of sensitivity to more basic emotions (fear, anger, jealousy, happiness) and approach self-management of these emotions differently due to a range of factors such as family upbringing and other life experiences.

Box 21.10   Learning activity

Discuss with your peers:

1. How strongly do you feel emotions?
2. What factors impact how likely you are to have larger fluctuations in emotions (positive or negative)
3. What strategies do you use when you feel your emotions may be maladaptive? Are there any new strategies you can think of to try?
4. How could you best structure an intervention session to ensure maintained motivation from your client? What might that look like for Xavier?

Individuals post-stroke often report an increased ability to be present in the most mundane of life events and appreciation for those around them. This may be a result of taking their time to accomplish tasks, a shifting life focus, or a greater reflectiveness of how to approach tasks generally. It is important as clinicians to not only take note of what our clients can do, but what they can do with the right supports in place.

Box 21.11   Learning activity

With your small group, complete the table in the Appendix about how Xavier can be enabled to complete his personal hygiene independently.

Further reading

Baars, B., & Gage, N. M. (2018). *Fundamentals of cognitive neuroscience: a beginner's guide.* Academic Press.
Lundy-Eckman, L., (2018). *Neuroscience: Fundamentals for rehabilitation*, 5th ed. Elsevier.
National Aphasia Association. (n.d.). *Aphasia definition.* www.aphasia.org/aphasia-definitions/
Wolf, T. J. & Nilsen, D. (2015). *Occupational therapy practice guidelines for adults with stroke.* AOTA Press.

References

Ayerbe, L., Ayis, S., Rudd, A. G., Heuschmann, P. U., & Wolfe, C. D. (2011). Natural history, predictors, and associations of depression 5 years after stroke: the South London Stroke Register. *Stroke, 42*(7), 1907–1911.
Ayerbe, L., Ayis, S., Crichton, S., Wolfe, C. D., & Rudd, A. G. (2013). The natural history of depression up to 15 years after stroke: the South London Stroke Register. *Stroke, 44*(4), 1105–1110.
Baars, B., & Gage, N. M. (2018). *Fundamentals of cognitive neuroscience: a beginner's guide.* Academic Press.
Bonilha, L., & Fridriksson, J. (2009). Subcortical damage and white matter disconnection associated with non-fluent speech. *Brain, 132*(6), e108.
Broca, P. (1861). Remarks on the seat of the faculty of articulated language, following an observation of aphemia (loss of speech). *Bulletin de la Société Anatomique, 6,* 330–357.
Chanes, L., & Barrett, L. F. (2016). Redefining the role of limbic areas in cortical processing. *Trends in Cognitive Sciences, 20*(2), 96–106.
Chen, P., Chen, C. C., Hreha, K., Goedert, K. M., & Barrett, A. M. (2015). Kessler Foundation Neglect Assessment Process uniquely measures spatial neglect during activities of daily living. *Archives of Physical Medicine and Rehabilitation, 96*(5), 869–876.
Cooper, C. L., Phillips, L. H., Johnston, M., Radlak, B., Hamilton, S., & McLeod, M. J. (2014). Links between emotion perception and social participation restriction following stroke. *Brain Injury, 28*(1), 122–126.
Corbetta, M., & Shulman, G. L. (2011). Spatial neglect and attention networks. *Annual Review of Neuroscience, 34,* 569.
de Schotten, M. T., Dell'Acqua, F., Forkel, S., Simmons, A., Vergani, F., Murphy, D. G., & Catani, M. (2011). A lateralized brain network for visuo-spatial attention. *Nature Proceedings, 14*(10), 1245–1246. doi:10.1038/nn.2905.
Escher, A. A., McKinnon, S., & Berger, S. (2022). Effective interventions within the scope of occupational therapy practice to address participation for adults with aphasia: A systematic review. *British Journal of Occupational Therapy, 85*(2), 99–110.
Etkin, A., Büchel, C., & Gross, J. J. (2015). The neural bases of emotion regulation. *Nature reviews neuroscience, 16*(11), 693–700.
Flowers, H. L., Skoretz, S. A., Silver, F. L., Rochon, E., Fang, J., Flamand-Roze, C., & Martino, R. (2016). Poststroke aphasia frequency, recovery, and outcomes: a systematic review and meta-analysis. *Archives of physical medicine and rehabilitation, 97*(12), 2188–2201.
Hilari, K. (2011). The impact of stroke: are people with aphasia different to those without? *Disability and rehabilitation, 33*(3), 211–218.
Hillis, A. E., Work, M., Barker, P. B., Jacobs, M. A., Breese, E. L., & Maurer, K. (2004). Re-examining the brain regions crucial for orchestrating speech articulation. *Brain, 127*(7), 1479–1487.
Intercollegiate Stroke Working Party. (2015). *Sentinel stroke national audit programme: Post-acute organisational audit public report.* London: Royal College of Physicians.
Kragel, P. A., & LaBar, K. S. (2016). Decoding the nature of emotion in the brain. *Trends in Cognitive Sciences, 20*(6), 444–455.
Lee, Y., Nicholas, M. L., & Connor, L. T. (2021). Identifying emotional contributors to participation post-stroke. *Topics in Stroke Rehabilitation,* 1–13.

Mesulam, M. M. (1981). A cortical network for directed attention and unilateral neglect. *Annals of Neurology, 10*(4), 309–325.

Navarro-Orozco, D., & Sánchez-Manso, J. C. (2021). Neuroanatomy, middle cerebral artery. StatPearls Publishing.

Shapiro, M., Raz, E., Nossek, E., Chancellor, B., Ishida, K., & Nelson, P. K. (2020). Neuroanatomy of the middle cerebral artery: implications for thrombectomy. *Journal of Neurointerventional Surgery, 12*(8), 768–773.

Tatu, L., Moulin, T., Bogousslavsky, J., & Duvernoy, H. (1998). Arterial territories of the human brain: cerebral hemispheres. *Neurology, 50*(6), 1699–1708.

Tsao, C. W., Aday, A. W., Almarzooq, Z. I., Anderson, C. A., Arora, P., Avery, C. L.,... & American Heart Association Council on Epidemiology and Prevention Statistics Committee and Stroke Statistics Subcommittee. (2023). Heart disease and stroke statistics—2023 update: a report from the American Heart Association. *Circulation, 147*(8), e93–e621.

Schöttke, H., & Giabbiconi, C. M. (2015). Post-stroke depression and post-stroke anxiety: prevalence and predictors. *International Psychogeriatrics, 27*(11), 1805–1812.

Schöttke, Henning, Leonie Gerke, Rainer Düsing, and Anne Möllmann. (2020). Post-stroke depression and functional impairments–A 3-year prospective study. *Comprehensive Psychiatry, 99*, 152171.

Skidmore, E. R., Whyte, E. M., Holm, M. B., Becker, J. T., Butters, M. A., Dew, M. A.,... & Lenze, E. J. (2010). Cognitive and affective predictors of rehabilitation participation after stroke. *Archives of Physical Medicine and Rehabilitation, 91*(2), 203–207.

Wernicke, C. (1874). *The aphasic symptom complex: A psychological study on an anatomical basis.* Breslau: Cohn & Weigert.

Wray, F., & Clarke, D. (2017). Longer-term needs of stroke survivors with communication difficulties living in the community: a systematic review and thematic synthesis of qualitative studies. *BMJ Open, 7*(10), e017944.

22 Natalie wants to drive her car and has a traumatic brain injury

Neuroscience facilitates our understanding of driving a car

Jessica L. Petersen, Stephanie N. Ritter, Calli M. Palmquist, and Thomas F. Bergquist

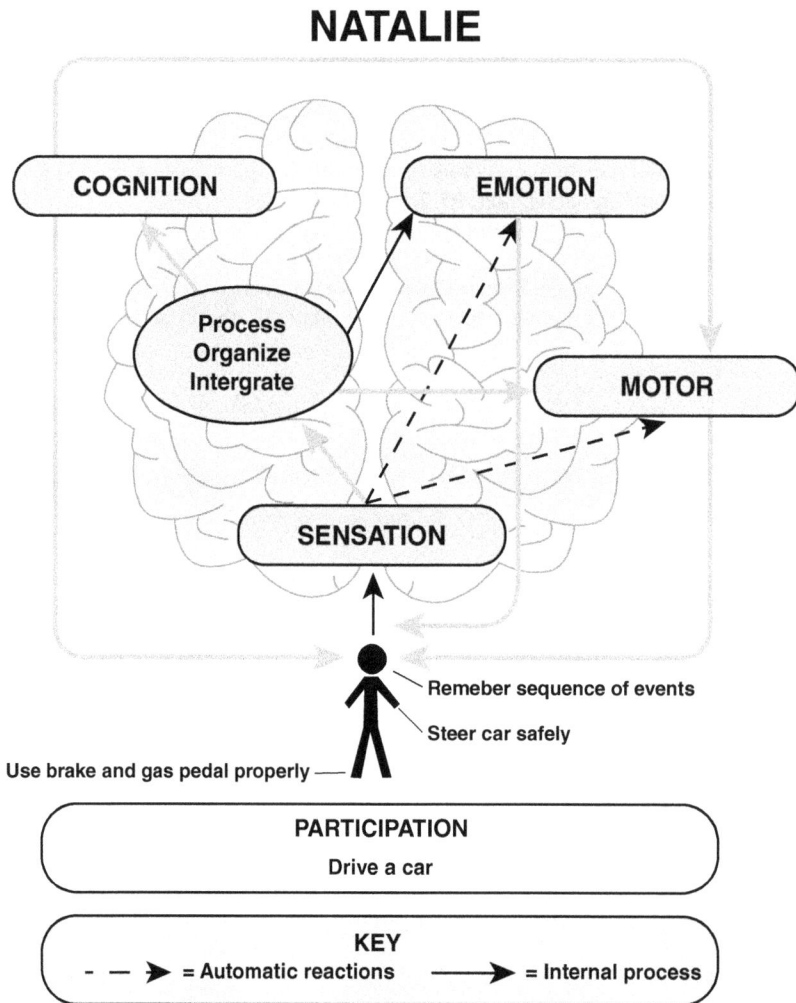

Figure 22.1 Natalie brain figure

DOI: 10.4324/9781003524380-27

Purpose of this chapter

This chapter illustrates the impact of a specific medical condition, in this case traumatic brain injury (TBI), on various aspects of a lived experience (driving a motor vehicle). To understand this better, we will look at the neuroscience behind some of the common cognitive, sensory, behavioral and physical changes that can occur after TBI. Although every TBI is unique in presentation, we can use an example from someone who has experienced this type of trauma to learn more about the neurologic functions that regulate one's ability to engage in the occupation of driving. We'll learn more about Natalie's experience with TBI and the impact that it has on occupational performance.

The key neuroscience concepts we will explore in this chapter include integration of the higher order brain areas (frontal, parietal, temporal and occipital lobes) with other internal processing centers. As with all the chapters, these components of the nervous system work with other systems to support overall human function.

Keywords for this chapter are listed in the box below. Be sure to learn what these key features are so you can get the most out of the chapter.

Keywords for this chapter

acquired brain injury (ABI)	judgement	reasoning
awareness	organization and planning	traumatic brain injury (TBI)
attention	prefrontal cortex	visual field
executive functions	processing speed	visuospatial

Let's find out about Natalie so we have a context for understanding the impact of her distinct nervous system on her life. As with all the chapters in this text, we learn these relationships from people who have distinct personal experiences in their lives.

Natalie, a 57-year-old who wants to drive

Natalie is a 57-year-old retired teacher. Recently widowed, Natalie now lives alone in a suburban area. She attends church regularly, volunteers there several days each week, and is an active member of a women's Bible study group. Natalie has two adult children both of whom live over three hours away.

About one month ago Natalie slipped and fell backward on an icy sidewalk and struck the back of her head. She suffered a TBI including a subdural hemorrhage. She has been home from the hospital for about one week. She was hospitalized for two weeks and spent six days in the inpatient rehabilitation unit where she received physical therapy (PT), occupational therapy (OT), and Speech Language Pathology services. About three weeks after her injury, Natalie was discharged and returned to her one-level home and is independent with most basic activities of daily living. Home healthcare is scheduled to come in twice per week to assist her with showering due to balance concerns and also with setting up medications. Her daughter was able to be with her for the first few days at home and feels that Natalie is able to safely use the microwave for light cooking, but is concerned about her use of the oven and stove because she forgot to turn the stove off after using it. Her daughter had to remind Natalie that she had already taken her medications each day, and Natalie is learning to use a weekly pill box. Her daughter also observed some unsteadiness when Natalie was walking across thresholds and when carrying something, so she now has a four wheeled walker to reduce her risk of falling. Due to concern about her memory and her balance, her children plan to be with her one to two times per week to help with activities including heavy cleaning, yardwork, paying bills, and shopping. Once she has completed in home therapy, the plan is for her to start outpatient therapies once per week and will rely on friends to drive her to appointments.

Natalie's daily activities have changed since returning home from her hospital stay due to her fall related injuries. She has stopped reading and watching television because it now gives her a headache. She tells her daughter that she doesn't enjoy reading anymore because she can't follow the storyline. She also tells her that she is having trouble finishing tasks at home because she loses track of what she is doing and starts something new. Natalie's inpatient OT encouraged her to use a daily planner and make lists, which she continues to use to help her keep track of her appointments and other day-to-day information.

Natalie would really like to return to volunteering at her church but needs to be able to drive to get there because her small town has limited public transportation. She also wants to be able to drive herself to church services and Bible study so she doesn't have to rely on friends. Considering the other changes they have observed, her kids have expressed concern about her ability to return to driving.

Box 22.1   Learning activity

Discuss with your peers:

1. Having read the narrative, what are you curious about?
2. What do you need to know more about?

Before you continue reading the chapter, work with your small group to discuss what you already know.

Box 22.2   Learning activity

1. What parts of the brain and associated cognitive skills support driving ability?
2. What are the various information processing and cognitive demands of driving?
3. What other factors in this case beyond the brain injury itself may impact the Natalie's goal of returning to driving?

With these ideas in mind, let's take a closer look at how the brain carries out functions that are needed for safe driving.

Neuroscience information to guide your thinking about Natalie

Traumatic brain injury

Acquired brain injury (ABI) encompasses a broad range of both traumatic and nontrau-matic injuries to the brain that can produce neurological and neurocognitive changes. Multiple conditions can result in ABI, including cerebrovascular accident (stroke), brain tumors, traumatic brain injury (TBI), and autoimmune or infectious encephalopathies among others. In the case of TBI, damage often occurs via diffuse injury impacting struc-tural integrity of brain tissue and is associated with multiple changes, including white matter shearing, glial injury, and disrupted synaptic communication (Blennow et al., 2012; Hemphill et al., 2015). The natural course of recovery and presentation of injury differs greatly between persons leading to the phrase, "If you have seen one TBI, you have seen one TBI." Recovery from TBI depends on multiple factors including severity of injury, duration of loss of consciousness, and the involved brain regions, but it can also be im-pacted by psychological factors such as comorbid depression (Powell et al., 2019). In TBI, maximal recovery often occurs early in the first year, but improvement can still be seen years post injury (Walker et al., 2018). This variability of brain injuries can make it more challenging to determine what types of impairments will be present. While it cannot be overstated that each TBI has unique features, this text will focus on how the neuroscience guides our thinking about the brain structures and functions that relate to driving.

Changes in driving patterns after TBI

Knowing that TBI recovery and presentation can vary greatly, let's briefly look at what the literature indicates about potential changes in driving ability. TBI is commonly associ-ated with changes in functional skills including driving patterns. Given the importance that independently operating a motor vehicle has for many individuals, returning to driv-ing and driving safely following injury can be a major focus of rehabilitation efforts. A review of recent literature on driving after TBI reveals very mixed findings ranging from no increased risk of motor vehicle crashes (MVC), to persons with TBI being 1.5 times more likely to be involved in MVCs compared with matched controls (Novack et al., 2022). These variations between studies could be due to differences in the sample size, information sources, and severity of injury. Thus, it was the conclusion of the authors that while crash risk is higher following TBI compared with national statistics, the results do not adequately justify restricting people from driving after TBI, given that most persons who resumed driving did not report experiencing any crashes (Novak et al., 2022). This does, however, provide rationale for an individualized assessment of the performance skills necessary for driving. For Natalie, who is experiencing new functional limitations, it's important that we take a closer look to determine what, if any, impairments are present that could affect her ability to drive.

A wide variety of cognitive, sensory, behavioral, and physical changes can occur after TBI which can impact safe driving. The following sections look at these in greater detail.

Cognitive functions

There are a number of cognitive skills that are crucial to the task of driving. These in-clude processing speed, attention, visuospatial ability and executive functions. Process-ing speed, or the ability to take in and quickly act on information from the environment, is a common area of concern following TBI (Dikmen et al., 2009). Tate et al. (1991), noted that slowed processing speed was identified in 34% of patients with a history of ABI. In their meta-analysis, Mathias and Wheaton (2007) found that participants with a history of severe TBI consistently performed approximately one standard deviation below their peers on tests of reaction time. Difficulties in processing speed and attention can also result in worse performance on higher order executive functioning, language, and memory tasks, which can lead to greater impairments across multiple domains following injury. Because of their impact on multiple cognitive and functional domains, attentional impairments are an important area of focus for return to driving.

Visuospatial impairments, including full or partial visual field loss and visuospatial neglect, can cause significant problems with navigational abilities, mobility, can limit functional independence, and negatively impact quality of life. Visuospatial neglect (also called hemispatial neglect) results in inattention or unawareness of stimuli presented to the visual field contralateral to the lesion location (Heilman & Valenstein, 2010). Visual field cuts can involve full or partial loss of vision for a particular portion of the visual field, depending on where the lesion occurred. While visual symptoms can resolve spontaneously, many patients continue to suffer from visuospatial difficulties months to years after the injury that can cause notable challenges for recovery of functioning, including driving. If you want to learn more about vision, see Chapter 8.

Executive functions have been defined as "capacities that enable a person to engage successfully in independent, purposive, self-directed, and self-serving behavior" (Lezak et al., 2012, p. 37). Executive dysfunction, common after TBI, encompasses a wide range of impairments including problems with self-monitoring; shifting between different tasks; the ability to correctly sequence, plan, or complete a task; maintaining drive or motivation; inhibiting automatic responses and goal management. In addition, anosognosia, or diminished self-awareness, is also common and can be very limiting of functioning following TBI (Vanderploeg et al., 2007). Caregivers of patients with executive dysfunction often report problems with goal-directed behaviors, socially inappropriate behavior, difficulty controlling emotional responses, difficulty with self-awareness about these changes, and difficulty maintaining functional independence. Other challenging behaviors include impulsivity, perseveration, rigidity, and/or disinhibition. Additionally, they may have trouble with abstract reasoning, problem solving, and/or organization. Given the role of executive functions in mediating other cognitive abilities (including attention, learning and memory, and language), as well as the impact these factors can have on day-to-day activities including driving, impairments in executive functions are, understandably, an important area to target as part of any rehabilitation effort.

Other areas of cognition are important for driving for the roles they play in interpreting, analyzing and responding to sensory input based on a person's memories and previously learned information. This includes judgment and reasoning skills.

Most of the decisions made while driving are based on a person's ability to judge a situation ("It looks like traffic is slowing down up ahead") and reason out a plan ("I should press on the brake").

Components of judgment:

- **Decision making** is the process and/or steps used to make a decision and/or choice.
- **Response inhibition** is the "suppression of actions that are inappropriate in a given context and that interfere with goal-driven behavior" (Mostofsky & Simmonds, 2008, p. 1).

- **Awareness** is the state of being conscious and the perception or knowledge of events, objects, or things. Awareness can be further classified into three interdependent types: intellectual awareness, emergent awareness, and anticipatory awareness (Crosson et al., 1989).

TBI can impact one or all components of judgment. Judgment changes can be seen in decision-making, where it can take a longer time to make decisions (Rogers et al., 1999; Rabinowitz & Levin, 2014). On the other hand, persons may be quick to make decisions leading to risky and impulsive actions (Neumann & Lequerica, 2015). Additional changes in judgment are seen with, "diminished capacity to appreciate the degree or extent of their deficits and anticipate the impact it is likely to have on their future performance despite previous failure" (Scott & Schoenberg, 2010, p. 233). Failure to recognize impairments that could create safety concerns with driving can lead to poor buy-in with the plan of care and limited ability to compensate or unsafe decisions such as driving against medical advice.

Like judgment, there are different forms of reasoning, all of which may be impacted after TBI.

- **Divergent reasoning**, a form of reasoning that involves generating as many possible outcomes and solutions, tends to be a form of reasoning that is heavily affected by TBI (Scott & Schoenberg, 2010). An example of divergent reasoning is the ability to describe multiple routes to get from one location to another.
- **Sequential reasoning** is used in common day-to-day activities such as cooking, driving, bathing, and dressing. Changes in sequential reasoning can impact problem solving. For example, persons may have a difficult time identifying the steps that are needed to solve a specific problem, or even have an inability to recognize that a problem exists (Scott & Schoenberg, 2010; Neumann & Lequerica, 2015).

As was noted earlier, driving requires quick judgment, and TBI can affect the timing of decision-making. When judgment is impaired after TBI, "drivers may be prone to more risk-taking behaviors, demonstrate poor awareness of driving problems or accidents, or be unable to recognize driving errors" (Schultheis & Whipple, 2014, p. 4). If a person reacts too quickly to an obstacle on the road, this could result in unsafe driving. Conversely, reacting too slowly while driving can also be unsafe.

Box 22.3   Learning activity

1. What types of problems could occur while driving?
2. What would happen if we didn't respond to that problem?
3. Share examples of how sequential reasoning is used in driving. What aspects of driving might be difficult if this type of reasoning is impaired?

Sensory functions

TBI can cause any number of changes to brain structures and functions, so we need to understand areas of the brain that are key players in both sensory input (how we receive, process, interpret and integrate sensory information) and output (our responses or actions) (Carron et al., 2016).

After TBI, it is possible to see changes in sensory systems, including visual, auditory and somatosensory. Each of these sensory systems plays a role in driving.

- **Visual.** When driving, a person is constantly and simultaneously scanning, focusing on objects, moving their eyes between cars, signs, and objects in their visual field and then making frequent decisions about how to respond to what they see. The visual field is what the brain sees and processes (Mason & Kandel, 1991). The entire process of receiving visual information, creating a picture, knowing what the objects are, determining spatial relationships of those objects in space and to the body, and finally deciding how to respond to the objects is a highly complex process and happens throughout various regions of the brain.
- **Auditory.** In addition to visual information, auditory information helps with making safe and accurate decisions while driving. When driving, a person listens for traffic around them as well as sounds from their own car to help guide decisions. Auditory information travels across the auditory pathways to the primary auditory cortex in the temporal lobe, where it is processed and compared with information in the brain responsible for storing past memories and integrated into the decision-making process (Burkhardt & Gillen, 1998).
- **Somatosensory.** The final sensory information needed for driving is somatosensory. Grasping the steering wheel, gear shifter or other car controls and feeling the pedals on your feet are all examples of tactile input. Additionally, moving across space in the car, going over bumps, and going around turns is providing proprioceptive information. Somatosensory information is processed in the primary and secondary sensory cortex within the parietal lobe, which in turn is integrated with auditory and visual information in the tertiary association cortex (Burkhardt & Gillen, 1998).

Box 22.4　Learning activity

How does one use the following sensory systems while driving to make safe and accurate decisions?

1. Visual.
2. Auditory.
3. Somatosensory.

Since Natalie hit the back of her head on the ground when she fell, we will want to explore what focal damage, or direct damage, may have occurred in that area of her brain, and more specifically, if any sensory changes are involved. The posterior-located occipital lobe houses the primary visual sensory area. Vision is obviously crucial for safe driving, therefore deserves thorough assessment. A TBI can cause problems with the oculomotor system if damage occurs in the parietal lobes, occipital lobe, prefrontal lobes, cerebellum, or brainstem (Scheiman, 1997). To learn more about the visual pathways, see Chapter 8. Let's take a closer look at the role of the occipital lobe.

Within the occipital lobe, the primary visual area receives information from the visual fields. This area combines visual information, makes sense of visuospatial relationships and has a role in visual memory. The brain does most tasks in an integrated manner with various parts of the brain working together. It therefore should not be surprising that the process of receiving, interpreting and responding to sensory information, including visual input, is not confined to one area of the brain. In other words, the occipital lobe does not work alone; other areas of the brain help to integrate and process visual and other sensory information as well.

- The **frontal lobes** contain the frontal eye field which controls voluntary eye movements.
- The **parietal lobes** are responsible for processing information such as depth, distance, spatial concepts, position in space and the difference between foreground and background.
- The **temporal lobes** deal with learning higher order visual tasks.

Luria (2012) described three areas of the brain that integrate sensory information for function. Damage to these units could cause problems with processing sensory information, such as what a person sees and hears while driving, or a person's motor response to that sensory information. These units are:

- The **arousal unit** regulates cortical tone and is housed in the brainstem. Information from the skin, muscles and joints is processed here. At the most basic level, this is where more automatic, stereotyped movements come from such as reflexes and basic mobility (Machado et al., 2010).
- The **sensory-input unit** receives, analyzes and stores information and includes the diencephalon, pituitary gland, limbic structures and basal ganglia (Vasković, 2022).
- The **organization and planning unit** is where the integration of the sensory information and planning for motor output occurs, and this unit, the prefrontal cortex, is housed in the anterior aspect of the cerebral cortex. The prefrontal cortex is "involved in memory formation, planning, execution, higher-order information processing and suppression of unwanted behaviors" (Hika & Al Khalili, 2023).

Box 22.5   Learning activity

Locate on a brain diagram the brainstem, diencephalon, pituitary gland, limbic structures, and basal ganglia.

Sensory motor integration

We know the significance of sensory input for driving, not only what we see, hear, or feel but also how the brain integrates and interprets that information to respond or make decisions. Cognitive functions such as attention, memory, emotions and executive functioning are integrated with the sensory information and previous life experiences. If all of these areas, tracts and processes are operating and integrating accurately, an appropriate motor response is generated. When driving, a person has to continuously make frequent adjustments and decisions based on sensory input. Ideation, initiation and preparation of a plan are happening all at the same time as well. A person's movement is continuously being modified by the sensory information being provided (Arnadottir, 1990).

Impairments in the sensory motor system can result in perceptual disorders which may affect skills needed for safe driving. This may include spatial relations (constructional abilities, figure/ground discrimination, form discrimination, depth perception, unilateral spatial attention and topographical orientation) and body scheme (anosognosia, somato-agnosia, unilateral body neglect, impaired right/left discrimination, finger agnosia) (Unsworth, 1999). Persons with TBI who experience perceptual disorders may have difficulty recognizing road signs, pedestrians, or safe following distances, for example.

As mentioned earlier, we need to keep in mind that TBI can result in diffuse injury, impacting multiple brain areas and there may be other impairments that could affect Natalie's ability to return to driving. Earlier, we mentioned that the frontal, parietal and temporal lobes assist the occipital lobe with processing visual information. Let's take a closer look at these areas of the brain again and see how they receive and integrate other sensory input as well.

- The **frontal lobes** house the primary motor areas that execute movement. Within the frontal lobes is the premotor cortex, responsible for planning, sequencing, timing, and organizing movement, as well as the intention of movement. There we will also find areas which control functions such as sequencing, timing, organization of action, initiation and planning, judgment, attention, alertness and working memory, among others. The information gathered and integrated in the sensory processing stages is sent to the primary motor cortex and supplementary motor areas in the frontal lobes. The left premotor cortex plans and sequences the movement and then that information is sent to the primary motor cortex where the movement is initiated.
- The **parietal lobes** house the primary sensory areas, including those responsible for fine touch sensation, proprioception and kinesthesia. Here we also find association areas responsible for coordination, integration, and refinement of sensory input, as well as functions of gnosis, praxis, body scheme and spatial relations.
- The **temporal lobes** house the primary auditory sensory area in the superior temporal gyrus responsible for auditory reception (Arnadottir, 1990).

Box 22.6 Learning activity

Review the sensory areas and the functions that they support. Which of these could have the biggest impact on driving?

Motor skills

TBI can result in a number of physical impairments such as paralysis or paresis of one or more limbs, spasticity, or impaired coordination, to name a few. Changes to body structures and functions can impact a person's ability to maneuver the steering wheel or operate other controls, as well as move from the accelerator to the brake pedal or vice versa. The primary motor cortex, located in the rear portion of the frontal lobe, is most involved in controlling voluntary movement; however, as with cognition and sensory function, in order to perform desired movements, the motor cortex must be able to receive information from other areas in the brain.

Box 22.7   Learning activity

What potential motor deficits could have resulted from Natalie's brain injury that would affect driving?

Neuroscience helps us understand adaptation and compensation

The World Health Organization (WHO) has developed the International Classification of Functioning model to understand how changes associated with known medical conditions (including brain injury) are associated with changes in functioning (Chan et al., 2009). This model classifies changes associated with brain injury into changes in (a) body functions and structures, (b) activity, and (c) participation. In the first of these categories, body functions and structures are measured by assessment of physical or mental functions, including the presence and degree of deviation from expected levels of performance. Activity limitations are an individual's inability to complete a basic or instrumental activity of daily living (ADL/IADL) (e.g., inability to recall appointments, follow a recipe while cooking, follow a medication regimen, balance a checkbook). Participation restrictions are a loss or change in social roles (e.g., loss of a job or inability to parent children) due to changes in body functioning and associated activity limitations.

The ICF model provides a framework and common language to help describe the overall health state and functional status of an individual (Chan et al., 2009). In Natalie's case, it can be used to both distinguish between and establish a connection among impairments (impaired visual perception, for example), activity limitations (driving), and participation restrictions (inability to attend church). With TBI, neuroscience helps us understand the function of neurologic structures, but also guides our understanding of the integrated processes that allow a person to perform activities. This complex network of neural connections that people possess helps determine the capacity to adapt and to compensate when body functions are impaired. Persons with TBI often identify their participation restrictions and activity limitations, much like Natalie whose goal is to return to driving, as the reason for which they are participating in rehabilitation. The clinician can use an understanding of neuroscience to help identify underlying impairments as well as areas of preserved function that can be used to create adaptations or compensation strategies and help people like Natalie reach their goals.

Box 22.8   Learning activity

Go to the WHO website and learn more about the elements of the ICF model. According to the ICF Model list what elements are relevant for Natalie within the following areas:

1. Body structure/function.
2. Health condition.
3. Activity.
4. Participation.
5. Environmental (positives and negatives).

> **Box 22.9   Learning activity**
>
> In small groups, discuss how these changes which occur after TBI would affect your day-to-day life. How would your life change if you were not able to drive? How would this change impact others around you? How would your future goals be impacted if you were not able to drive independently? Would you be open to alternative means of transportation (if available) if you were not able to drive?

Daily life routine: Driving a car in day-to-day life

The activity of driving is not only valued for its inherent implications of independence, but it also provides access to a wide range of activities occurring outside the home. Driving is important for community integration and participation. The ability to return to driving after brain injury has positive associations with return to work, social engagements, and participation in recreational activities. Perna et al. (2021) found that after moderate to severe TBI, the ability to drive is associated with more community participation, improved functional outcomes, less depressive symptoms, and greater life satisfaction. The ability to drive is of even greater value for those who live alone and/or in areas where public transportation is scarce. Driving not only improves access to social and vocational activities but increases independence with many instrumental activities of daily living such as grocery shopping, banking, and attending appointments.

> **Box 22.10   Learning activity**
>
> With your small group, complete the table in the Appendix about Natalie's goal of return to driving, which includes addressing what steps to take if driving is ultimately not an achievable goal.

Back to the person's life: Natalie wants to drive her own car to church

With the information that has been discussed regarding areas of the brain responsible for functions related to driving, consider the following:

> **Box 22.11   Learning activity**
>
> 1. In class or small groups, if necessary, what accommodations and compensation strategies may help Natalie return to driving? Use your neuroscience knowledge and what you know about Natalie to guide your idea generation.
> 2. What skills/abilities would you want to evaluate when you see Natalie?
> 3. Briefly explore assessment tools and treatment ideas appropriate for Natalie's potential areas of need.

What do we know about ourselves and the population at large from Natalie's story and brain injury?

There are many brain functions which work together so that we can successfully perform everyday activities. Under normal conditions we may take these for granted, but when one of more of these brain functions is impaired, activity limitations can result. In this chapter, we have described the many different functions necessary to safely drive a motor vehicle.

As we know, the nature and severity of challenges which a person may experience after TBI depends upon their own unique personal history, the environment in which they perform tasks, and the location and extent of their TBI. Knowing what functions are controlled by specific areas of the brain and how they each interact with each other can help us determine the best way to help a person who has had a TBI and their family.

Further reading

If interested in further reading about the lived experience of TBI:

Osborn, C. L. (2000). *Over my head: A doctor's own story of head injury from the inside looking out*. Andrews McMeel Publishing.

Siles, M., & Beuret, L. J. (2006). *Brain, Heal Thyself: A Caregiver's New Approach to Recovery from Stroke, Aneurysm, and Traumatic Brain Injuries*. Hampton Roads Publishing.

References

Arnadottir, G. (1990). *The brain and behavior: Assessing cortical dysfunction through activities of daily living*. St. Louis: Mosby.

Blennow, K., Hardy, J., & Zetterberg, H. (2012). The neuropathology and neurobiology of traumatic brain injury. *Neuron, 76*(5), 886–899. https://doi.org/10. 1016/j.neuron.2012.11.021

Burkhardt, A and Gillen, G. (1998). *Stroke rehabilitation: A function-based approach*. Mosby.

Carron, S. F., Alwis, D. S., & Rajan, R. (2016). Traumatic brain injury and neuronal functionality changes in sensory cortex. *Frontiers in Systems Neuroscience, 10*, 47.

Chan, F., Gelman, J. S., Ditchman, N., Kim, J.-H., & Chiu, C.-Y. (2009). The World Health Organization ICF model as a conceptual framework of disability. In F. Chan, E. Da Silva Cardoso, & J. A. Chronister (Eds.), *Understanding psychosocial adjustment to chronic illness and disability: A handbook for evidence-based practitioners in rehabilitation* (pp. 23–50). Springer Publishing.

Crosson, B., Barco, P. P., Velozo, C. A., Bolesta, M. M., Cooper, P. V., Werts, D., & Brobeck, T. C. (1989). Awareness and compensation in postacute head injury rehabilitation. *Journal of Head Trauma Rehabilitation, 4*(3), 46–54. https://doi.org/fv6fw2

Dikmen, S. S., Corrigan, J. D., Levin, H. S., Machamer, J., Stiers, W., & Weisskopf, M. G. (2009). Cognitive outcome following traumatic brain injury. *Journal of Head Trauma Rehabilitation, 24*(6), 430–438. https://doi.org/fdxp9v

Heilman, K. M., & Valenstein, E. (2010). *Clinical neuropsychology*. Oxford University Press.

Hemphill, M. A., Dauth, S., Yu, C. J., Dabiri, B. E., & Parker, K. K. (2015). Traumatic brain injury and the neuronal microenvironment: A potential role for neuropathological mechanotransduction. *Neuron, 85*(6), 1177–1192. https://doi.org/10.1016/j.neuron. 2015.02.041

Hika, B., & Al Khalili, Y. (2023). Neuroanatomy, prefrontal association cortex. In StatPearls [Internet]. StatPearls Publishing.

Lezak, M. D., Howieson, D. B., Bigler, E. D., & Tranel, D. (2012). *Neuropsychological assessment* (5th ed.). Oxford University Press.

Luria, A. R. (2012). *Higher cortical functions in man*. Springer Science & Business Media.

Machado, C., Estevez, M., Redriguez, R., & Perez-Nellar, J. (2010). Wakefulness and loss of aware-ness: brain and brainstem interaction in the vegetative state. *Neurology, 75*(8), 751–752.

Mason, C. & Kandel E.R. (1991) Central visual pathways. In Kandel ER, Scwartz TH, Tessel TM, editors: *Principles of neural science* (3rd ed.). Appleton and Lange.

Mathias, J. L., & Wheaton, P. (2007). Changes in attention and information-processing speed following severe traumatic brain injury: A meta-analytic review. *Neuropsychology, 21*(2), 212–223. https://doi. org/10.1037/0894–4105.21.2.212

Mostofsky, S. H., & Simmonds, D. J. (2008). Response inhibition and response selection: two sides of the same coin. *Journal of Cognitive Neuroscience, 20*(5), 751–761. https://doi.org/10.1162/jocn.2008.20500

Neumann, D., & Lequerica, A. (2015). Cognitive problems after traumatic brain injury. *Archives of Physical Medicine and Rehabilitation, 96*(1), 179–180. https://doi.org/10.1016/j.apmr.2013.06.003

Novack, T., Zhang, Y., Kennedy, R., Rapport, L. J., Bombardier, C., Bergquist, T.,... & Brunner, R. (2022). Crash risk following return to driving after moderate-to-severe TBI: A TBI model systems study. *The Journal of Head Trauma Rehabilitation, 10,* 1097.

Perna, R., Pundlik, J., & Arenivas, A. (2021). Return-to-driving following acquired brain injury: A neuropsychological perspective. *NeuroRehabilitation, 49*(2), 279–292.

Powell, M. R., Brown, A. W., Klunk, D., Geske, J. R., Krishnan, K., Green, C., & Bergquist, T. F. (2019). Injury severity and depressive symptoms in a post-acute brain injury rehabilitation sam-ple. *Journal of Clinical Psychology in Medical Settings, 26,* 470–482.

Rabinowitz, A. R., & Levin, H. S. (2014). Cognitive sequelae of Traumatic Brain Injury. *Psychiatric Clinics of North America, 37*(1), 1–11. https://doi.org/10.1016/j.psc.2013.11.004

Rogers, R. (1999). Dissociable deficits in the decision-making cognition of chronic amphetamine abusers, opiate abusers, patients with focal damage to prefrontal cortex, and tryptophan-depleted normal volunteers evidence for monoaminergic mechanisms. *Neuropsychopharmacology,* 20(4), 322–339. https://doi.org/10.1016/s0893-133x(98)00091-8

Scheiman M. (1997). *Understanding and managing vision deficits: A guide for occupational thera-pists.* Thorofare, NJ: Slack Inc.

Scott, J. G., & Schoenberg, M. R. (2010). Frontal lobe/executive functioning. *The Little Black Book of Neuropsychology,* 219–248. https://doi.org/10.1007/978-0-387-76978-3_10

Schultheis, M. T., & Whipple, E. K. (2014). Driving after traumatic brain injury: evaluation and rehabilitation interventions. *Current Physical Medicine and Rehabilitation Reports, 2,* 176–183.

Tate, R. L., Fenelon, B., Manning, M. L., & Hunter, M. (1991). Patterns of neuropsychological im-pairment after severe blunt head injury. *Journal of Nervous and Mental Disease, 179*(3), 117–126. https://doi.org/cdt4k6

Unsworth, Carolyn. (1999). *Cognitive and perceptual dysfunction: A clinical reasoning approach to evaluation and intervention.* F.A. Davis Company.

Vanderploeg, R. D., Belanger, H. G., Duchnick, J. D., & Curtiss, G. (2007). Awareness problems following moderate to severe traumatic brain injury: Prevalence, assessment methods, and injury correlates. *Journal of Rehabilitation Research and Development, 44*(7), 937–950. https://doi.org/10.1682/JRRD.2006.12.0163

Vasković, J. (2022). Subcortical structures. www.kenhub.com/en/library/anatomy/subcortical-structures-anatomy

Walker, W. C., Stromberg, K. A., Marwitz, J. H., Sima, A. P., Agyemang, A. A., Graham, K. M., Harrison-Felix, C., Hoffman, J. M., Brown, A. W., Kreutzer, J. S., & Merchant, R. (2018). Predict-ing long-term global outcome after traumatic brain injury: Development of a practical prognostic tool using the Traumatic Brain Injury Model Systems National Database. *Journal of Neurotrauma, 35*(14), 1587–1595. https://doi.org/10.1089/neu.2017.5359

23 Antoine wants to play with his grandchildren and has Parkinson's disease

Neuroscience facilitates our understanding of playing with grandchildren

Whitney Henderson

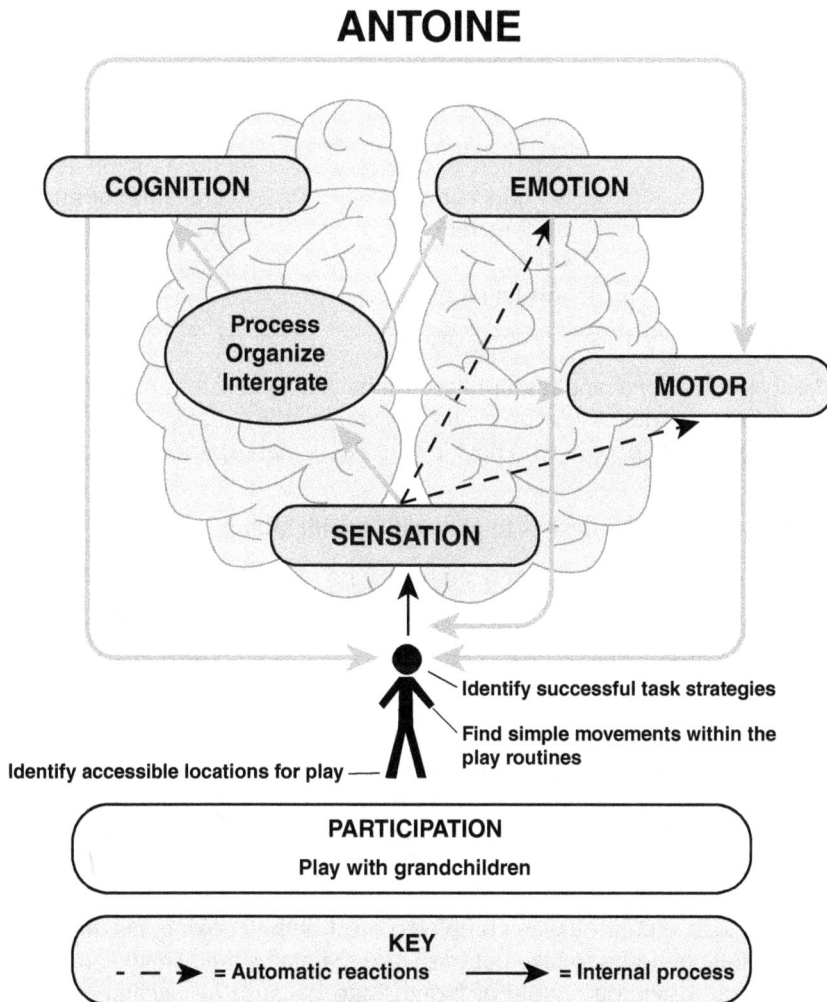

Figure 23.1 Antoine brain figure

DOI: 10.4324/9781003524380-28

Purpose of this chapter

In this chapter, we highlight the neuroscience underpinnings of how motor and cognitive interactions influence leisure occupations. Individuals with Parkinson's disease (PD) experience a wide variety of motor and non-motor symptomology which greatly impact their ability to participate in their valued occupations and their quality of life. We will meet Antoine and his family and explore his desired leisure occupations to increase understanding of motor and cognitive connections in the brain.

The key neuroscience concepts we will explore in this chapter include how the cortex, subthalamic nucleus, globus pallidus, basal ganglia, and thalamus integrate information for use in everyday experiences. As with all the chapters, these components of the nervous system work with other systems to support overall human function.

Keywords for this chapter are listed in the box below. Be sure to learn what these key features are so you can get the most out of the chapter.

Keywords for this chapter

basal ganglia	putamen	subthalamic nucleus
caudate nucleus	SN pars compacta	ventral anterior nucleus
globus pallidus	SN pars reticula	ventral lateral nucleus
hyperdirect pathway	striatum	
indirect pathway	substantia nigra	

Let's find out about Antoine and his family so we have a context for understanding the impact of his distinct nervous system on his life. As with all the chapters in this text, we learn these relationships from people who have distinct personal experiences in their lives.

Antoine, a 67-year-old who desires to play with grandchildren

Antoine is a 67-year-old, African American male who received a diagnosis of PD approximately six years ago. He has been married to his wife, Paula, for 45 years and they have four children (three daughters and one son) and nine grandchildren. His children and grandchildren live within a 50-mile radius of their small town and are very supportive. Prior to retirement at age 62, Antoine worked full time as an electrician for 39 years at a local university. He has an associate's degree.

Antoine remains independent in basic activities of daily living such as dressing, showering, grooming and toileting. He does require extra time to complete these tasks due to bradykinesia (slowness of movement) and fatigues easily. He can walk independently but does have mild rigidity throughout trunk and neck and demonstrates hypokinesia (small movement) in gait pattern. He also displays a resting tremor in bilateral upper extremities.

Prior to diagnosis, Antoine's wife completed most of the cooking, cleaning, and laundry tasks. Antoine continues to take out trash and maintains their small yard and garden. He elected to quit driving a couple of months ago because he became concerned for safety. His wife has started to assist with financial and medication management because Antoine is having more difficulty with his concentration and memory.

Antoine and his wife remain active. They walk several times a week at the local YMCA. They are very involved in the grandchildren's activities and frequently attend their musical concerts, sporting events, and celebratory parties. Antoine and Paula frequently watch their grandchildren. Antoine enjoys playing card and board games, fishing, completing woodworking projects, and watching sports when they visit. Lately, his family has noticed a lack of interest in and motivation (apathy) for these activities and reports more daytime sleepiness. When he was playing a game with his family last week, his daughter noticed that Antoine was "not paying attention" and had to "always remind him of his turn and give him extra time to play his cards (slowed thinking)." His son also noticed while they were fishing with grandchildren that he had a lot of difficulty starting (initiating) his cast and appeared to be stuck (freezing gait) while walking around the pond. It became worse when he had to do two things at once, such as casting while listening to one of the grandchild's stories or walking while trying to figure out the issue with the fishing rod (simultaneous tasks).

Antoine's strengths include large network of support from family and friends, engagement in a local PD support group, strong faith and an active participation in church activities, desire to remain as independent as possible, and willingness and ability to learn new or modified strategies.

Box 23.1   Learning activity

Discuss with your peers:

1. Now that you have met Antoine, what are you curious about related to symptomology and occupational performance?
2. What do you believe you need to know more about in order to help Antoine?

Box 23.2   Learning activity

In the section above there are many words relevant to the signs and symptoms individuals with PD experience. Take a moment to locate videos demonstrating those terms so you can begin to think about and apply the motor and cognitive interactions to Antoine.

Before you continue reading the chapter, work with a peer or small group to discuss what you already know and what you learned from the videos.

Keywords: globus pallidus, bradykinesia, rigidity, hypokinesia, resting tremor, Parkinson's disease, apathy, freezing gait

---

Box 23.3   Learning activity

1. What do you currently know about PD?
2. During leisure activities, what parts of the brain would you expect to support:

   a. Motor performance.
   b. Cognitive performance.
   c. Emotion and motivation.

2. How do the motor and cognitive systems interact to enhance engagement in leisure?
3. What other sensory mechanisms contribute to participation in leisure?
4. How might the context influence participation in leisure?

Now that you have reviewed important information and engaged in discussion, we can begin to explore what leisure occupations require from the nervous system.

Neuroscience information to guide your thinking about Antoine

Traditionally, when we think about PD, we often turn our attention to the motor concerns impacting an individual's life. However, it is often the non-motor concerns (e.g. cognition, fatigue, anxiety) that have a greater impact on an individual's ability to participate and quality of life (Eisinger et al., 2018; Wood et al., 2022). We will use Antoine's story to understand how many areas of the brain interact and impact participation in leisure tasks.

In the central nervous system, there are three hierarchical levels of control: high, middle, and low (Bear et al., 2016). We will discuss these three levels as each applies to Antoine and his engagement in leisure activities. The highest level of this system is the association areas of the cortex and the basal ganglia of the forebrain (both of which we will discuss later in this chapter). It is in these areas of the brain that Antoine would develop a strategy—a goal for movement (motor) and a plan to best achieve that goal (cognition). The cortex contributes an abundance of valuable information for participation in leisure activities. For example, let's consider Antoine is playing a card game with his grandchildren. Using information from a variety of senses, the cortex provides details to assist to produce movement when reaching to play a card in the center of the table. He may see (vision) that his grandchild is also going to play a card, hear (audition) a grandchild giggling about what card he may be playing, or feel where and how his arm is in space (proprioception/kinesthesia). Based on this incoming information, Antoine must create a strategy to move the best card from his hand to the best location in center of the table. He considers multiple options (e.g. which card to play and which stack to place the card), which are filtered through the basal ganglia and back to the cortex until he decides on the best move.

The middle level includes the motor cortex and cerebellum and involves tactics—the sequences and timing of motor movements in space to achieve the desired goal accurately and efficiently. Once Antoine has a strategy or goal for playing a card, the motor cortex and cerebellum make the decision about how to move and provide instructions to the brain stem and spinal cord (e.g. the lowest level). This lower level is focused on the execution of movement in which neurons fire to produce and adjust movement (see Chapters 4, 5, and 6). The motor neurons in Antoine's spinal cord produce coordinated movement of his shoulder, elbow, forearm, wrist and fingers while the brainstem and cerebellum provide crucial information for postural adjustments as he reaches out of base of support to place the card.

Important brain structures and functions

To best understand the cognition and motor interface in leisure tasks, we will examine the highest level in greater depth. Returning to our example, Antoine needs somatosensory information before he can calculate a motor plan (strategy) to play a card. The posterior parietal cortex and the prefrontal cortex play a large role in regulating the flow of this valuable information. The parietal and anterior lobes are heavily interconnected and is where decisions are made about which strategy to use and the outcome of that strategy. This information is filtered through the basal ganglia and back to the motor cortex (see Chapters 4, 5, and 6).

Basal ganglia

As briefly mentioned earlier in chapter, the basal ganglia is also involved as part of the network of high level of motor control and is an important structure to understand when thinking about the ability of individuals with PD to participate in their desired occupations. We will begin our discussion with the anatomy and function of the basal ganglia.

Box 23.4   Learning activity

Find a picture of the basal ganglia, so you have a visual reference as you read this section.

Keywords: basal ganglia, caudate nucleus, putamen

As previously discussed, the basal ganglia receives input from all regions of the cortex (frontal, parietal, and temporal lobes) and has several important components. On your picture, locate the C-shaped caudate nucleus and putamen. The caudate nucleus and the putamen form the striatum. The striatum receives incoming information from the mentioned cortical areas and the substantia nigra (discussed later) and sends it to the globus pallidus. Locate the globus pallidus on your picture and place an active [+] sign on it. It will be important for you to note that the globus pallidus is active [+] at rest. The globus pallidus outputs this information to the nuclei of the thalamus. Therefore, the primary function of the basal ganglia is to integrate inputs from many areas of the brain and funnel information through the thalamus to the motor cortex to influence movement. Therefore, its function is often described as a brake hypothesis. When Antoine is sitting still waiting to play a card during a game, he must "put the brakes on" movement except for the postural reflexes that help him maintain an upright position. When Antoine is ready to play a card, he must "put the brakes on" the postural reflexes and "release the brakes" on movement so that he can participate in the leisure task.

Scientists and scholars previously viewed the basal ganglia as the main structure for the regulation of voluntary movement. However, we now know it is highly involved in regulating higher cerebral functions for cognition, such as decision-making and planning, which we will further discuss later in this chapter.

Thalamus

Box 23.5   Learning activity

Find a picture of the thalamus, so you have a visual reference as you read this section.

Keywords: thalamus, ventral anterior nuclei of thalamus, ventral lateral nuclei of thalamus

---

The ventral anterior and the ventral lateral nuclei are important structures that reside within the thalamus to aid in the learning, coordination, and planning of movement. It receives input from the basal ganglia (specifically the GP) and sends output to the motor cortex. At rest, these nuclei are inactive [–] because it is inhibited by the active nature of the globus pallidus. In this state, no movement is produced.

In this chapter, we primarily discuss the role of the thalamus from a motor perspective. However, we want to highlight its cognitive features. Historically, the thalamus was considered a passive, triage center in which it determined and filtered information to other regions of the brain for processing. In the past few decades, studies demonstrate that the thalamus is an active contributor to cognitive thought processes, particularly attention, processing speed, and memory. Early studies discussed its important role in selective attention and filtering of visual information (Bonelli & Cummings, 2007; Fama & Sullivan, 2015). For Antoine, this would include focusing on a card game in a loud, crowded room or visually sifting through various cards on table to determine the next play.

The direct pathway

Now that you know more about the relevant structures, we can begin to examine how these components interact to form a circuit or pathway. It may be helpful to have your pictures available. Within this pathway, there are both excitatory and inhibitory neurons. Information from the cortex (frontal, temporal, and parietal lobes) projects onto the striatum (caudate nucleus and putamen) and creates an excitatory response. Draw an arrow from the cortex to the striatum and place an active [+] sign by the arrow. Within the basal ganglia, the striatum sends information to the globus pallidus (specifically the internal division). Draw an arrow from striatum to the globus pallidus. Remember the globus pallidus is active [+] at rest. However, when the striatum receives input from the cortex it creates an inhibitory response to the globus pallidus which inhibits ("turns down") its activity. Therefore, you can place a negative sign [–] by this arrow to show reduction in or no activity of the globus pallidus. The globus pallidus sends information to the nuclei of the thalamus. Draw a line from the GP to the nuclei of the thalamus. Remember from the previous section that these nuclei are inactive [–] at rest because of the active nature of the GP. Therefore, when the GP becomes inactive, the thalamic nuclei become active (excited) because it is no longer inhibited by the GP. You can draw an active [+] sign next to that arrow. The thalamic nuclei send information back to the cortex to close the circuit. Draw a line back to the cortex to close the loop. You can also place an active [+] sign next to that arrow as that is an excitatory, active response to facilitate movement. In conclusion, the direct pathway produces an excitatory effect on movement (Figure 23.2).

Box 23.6   Learning activity

This is a complex pathway. Take a moment to pause and check your understanding. You can do this in many ways:

1. Find a blank piece of paper or whiteboard and draw the pathway.
2. Describe the pathway out loud to yourself or to a peer.
3. Find and review a video explaining the direct pathway.

Keywords: direct pathway of basal ganglia

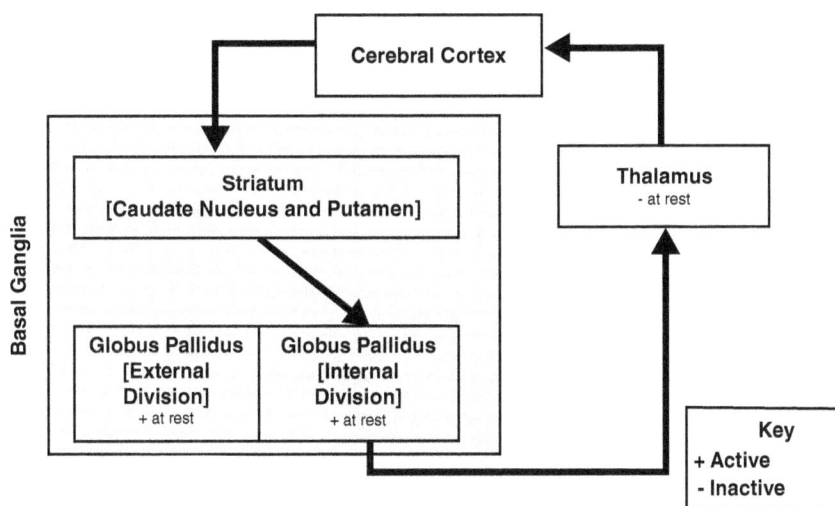

Figure 23.2 The direct pathway for facilitation of movement

The indirect pathway

The basal ganglia also has an indirect pathway. The indirect pathway incorporates many of the same structures discussed in the direct pathway, but also includes the subthalamic nucleus. Locate the subthalamic nucleus on a picture as it sits just below the thalamus.

This pathway begins the same way as the direct pathway in that the cortex projects excitatory information to the striatum. However, in the direct pathway the striatum sends information to the internal division of the GP, but in the indirect pathway the striatum sends information to the external division of the GP. The response is the same in that the GP is inhibited. The external division of the GP sends projections to the subthalamic nucleus (not the nuclei of thalamus in the direct pathway). Because the GP is inhibited, the subthalamic nucleus becomes excited. The subthalamic nucleus sends excitatory, active [+] neurons back to the internal division of the GP which joins back to the direct pathway to send information to the thalamus. However, if you recall from the previous section that when GP is active, the nuclei of the thalamus are not. Therefore, the result of the indirect pathway is inhibition of movement (Figure 23.3).

Box 23.7   Learning activity

1. Check your understanding of the indirect pathway. You can:

   a. Add the indirect pathway to your drawing of the direct pathway.
   b. Describe the differences between the direct and indirect pathways out loud to yourself or to a peer.

2. Watch a video of the indirect pathway.

Keywords: indirect pathway of basal ganglia

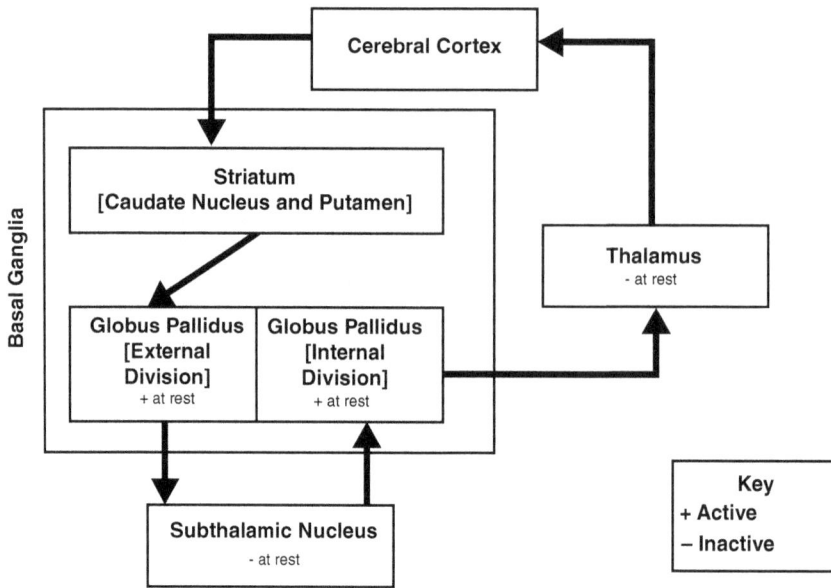

Figure 23.3 The indirect pathway for inhibition of movement

When the basal ganglia functions properly, there is a balance between these two pathways. When it is not balanced, it results in motor dysfunction. Let's apply this information to Antoine's engagement in leisure tasks. Antoine is playing a card game with his grandchildren. It is his turn. He looks at the table to determine what card was played (vision) and looks at his hand to decide which of his cards to play (decision making). At this time, the frontal (cognition) and parietal (perceptual) lobes of the cortex are providing input to the basal ganglia to use the indirect pathway to inhibit movement until the cognitive decision and motor plan has been made about which card to play and where to play it. After careful consideration, Antoine elects to play the Queen of hearts on the fourth pile of cards. The cortex sends the plan to the basal ganglia to activate the direct pathway to execute the movement.

The hyperdirect pathway

We will add a third pathway to our discussion—the hyperdirect pathway. In this pathway, the cortex bypasses the striatum of the basal ganglia and directly connects to the subthalamic nucleus. Neurons from the cortex send excitatory information to the subthalamic nucleus, which sends excitatory information to the internal division of the GP. As we saw in the indirect pathway, the GP (internal division) has an inhibitory effect on the motor cortex when it becomes excited. Therefore, the hyperdirect pathway also inhibits movement. However, because this pathway bypasses the striatum (the caudate nucleus and putamen), it is believed to play a role in quickly preventing or stopping movement that the direct pathway is initiating. We can apply this information to Antoine's leisure task of playing "Slapjack" with his grandchildren. Antoine is currently waiting to play a card (indirect pathway, no movement). One of his grandchildren plays a card and Antoine thinks it is the jack of clubs. Therefore, the direct pathway signals Antoine to move his hand to "hit" the card before his grandchild. However, he suddenly realizes that it is the king of clubs and quickly stops the movement of his hand to prevent hitting the card. In this case, perceptual information from the cortex directly goes to the subthalamic nucleus in the hyperdirect pathway to quickly stop the movement of the direct pathway (Figure 23.4).

Substantia nigra

Another important structure to understand when learning about the motor and cognitive interaction is the substantia nigra ("black substance"). Locate this structure on a picture. Because of the high levels of dopamine neurons, this area appears darker than neighboring areas (hence the name). This area of the brain is the most affected in Parkinson's disease. Therefore, many challenges impacting Antoine's ability to engage in leisure occupations stem from a loss of dopaminergic neurons in the substantia nigra.

The substantia nigra is primarily responsible for initiating and controlling movement but also plays a valuable role in cognition and emotion. As we previously discussed, the direct and indirect pathways influence movement. However, both pathways rely heavily on the neurotransmitter dopamine to function successfully. It is the substantia nigra that provides dopaminergic neurons to the striatum of the basal ganglia. Therefore, you could draw a line from the substantia nigra to the striatum of the basal ganglia (Figure 23.5). We can further break down the substantia nigra into two portions: the SN pars reticula and the SN pars compacta.

The SN pars reticula has a complex role in eye and head movement (motor) and the ability to learn and think (cognition). It uses a chemical, GABA, and primarily projects to the thalamus to control aspects of movement and behavior. However, the SN pars compacta has a greater impact on the pathways discussed above as it is the portion containing dopamine.

In PD, there is a decrease in dopaminergic neurons in the SN pars compacta which disrupts the pathway to the striatum. As a result, individuals with PD may experience motor

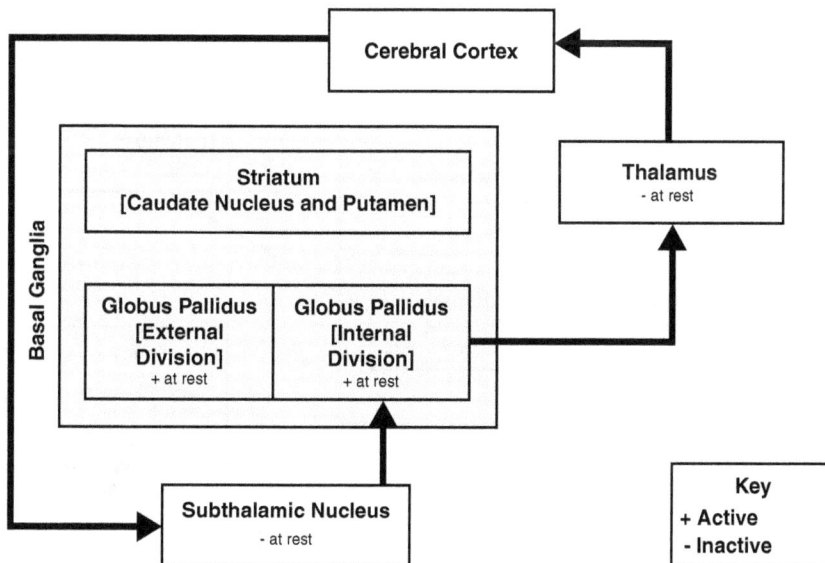

Figure 23.4 The hyperdirect pathway for inhibition of movement *quickly*

difficulties, such as initiating movement, developing tremors, or having limb rigidity and slowness of movement. In addition, dopamine plays an important role in motivation and reward. Our willingness to engage in cognitive and physically demanding tasks is central to human behavior. Dopamine influences our motivation to invest physical and cognitive effort in exchange for a reward, which in turn, affects our performance and participation. Therefore, when dopamine is reduced, individuals may be less motivated to engage in tasks that require effort and energy. It is estimated that approximately 40% of individuals with PD experience apathy (lack of interest or enthusiasm) as a result of the dopaminergic dysfunction (McGuigan et al., 2019). In our example, Antoine's family reported a lack of motivation for leisure tasks. His lack of interest in the physically demanding task of fishing or cognitively demanding task of a card game is likely the result of reduced dopamine to incentivize his effort for participation in these tasks.

Multiple pathways

Now that you have a basic understanding of the motor pathway, it is important to note that the basal ganglia participates in many circuits or loops. However, only a few of the circuits are entirely motor with many other circuits involved in important cognitive functions. There are five major frontal-subcortical circuits (one limbic, two associative (prefrontal), one oculomotor, and one motor) (Table 23.1). In recent literature, the non-motor aspects of PD are receiving attention; particularly the cognitive changes that are relatively common with this population (Eisinger et al., 2018; Prakash et al., 2016; Watson & Leverenz, 2010; Wood et al., 2022). Therefore, we will provide a brief overview of the five basal ganglia circuits to increase understanding of the structure's impact on multiple functions.

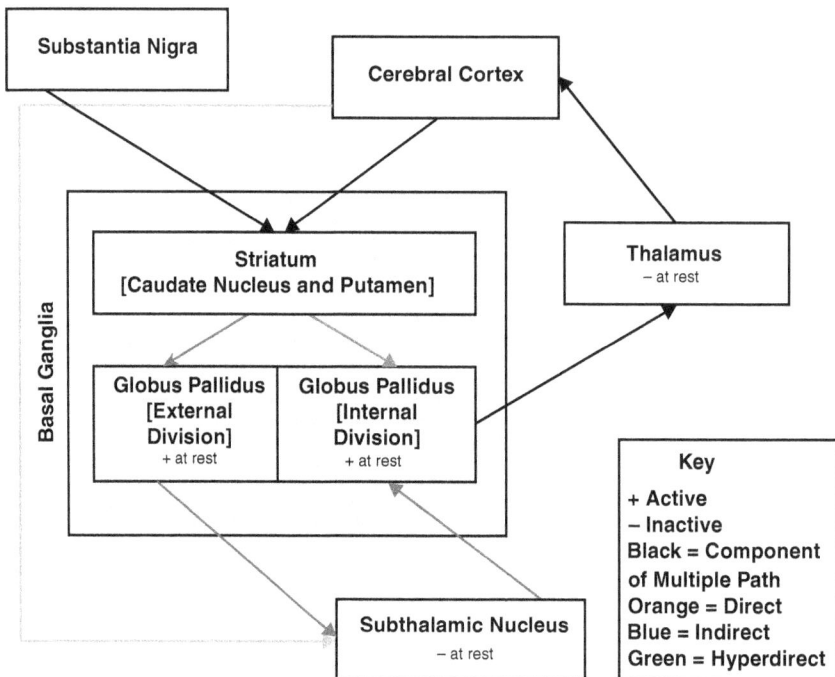

Figure 23.5 Pathways with *substantia nigra*

These five circuits share common structures and routes that we previously discussed (e.g. cortex, basal ganglia, thalamus). The circuits run adjacent to each other and project onto different areas of the basal ganglia, thalamus, and cortex. Each circuit is anatomically segregated but maintains the same parallel arrangement throughout the loop. Because of their similar pathways, we will not go in-depth to the specifics of each circuit but will provide an overview of their roles so you can appreciate the motor and cognitive interface. In addition, each of these circuits connects with other areas of the brain to further influence motor and cognitive performance and each possess a direct and indirect pathway. These circuits integrate information to produce a response.

Many new studies are investigating the relationship between cognitive and motor symptoms with individuals with PD with findings suggesting potential overlap of these processes and functions. For example, Schneider et al. (2015) found that participants with PD that had more posture, balance, and gait concerns had the highest number of adverse cognitive and visuospatial outcomes. In addition, researchers found an association between bradykinesia and executive functions. Each of the examples highlights the motor-cognitive interface suggesting involvement and connections in similar circuits.

To further highlight the cognitive and motor interface, we can turn our attention to Antoine an additional time. Literature consistently notes that individuals with PD experience difficulty coping with complex cognitive and motor demands. It is challenging for these individuals to dual task—carry out two tasks simultaneously. Antoine may experience reduced attention to grandchildren while attempting to navigate a rough terrain while

Table 23.1 Five basal ganglia circuits

Circuit (motor or non-motor, type of circuit)	Description	How might appear in Antoine's leisure task
Motor (motor, motor)	Motor performance optimization in tasks (described in previous section)	Decreased initiation to reach for card or cast fishing rod; slow and small movement during board game and fishing
Oculomotor (motor, oculomotor)	Motor control of eye movements	Reduced saccades when searching for a card; lack of smooth eye movements when scanning the pond; eyes don't reach visual target
Dorsolateral Prefrontal (non-motor, associative)	Mediates executive functions (e.g. the cognitive loop—attention, working memory, planning)	Difficulty sustaining attention during card game or shifting attention in response to cognitive and motor demands of fishing; difficulty remembering rules of a new board game
Anterior Cingulate (non-motor, associative)	Participates in motivation and emotion	Apathy; lack of motivation to participation in leisure tasks; decrease initiation of move [motor] or respond to questions [cognitive] in leisure occupations; emotional lability
Orbitofrontal (2 portions) (non-motor, limbic)	Medial: integrates visceral-amygdala functions (internal state) Lateral: ingrates limbic and emotional information into behavioral responses	Increased irritability and frustration in leisure tasks (e.g. when grandchildren speak loudly, not following rules); decreased inhibition (yells at grandchildren when frustrated)

328 The Neuroscience of Everyday Life

fishing. Similarly, while playing a very cognitively demanding card game, he may move slower or smaller during game play.

Daily life routine: Playing with grandchildren

Individuals across the lifespan are intrinsically motivated to engage in a variety of leisure activities in and with their various contexts (physical, social, technological, etc.). They may participate in a variety of low demand (e.g. reading, knitting) or high demand (e.g. pickleball, hiking) leisure tasks. Evidence suggests that when individuals participate in leisure occupations, they have more positive health and well-being outcomes (Reilling Ott & Kolodziejczak, 2020). For individuals with PD, motor and cognitive symptomology can impact their ability to engage in this meaningful occupation as their brain experiences many neuroanatomical changes as a result of this chronic condition.

Box 23.8   Learning activity

In a small group, discuss how the neuroscience may affect Antoine's performance and participation in other valued leisure occupations. Consider:

1. Motor.
2. Cognition.
3. Emotional.
4. Integration of these three areas into the occupation.

Back to the person's life: Antoine wants to play with his grandchildren when they visit

Now that you know more about brain functioning in individuals with PD, how can you use scientific reasoning to support Antoine's participation in leisure occupations? You will certainly learn more about potential strategies in other courses, but knowing the foundational neuroscience information will provide the foundation for your professional reasoning.

Box 23.9   Learning activity

In a small group, discuss these questions.

1. How might a cognitive strategy foster motor performance during leisure?
2. How might a task or environmental adaptation for motor concerns contribute to Antoine's motivation to engage in leisure?
3. How might a task or environmental adaptation for cognitive concerns contribute to Antoine's motivation to engage in leisure?
4. How might you reduce motor demands to promote cognitive performance? How might you reduce cognitive demands to promote motor performance?

What do we know about ourselves and the population at large from this brain condition and this family story?

Even though we learned about this information in relation to individuals with PD, everyone uses motor and cognitive processes to engage in desired occupations. Furthermore, individuals in the general population may experience subtle similarities discussed throughout this chapter. For example, some individuals may require more time to initiate a task, have more difficulty doing two tasks at once, or lack motivation to do a task that is cognitively or motorically demanding. However, we all have the ability to use our unique strengths to make tasks and contextual adaptations to foster performance and participation in valued occupations.

Box 23.10   Learning activity

With your small group, complete the table in the Appendix about how Antoine can be enabled to play with his grandchildren while managing his Parkinson's disease.

Further reading

If interested in further reading about the lived experiences of Parkinson's disease or caring for someone with Parkinson's disease:

Marie, L. (2020). *Everything you need to know about caregiving for Parkinson's disease*. CreateSpace Independent Publishing.

Okun, M. S., Malaty, I. A., & Deeb, W. (2020). *Living with Parkinson's disease: A complete guide for patients and caregivers*. Robert Rose.

Ritscher, G., Dean, J., & Robert, M. (2020). *Rising above Parkinson's: Take on life's greatest challenges and learn to thrive*. Delphi Publishing.

Soundy, A., Stubbs, B., & Roskell, C. (2014). The experience of Parkinson's disease: A systematic review and meta-ethnography. *The Scientific World Journal, 2014*, 613592.

Stephenson, C., Flynn, A., Overs, A., Stickland, K. (2023). Support needs of people with younger onset Parkinson's disease: An interpretative phenomenological analysis. *Collegian, 30*(2), 335–342.

Horne, J. & Tagliati, M. (2022). *Parkinson's disease for dummies* (2nd ed.). Wiley Brand.

Visit:

- www.parkinson.org
- www.michaeljfox.org

References

Alexander, G. E., Crutcher, M. D., DeLong, M. R. (1990). Basal ganglia-thalamocortical circuits: parallel substrates for motor, oculomotor, "prefrontal" and "limbic" functions. *Progress in Brain Research, 85*, 119–146.

Bear, M. F., Connors, B. W., & Paradiso, M. A. (2016). *Neuroscience: exploring the brain* (4th ed.). Jones & Bartlett Learning.

Bonelli, R. M., & Cummings, J. L. (2007). Frontal-subcortical circuitry and behavior. *Dialogues in Clinical Neuroscience, 9*(2), 141–151. doi: 10.31887/DCNS.2007.9.2/rbonelli

Eisinger, R. S., Urdaneta, M. E., Foote, K. D., Okun, M. S., & Gunduz, A. (2018). Non-motor characterization of the basal ganglia: evidence from human and non-human primate electrophysiology. *Frontiers in Neuroscience, 12*, 385. doi:10.3389/fnins.2018.00385

Fama, R., & Sullivan, E. V. (2015). Thalamic structures and associated cognitive functions: relations with age and aging. *Neurosci Biobehav Rev., 54*, 29–37. doi: 10.1016/j.neubiorev.2015.03.008

Marinelli, L., Quartarone, A., Hallett, M., Frazzitta, G., & Ghilardi, M. F. (2017). The many facets of motor learning and their relevance for Parkinson's disease. *Clinical Neurophysiology, 128*, 1127–1141. http://dx.doi.org/10.1016/j.clinph.2017.03.042

McGuigan, S., Zhou, S. H., Brosnan, M. B., Thyagarajan, D., Bellgrove, M., A., & Chong, T. T-J. (2019). Dopamine restores cognitive motivation in Parkinson's disease. *Brain, 142*(3), 719–732. https://doi.org/10.1093/brain/awy341

Prakash, K. G., Bannur, B. M., Chavan, M. D., Saniya, K., Sai Sailesh, K., & Rajagopalan, A. (2016). Neuroanatomical changes in Parkinson's disease in relation to cognition: an update. *Journal of Advanced Pharmaceutical Technology and Research, 7*(4), 123–126. doi: 10.4103/2231–4040. 191416

Reilling Ott, K., & Kolodziejczak, S. (2020). *Interventions to improve and maintain the performance of and participation in leisure and social participation among adults with Parkinson's disease: Systematic review of related literature from January 2011–December 2018* [Critically Appraised Topic]. American Occupational Therapy Association.

Schneider, J. S., Sendek, S., & Yang, C. (2015). Relationship between motor symptoms, cognition, and demographic characteristics in treated mild/moderate Parkinson's disease. *PLoS ONE, 10*(4), 1–11. doi: 10.1371/journal.pone.0123231

Sousa, N. M. F., Macedo, R. C., & Brucki, S. M. D. (2021). Cross-sectional associations between cognition and mobility in Parkinson's disease. *Dementia & Neuropsychologia, 15*(1), 105–111. https://doi.org/10.1590/1980-57642021dn15-010011

Watson, G. S., & Leverenz, J. B. (2010). Profile of cognitive impairment in Parkinson's disease. *Brain Pathology, 20*(3), 640–645. https://doi.org/10.1111/j. 1750–3639.2010. 00373.x

Wood, J., Henderson, W. & Foster, E. R. (2022). Occupational therapy practice guidelines for people with Parkinson's disease. *American Journal of Occupational Therapy, 76*(3), 7603397010.

Appendix

Table template for analysis of participation features with nervous system functions

This template is also available for free download from the Routledge website: www.routledge.com/9781638221265.

Date: _____

Name of person being analyzed: _____ from Chapter _____

Daily life activity of interest in this analysis: _____

Student(s) names for assignment: _____

What are the MOST LIKELY neuroscience factors affecting this person's ability to participate?

Nervous system functions	How the nervous system function shows up in this task	Nervous system areas/processes that support this function	What is most likely to be affecting with the person's ability to participate in the activity of interest?
Sensory processing	**Visual:**	Eyes, visual pathways, visual cortex	
	Auditory:	Ears, auditory pathways, auditory cortex	
	Vestibular:	Vestibular organ, vestibular pathways, sensorimotor cortex	
	Proprioceptive:	Proprioceptors, spinal cord and brainstem pathways, sensorimotor cortex	
	Somatosensory:	Touch receptors, spinal cord and brainstem sensory pathways, autonomic pathways, sensorimotor cortex	

Chemical senses [smell, taste]: Olfactory and gustatory receptors, pathways

Interoception: Gut receptors, amygdala, limbic system

Motor processing

Coordination: Sensorimotor pathways, cerebellum, basal ganglia, autonomic pathways

Planning: Sensorimotor cortex
All the association areas

Execution: Sensorimotor pathways, autonomic pathways, cerebellum, basal ganglia

Cognitive processing Integrating areas of brain such as Wernicke's and Broca's areas in auditory cortex, thalamus, prefrontal, frontal cortex

Social-emotional processing Integrating areas of the association areas of the parietal and temporal lobes

Language processing Wernicke's and Broca's areas in auditory cortex, thalamus, limbic system

Index

Note: **Bold** page numbers indicate tables, *italic* numbers indicate figures.

For Product Safety Concerns and Information please contact our EU
representative GPSR@taylorandfrancis.com
Taylor & Francis Verlag GmbH, Kaufingerstraße 24, 80331 München, Germany

www.ingramcontent.com/pod-product-compliance
Lightning Source LLC
Chambersburg PA
CBHW081047220326
41598CB00038B/7013